LOVE YOUR SISTER

LOVE YOUR SISTER

HOW FAR WOULD YOU GO
FOR SOMEONE YOU LOVE...
ON A UNICYCLE?

CONNIE & SAMUEL JOHNSON

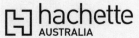

Hachette Australia will donate $1.00 for every copy sold of Love Your Sister *to the Garvan Research Foundation in support of the Connie Johnson Fellowship in Breast Cancer Research. Sales will be determined by actual sales of the print edition recorded through Nielsen Bookscan and actual ebook sales reported by ebook retailers to Hachette Australia.*

Note: Some names have been changed throughout this book.

Published in Australia and New Zealand in 2014
by Hachette Australia
(an imprint of Hachette Australia Pty Limited)
Level 17, 207 Kent Street, Sydney NSW 2000
www.hachette.com.au

10 9 8 7 6 5 4 3 2 1

Copyright © Connie Johnson and Samuel Johnson 2014

National Library of Australia
Cataloguing-in-Publication data

Johnson, Connie, author.
Love your sister/Samuel Johnson, Connie Johnson.

ISBN 978 0 7336 3324 9 (paperback)

Johnson, Connie.
Johnson, Samuel.
Breast – Cancer – Research – Australia.
Unicycles – Records – Australia.
Cycling – Records – Australia.
Fund raising – Australia.
Brothers and sisters – Australia.

Other Authors/Contributors: Johnson, Samuel, author.

616.994009

Cover design by Christabella Designs
Front cover image courtesy Gina Milicia/www.ginamilicia.com
Inside back cover image courtesy Paul Simmons
Internal photos from Connie and Samuel's family collection, additional photos courtesy Alistair Marks/alistairmarks.com
Text design by Bookhouse, Sydney
Typeset in 12/19.4 Goudy Old Style and Goudy Sans Std
Printed and bound in Australia by Griffin Press, Adelaide, an Accredited ISO AS/NZS 14001:2009 Environmental Management System printer

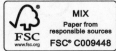

To my boys, big and small –
Mike, Willoughby and Hamilton.

In loving memory of Dad and Aunty Marg.

– Connie

CONTENTS

Every year in Australia alone over 14,000 women are diagnosed with breast cancer and every year nearly 3000 women die of advanced breast cancer.

But it isn't just women who are affected. Every time a woman is diagnosed her partner, her parents, her friends, her siblings, her children are all affected, even more so if she passes away of advanced breast cancer, so it is time for women to step up and take action.

Don't fall into the booby trap – be breast aware.

Men can help too, by learning how to do a breast check, and . . .

Save a life – grope your wife!

A little known fact about breast cancer is that men get it too. About 1 in every hundred cases of breast cancer is male, which means nearly 130 men are diagnosed every year and close to 30 will die.

So, no matter what your gender, be breast aware, and be proactive about your health, so you don't become a statistic like my sister.

– Samuel Johnson

A NOTE FROM CONNIE

Nowadays I often talk about my feelings about cancer – how cancer has shaped who I am today and what my relationship with cancer is like. I've had quite a few years to think about it and this is how I sum it up: me and cancer, we have a love–hate relationship. I hate cancer, but cancer loves me. It's pretty unusual to have cancer as a child, not many people have cancer in their twenties, and it isn't common to get cancer in your thirties. I had it when I was 12, then again when I was 22, and I was diagnosed with terminal cancer when I was just 33. All different, unrelated cancers, all unrelated to previous treatments. Just the luck of the draw.

But this time, with this last diagnosis, there is a difference. This time I won't be a cancer survivor. That is a hard thing to write down and an even harder thing to come to terms with, especially now that I'm a mum. Writing this book is one of the things I had on my bucket list (along with seeing my brother, Sam, finish the ride and scrapbooking memories for my kids).

Sam and I want to share our story to help others, to make sure women pay attention to their health and check their boobs regularly. We want people to remember our catchphrase, 'Don't fall into the booby trap, be breast aware.' I also want people to understand how Love Your Sister came about – how Sam stepped up to help me make a difference, to help me make my life mean something more permanent, to help me become somebody who made a difference to others. Dying of cancer is such a random, cruel and ultimately solitary experience and I wanted it to create a positive reaction in some way. I want people to think of me and smile. If telling my story, our story, can save just one woman from saying goodbye to her children too early then I'll feel that my death will not be meaningless. That is a comfort.

But there's something else I want to do with this book, too. I want to show how people can help their loved ones inflicted by this disease. If I can make someone think twice before uttering a comment like, 'Just be positive, you can beat this!' – as if cancer cells shrivel up and die if you are cheery – then that will be another great outcome. There is a big difference between a cancer diagnosis and a terminal cancer diagnosis. I know because I've experienced both. I can be as positive as Pollyanna and as cheery as The Wiggles but it won't help me this time around. I understand that people struggle to know what to say. I get that people want to help. Being positive definitely makes the life I have left more meaningful, but it won't extend it – it won't give me more time.

So, just remember this: don't be scared. You don't have to say something wise or witty or memorable. Be there for your friend or family member. Listen. Hold their hand when they need it, and give them space when they need that too.

There are no rules when it comes to dealing with cancer – for the person with the disease or for those who love them. We all have to find our own way. But thanks to my family and a promise Sam made, my cancer has meant $1.8 million (and counting) has been raised for breast cancer research, more women are getting their breasts checked, and we have one big story to tell.

We weren't sure how we should put it all down. There is so much to say and Sam and I have very different ways of seeing things and very different ways of telling the story. So we decided the best way was to mix it up a bit between us. This is our way. This is our story.

Connie xx ♡

PART I

THE NOT-SO-SECRET LIFE OF US

CHAPTER 1

DEAD LEG

22 NOVEMBER 1989

'Dad, *pleeease*, my leg is really sore, I can't ride to school. Can you give me a lift?'

My family often teased me about the way I counted my bruises, and I was always telling them something ached or that I felt sick. Dad called me 'the girl who cried wolf' so his response wasn't totally unexpected.

'Con, I can't drop everything just because you're a bit sore. I've got that important meeting and I'm running late. You're going to have to get yourself there. I'll see you this afternoon.' He straightened his tie, swept up his briefcase, and headed for the door. I was just being Connie.

None of us knew it, but that morning was the start of everything turning upside down. This time there really was a wolf hiding in the bushes, just out of sight. Dad had no idea I'd already tried to ride to school, but my left leg hurt so much I went back to ask him for a lift. Sam had rushed off without me, leaving me the bike; he didn't want to be late, which was fair enough. I listened to Dad's car pull out of the driveway and then screamed in my loudest, angriest voice. I threw my house keys across the room and they smashed into the wall and fell to the carpet with a thud. That didn't make it any better.

'Well if I can't *get* to school, then I'm just not going to *go* to school,' the inner rebel in me whispered, but the conscientious do-gooder I really am drowned her out. I had only ever missed class when I had chickenpox as a primary schooler and I had never missed one period of Year 7. I prided myself on my good grades, so the thought of skipping class was a first for me.

I knew if I didn't hurry I'd be late for first period Geography so I didn't really have time to debate with myself any longer. I grabbed my bag and limped out to the driveway where the bike I shared with Sam lay on its side. I hoisted my heavy school bag onto the pack-rack and strapped it on, swung my leg up over the crossbar, onto the pedal and pushed off.

Pain seared in the calf of my left leg and tears ran down my cheeks without me actually crying. I had to stop before I even got as far as the end of the driveway. I didn't know what to do. Walking hurt too much, pedalling hurt too much, so I ended up hopping on my good leg, while leaning on the bike, all the way to school.

It was a hot November morning already, even though it wasn't yet 9 am. It was surely going to be a sizzling summer. I was sweating and had to stop every hundred metres or so to have a little rest. I soon realised that there was no way I was going to make it in time for Geography. I wondered if anyone would notice and if Mr Castlemaine would wonder where I was. I didn't want to get into trouble. I decided I'd give up on getting to school on time and just aim to make it before the beginning of second period French. I started to cry properly, not from pain, but from frustration. I didn't like the feeling that I was wagging school – I just wanted to get to class and start working – and I certainly didn't want to face the embarrassment of walking into class long after everyone else. My French teacher, Mrs Raynor, was strict and I knew she'd have no sympathy for a latecomer.

Part hopping, part riding, part leaning on my bike – I finally made it to school. The bike shed had already been locked, so I chained my bike to the side of the fence and started hobbling in the direction of the classrooms. I was hot and sweaty and I was sure my face was red. When I cry I get a red mark on my right cheek that Sam calls my crying mark. He can always tell when I've been crying because it doesn't fade for hours. I limped up to the classroom and peered through the little glass panel in the heavy blue door of the French classroom. Class had already begun and as soon as I made eye contact with Mrs Raynor, the tears started again. I slid down the wall onto the floor like a sack of potatoes. I couldn't walk into the class and have everyone look at my red face, and my leg hurt so much I couldn't bear it.

When Mrs Raynor saw me through the window, her normally neutral expression became concerned. I heard her tell the class to go on with an exercise and she came out to where I was slumped on the floor. She squatted down and put an arm around me. This little kindness was too much for my fragile state and I just cried and cried. I eventually stuttered through the sobs that my leg was sore and that I was sorry for being late. She behaved just how I imagined a mum would act – she cuddled me, reassured me, and walked me to the office, letting me lean on her arm the whole way to reduce the pain and strain on my leg. Her kindness just made me cry even more.

When we got to the office, Mrs Raynor whispered something to the lady behind the sliding glass window and took me to the sick bay where a teacher I had never met came to see me. He explained that he was a science teacher and a medic and he took a look at my leg. He told me that it was very swollen and asked if I'd been bitten by anything on the way to school. With a concerned look on his face, he left the room with Mrs Raynor to go and call my dad.

I didn't want anyone to call Dad. He'd been working all year researching and writing a history for the Royal Melbourne Golf Club and this was the day he was presenting his first draft. It was a big deal. I sat in the sick bay and hoped that they wouldn't be able to get hold of him. I could hear the office lady on the phone asking for a Mr Joseph Johnson.

'Connie's leg is very swollen and she needs medical attention. Are you able to come and pick her up?' I heard the office lady say.

After a little while, Mrs Raynor came back in to the sick bay, sat beside me on the bed and put her arm around me again. 'I have to get back to class, Connie. The students will be wreaking havoc by now without me there. You take care now. Your dad is going to be here soon. He'll take you to see a doctor.'

I bit my lip trying not to cry again. She was being so nice, and my leg was so sore. Another tear escaped as she walked away.

I sat in the sick bay, swinging my leg back and forth over the side of the bed, waiting for Dad. It didn't hurt as long as I didn't touch it, or put weight on it. I started to think maybe there was nothing wrong with it at all. 'What if Dad arrives and I'm fine?' I worried. He would be furious. I jumped down off the side of the bed and as soon as I put weight on my left leg the pain burned again. I breathed a sigh of relief – at least I wasn't pulling Dad out of work for nothing.

It was so weird just waiting there, and time seemed to drag. A big clock hung on the wall above the bed, ticking loudly, and I could hear the office lady tapping away on a typewriter in the other room. The school seemed so quiet and eerie with everyone in class.

After what seemed like an eternity I heard the creaky clack of Dad's leather shoes on the lino in the school corridor. 'I'm Joe Johnson, here to collect Connie. You rang me.'

When the office lady escorted him into the sick bay he smiled at me. He grabbed my bag and walked out, my signal to go with him. I couldn't keep up so he slowed down and asked quietly, 'How's your leg?'

'It hurts so much,' I said.

'I'm sorry about this morning. I didn't realise it was so bad.'

There was a doctor's surgery just across the road from the school, so we drove there, and sat down in the waiting room. The room was brown – the walls were panelled with wood and the carpet was brown with orange stripes. There were two brown lounges and several brown plastic chairs lining the walls. It felt dark and dingy, and the silence made it seem even darker. There was an old woman with a walking frame sitting opposite us. I started playing with the toys that were in the corner of the waiting room. There was one of those wooden blocks with coloured twisted wires with beads on them. I started threading the beads along a wire and counting them.

The woman looked at me sideways and I realised I was too old to be playing with a toddler's toy like that, so I pushed it away and waited quietly.

'Constance Johnson?' the doctor called. His name was Dr Liefman. He had a calm smile and he patted me on the back as I limped in with Dad. I liked him right away. When he saw my leg, he pulled a piece of string out of his top drawer and held it around my right leg, then he threaded it around my left leg. He held the string up to Dad with his thumbs marking two points on the string about 10 centimetres apart.

'There is some significant swelling, and there is no evidence of a bite of any kind,' Dr Liefman said.

Dad tilted his head to one side slightly. 'So what do you think it is?'

'I can't tell at this point, but we need to do an X-ray. Right away, please. Tell them you need to bring the films with you and then report back to me immediately. Don't worry about an appointment. I will see you when you get back.'

As we left the doctor's surgery, Dad looked down the street and nodded towards the milk bar. 'Want a bag of mixed lollies, Con?'

'Nah, I can't walk that far. Let's just go,' I answered.

—

The hospital was busy; there were doctors and nurses walking around talking to each other, looking at files as they went. There were mums with crying babies, and lots of old people in the waiting room.

Dad tapped his foot impatiently as we waited for our turn. He folded his arms across his chest, leant back against the wall and glanced across at a man with an icepack wrapped around his hand. 'Guess the job,' he said, trying to get me to join in one of our favourite games. We guess what strangers do for a living, and make up stories about them.

'Definitely a tradie, look at those boots, and the shorts. I can't tell if he's a builder or a council worker,' I offered.

'I think he's a brickie. And he must have a dog that goes to work with him. I wonder where the dog is now? Probably in the back of the ute in the car park.'

'Yeah, his dog is called Jack, and it's one of those black and white sheepdogs – you know? A border collie. Do you reckon he's married?'

'Definitely. His wife's name is Janet and she's at home making him a stew for dinner tonight.'

We continued making up lives for all the people in the waiting room, inventing names, jobs, pets and children. I leant against Dad, he put his arm around me and we cuddled, still waiting for our turn.

When we finally got called, I had to go in by myself. It hurt as they twisted and bent my leg every which way to get the right pictures and, even though I tried not to, I cried out in pain.

Back at Dr Liefman's with the X-rays, the receptionist buzzed the intercom and he came out immediately and ushered us into his room. He read the report and held the X-rays up to the light. Then he asked if he could talk to Dad alone for a few minutes.

I went and sat back in the horrible brown room to do even more waiting. When Dad finally came out to get me, his face was this weird shade of grey and he walked with his shoulders stooped, his hands hanging limply by his sides. He held his arm out to me and I hobbled over into a cuddle as he helped me out to the car.

When I was sitting safely in the front seat, he said he'd be back in a minute, and walked away down the street. He came back a few minutes later holding one of the biggest bags of mixed lollies I'd ever seen. 'Let's share them, hey?' he said, and started the ignition.

CHAPTER 2

NO VICTIMS IN THIS FAMILY . . . BUT A SIX-YEAR-OLD CRIMINAL GETS AWAY WITH THE PRIZE

Every family has a black sheep, but my family is different – they are all black sheep except for me. I am the white sheep. I knew that I was better than my dad, better than my brother, better than my sister, from a very young age. I had proven it, time and time again.

How did I know? Well, for one, my bedroom was organised.

The teddies were arranged in a row from largest to smallest, colour graded, with the dark brown teddies fading into the light brown then grey to white, like a new tin of Derwent pencils. They sat at the end of my bed, which was covered with a mismatch of tatty old sheets and blankets pulled tight and tucked in. Dad might not have bought me age or gender appropriate bedding (no pink princesses for me), but the bedding I did have was perfectly presented.

My pink painted cane wardrobe was filled with clothes hanging on colour-matched coathangers. My favourite brown and pink woollen jumper hung on a pink hanger, with my brown cardie on one side on a brown hanger, and my pink windcheater on the other side on a pink hanger.

Under my perfectly hung clothes sat my summer shoes and my winter shoes, side by side, in pairs – the sandals under my summer clothes and the school shoes under the winter clothes, with my gumboots standing at the end after a small gap, because although they were footwear, they couldn't be categorised with the other shoes.

My desk was never messy. I was so proud of that desk. It had a map of the world on it, and I wanted anyone who might wander into my room at any given moment to be able to see it in all its splendour, so there was never any clutter there. My pens, pencils and textas, all in their separate pencil cases, were lined up with precision in the top drawer. The second drawer held paper and notebooks, and all of my paperwork was organised into manila folders in the bottom drawer – one for stories, one for drawings and one for the cards and letters I had received over the years. No matter what I was doing, or what stage my projects were at, I always tidied up afterwards, leaving my world map clearly visible.

Having a clean room illustrated to people, whomever they were, that I was clean, mature and responsible. This didn't matter to Sam. Things were strewn about all over his room – it was absolute chaos.

This is what Sam doesn't understand. Order matters.

—

Sam: There was Connie's way and then there was Connie's way. They were my choices. If I wanted to be the doctor, too bad, it was my job to be the patient, doctor's orders . . . every time. If we were playing Canasta, her 'pures' were way more pure than mine, and were relished as such. She was so good at her homework too. She worked meticulously and decorated her homework in a way that helped me see how she became an avid scrap-booker. When she coloured in a picture, she *never* went outside the lines. My concentration would drift and I breached the lines heaps, always realising too late. She always maintained authority, even when she was play-acting. She was older, smarter. And she was boss.

Now I think about it, maybe Connie had a part in my anti-authoritarian streak, which is still a big part of me today. She was a tempestuous girl and when she got that 'Connie' look, you most certainly didn't mess with her, or you'd be liable to cop a shoe in the head when you weren't looking.

—

Sam was three when our mum died. I was four. Dad brought us up. Our elder sister Hilde is eight years older than me and she left home when she was fifteen. We moved around a lot as kids, every year a different house, a different school. Dad was a writer, and anyone who writes for a living knows it can be feast or famine, so he was also a renovator. That's how he supported us after Mum died – writing at home, which allowed him to be with us – he'd fit writing and renovating around bringing up his kids. He had vision. He could see a palatial family home in an old rundown shack. He would buy something unfit for human habitation and turn it into something big and beautiful.

13

All with his own hands. And while he was getting up ladders and painting, knocking down walls and re-carpeting rooms, he was always thinking. Structuring sentences, moulding ideas and organising his thoughts so that at night, when we were asleep, he could sit down with a beer and write his books. He would sell the house for a profit and publish a book each year, earning enough money to buy another shack, and just enough money for us to live on.

Each time we left a place I was sad, because we were leaving a house I finally approved of and wasn't embarrassed to bring my friends to, but I was also excited. Excited that I would have a new start. A clean slate.

Once we were old enough, Dad would enlist our help to pack up at the end of each year, in preparation for the next move. Once Hilde moved out of home I was the boss as far as I was concerned. I would proudly help Dad. He could rely on me – unlike Sam, who would get bored and wander off. I worked hard and helped Dad stay organised. The kitchen was always my favourite room to pack. One box for glasses and mugs. One box for plates and bowls. One box for pots. One box for cutlery. And at the end, when there was a mismatch of kitchen items that didn't fit in their allocated boxes, I would seal up the final box and proudly label it 'Misc'. Everything is alright in the world if you just have some order.

I would also pack up my own room, sealing and marking each box with a permanent marker. I would leave the boxes in a neat pile, waiting for Dad or Sam to come and carry them for me. I wasn't strong, so I left the lifting to them. I didn't want to hurt myself or add to my already vast collection of bruises.

My list of injuries was wide and varied and when they happened, I'd make sure to tell Dad and Sam all about them. A paper cut on my finger, a bruise on my knee, a sore elbow; 'Could it be dislocated?' I'd ask. The thing was, nobody understood how fragile I was. They always laughed at me for gingerly presenting my latest wound or for not being able to catch a ball in case I hurt myself. They joked that I couldn't run a hundred metres without falling over. When I tried my hand at tennis, they were in hysterics: I'd swing my racquet through the air, so confident that this was going to be the shot that showed them I wasn't such a klutz, and then I'd miss the ball entirely and fall on my bum. (I didn't show them that bruise!) I wanted to be a part of their boys club. I wanted to be good at tennis like Dad and Sam. I wanted to be good at footy. I wanted to show them that I could be as good on the sports field as I was in the classroom.

That's what I was trying to do on the day we packed up the house in Williamstown. We were waiting for the removalists to come and Grandma (Mum's mum) had come over to say goodbye and wish us luck. I was sitting precariously on a pile of boxes, watching Dad and Sam play a bit of kick-to-kick. Eager to impress, I decided to join in and stood so that I would make a triangle with them and could be included. They didn't even notice I was there. I called out, 'Kick it to me, kick it to me,' and Dad kicked the ball my way. It was a little kick, he was being gentle with me but I was determined to prove myself and show him he didn't have to be. I was going to be more like Sam! The ball was sailing through the air, as if in slow motion, and I jumped up, arms held high, ready to make the mark and show them both what I could do. The ball hit the tip of my middle finger and I fumbled, the ball fell to the ground and I followed, screaming in pain. I'd broken my finger this time, I was sure of it.

Sam laughed and ran over to scoop up the ball, then ran back to his position to continue the game. Dad shouted out, 'Up you get, Con, you'll be right,' as he caught Sam's huge kick. Only Grandma understood the gravity of the situation. She pulled me into a hug and inspected my finger closely, asking me to move it and frowning when I couldn't.

Grandma insisted that Dad take me to the hospital for an X-ray and wouldn't listen when he tried to tell her I'd be fine. The X-ray proved quick smart what I already knew and I was sent home with a bandage on my hand, which I wore proudly as a badge of honour. I wasn't going to let Dad and Sam forget it.

I may not have been sporty like Sam, or as good at riding a bike, but I held the place as 'the smart one' in the family. This was a position I guarded fiercely because my hold on it was tenuous at best. Sam was superior to me in many ways, but as far as I was concerned I had the smarts, and with that knowledge I was able to maintain my grip on this disorderly world. That was my thing. Sam had his own way of making things okay and I'll let him tell his own story throughout this part. But I reserve the right to be the boss of it.

—

Sam: Connie may have had her ordered-universe thing going on but there was only ever one thing that truly suited me as a young boy, and that was my bike. It wasn't just a bike to me. It was my first true companion *and* a ticket to freedom. It was always there. Never did it tell me what to do or where to go or how to be – I told it and I was boss. My trusty bike might as well have had wings because, to me, riding actually felt like flying. Who needed a Magic Carpet or a Wishing Chair when you could glide through the air as smoothly as I did? I favoured laneways, shortcuts, tracks and driveway kerbs, as all boys do, but one thing I felt most sure of was that I loved whizzing down hills more than any other kid.

But the thing was, I didn't own a bike that was *meant* to fly. Mine was bought sixth-hand from the *Trading Post* and was heavy and ugly; re-sprayed into awfulness. I had to share it with Connie and, because we shared, I could dink better than anyone. My knack for physical trickery was born the day I realised I could escort Connie on my bike no matter where she wanted to place herself, school bags and all. I became a weight-distribution specialist. No one ever asked if they could have a turn on my heavy black bike, but that's only because they didn't know my bike was magic. It took Connie where she needed to be and me *wherever* I wanted to go. And it didn't need batteries because you don't need batteries to fly a bike.

Part of the reason I felt so free on my bike was that Dad rarely placed limits or boundaries on us, and when he did he did it for good reason. For example, during our stint in Gawler, in what was then the outskirts of Adelaide, I was never allowed to get off the train at Elizabeth Station. As an almost-nine-year-old, I knew exactly why. It was the murder capital of the state and poverty, crime, violence and drugs were everywhere. Although I didn't possess the capacity to even remotely comprehend the nuances of social discord, I did have enough Dickens up me to know that if I *did* get off at Elizabeth Station, some Fagin type would most certainly net me and force me to steal stuff and make my family ashamed of me. Dad's perfectly painted picture of peril prevailed against any desire I may have held to defy his clear and powerful brand of reasoning.

But, Elizabeth Station aside, I was pretty much allowed free rein and through this I developed my lust for independence – a desire which still burns obstinately within me today. If I had nowhere in particular to go and no one in particular to share my time with, I would play the left–right game with myself. I'd just get on my bike and take a left, then I'd take a right, then a left, and so on, until I happened upon something worth stopping for – like feathers. Not any old seagull discard; no, it took more than that, but an uncommon feather, however small, would be enough to stop me in my tracks, especially a spotted feather – they really took my fancy. A good skimming stone would also do the trick. A solid stick that could double as a scythe. A particularly odd or vivid flower. A centipede. A ball. (I was always surprised by the number of unattended balls lying around the place.) I even found my share of stray dogs. They loved following me because I loved dogs and dogs can tell who loves them. I'd lead them home and beg Dad to let me keep them. Curiosity led me forward; I just loved not knowing what was around the corner. I was at the very beginning of learning just how much there was to learn.

On my bike, playing the left–right game, I found so many good spots. There were two basic prerequisites that defined a good spot: it had to be hard to find *and* hidden from view. The bonus factor came into play if the good spot boasted a perch; somewhere from where you could more fully appreciate said good spot. These spots were rare and I was on constant lookout for them. When I found a fresh good spot I'd excitedly bank it away in my mind as a safe place to go, should I ever need it. I had no experience with the toughness of life at this point, but I definitely held with me a sense of general foreboding. My best friend, David Blosfelds, had a dad who was an ambo, and he was the first on the scene at the infamous Russell Street Bombings in Melbourne in 1986. Plus, Dad listened to ABC radio all the time so I knew that life would not always be good and that one day my luck would surely run out and I would probably inevitably need refuge from something, if not everything, statistically, perhaps. You just never know, *really*, do you?

I had at least 20 proper good spots on the go at any one time. Some of the better ones made such an indelible impression on me that I could even find them for you now, first try. If I was ever trailing with a friend I would delight in revealing my good spots, under an oath of secrecy of course, invariably evoking lashings of appreciation. I knew I was a better explorer than my friends. They had Lego and trampolines and things to distract them. I harboured no such frippery and just knew my hood. It was thanks not just to the curiosity that Dad had so carefully fostered in me, but also to my bike, which enabled me to discover worlds previously unknown. In an adult-free zone on a bike with wings, with nought for distraction, there was no way I *wasn't* going to stockpile a stash of earthly delights, and that's exactly what I did. If the aliens landed, or if everything got atomic again, or if the AIDS thing became more than a thing, or if the Ozone went to *every* zone, then I would perhaps end up being feted as the Official Master of Safe Spots — of that I could be unsure.

—

Sam's right. Dad didn't put limits on us. He trusted us. And, let's be honest, how hard is it to trust someone who colour-codes their clothes? Sam was another story, and I wasn't going to let him forget it. When he was six and I was seven we went shopping with Dad after school. Dad shopped in small quantities every day — to the bakery for a loaf of bread, to the greengrocer to get the fruit for our lunches the next day and the vegies for dinner, then off to the butcher for the meat for dinner that night and the cold meats for our sandwiches. He'd go to the supermarket to get biscuits. Dad always bought gingernuts, because neither Sam nor I liked them, and so we wouldn't eat them and leave him with nothing to have with his cup of tea. At the supermarket counter one day I saw Sam's arm shoot out quickly and then his hand disappeared into his pocket. I didn't think much of it until we got outside. Dad was walking ahead of us to the car and Sam pulled out a pack of chewy and offered me a piece.

The look on his face gave it away and I knew what he'd done. He was so happy to have something to share, that he didn't even consider I'd be worried. I refused to take a piece but waited until he had chewed the entire pack before telling him that he shouldn't have shoplifted. I allowed him to dig himself into a hole. Once he had his mouth full of a huge wad of gum there was no chance of redemption. I now had a weapon, and I wasn't afraid to use it. Often.

For the next five years every time Sam threatened to dob on me for something or did something I didn't like, the threat came out.

'Stop teasing me, Sam, or I'll tell Dad about the chewy.'

It had immense power and I wielded it with neither shame nor pity.

'Stop copying me. I'll tell Dad about the chewy.'

'Give me some of your lollies, or I'll tell Dad.'

Sometimes I didn't even need to say it, I just looked at him in a certain way and he acquiesced.

One night we were up late, way after bedtime. Dad was in the bath so we went to the kitchen to grab a snack. Sam poured himself some cornflakes and I did the same. He poured on the milk and sprinkled on some sugar, with *my* favourite spoon. I loved that spoon. It had a black plastic handle and was the only one like it we had. It didn't match the silverware we inherited from Nanna (Dad's mum) when she died. It was a stray.

I asked Sam politely for 'my' spoon back and he said no, he was using it. Then he told me it was, in fact, 'his' spoon.

After a heated argument I pulled out my well-worn weapon: 'Give me my spoon or I'll tell Dad about the chewy.'

He looked me straight in the eye and said, 'So, tell him. I don't care.'

My shock was profound. This had always worked! I called his bluff, walked confidently to the bathroom door and knocked boldly. He didn't seem worried at all. I mouthed 'I *will* tell' and he just shrugged in a completely infuriating way.

I had no alternative. I either had to use my ammo and lose it forever, or walk away and accept that Sam had won the favoured black spoon. I wasn't giving up so easily.

'Dad, do you want to know what Sam did?' I called through the bathroom door.

'Oh, Con, you should be in bed. You should both be in bed. And don't be a dobber, people don't like dobbers,' Dad replied.

I ignored that and ploughed on.

'But Dad, it's important, you really need to know about this, it's really bad.' I took a deep breath and blurted it out, 'Sam stole some chewy from the supermarket.' I was filled with confidence, sure that Sam was well and truly busted.

'When did this happen, Con?' my dad asked from the other side of the door, sounding bored and irritated.

My confidence slipped a notch. 'When he was in Grade One.'

'Oh, don't be silly. It happened years ago. Why would I be worried about that?'

The victory was Sam's and he walked away, holding the spoon up proudly, waving his hand from side to side. I knew I was never going to use 'my' spoon again.

CHAPTER 3

A FLOCK OF SEAGULLS WINS THE DAY AND THE CROWN SLIPS AWAY

I've heard it said that families are defined by big, dramatic moments, and I guess that's true to a degree. Every family, every person, faces sorrow, loss, death and dysfunction at different times and we all learn to cope with it in different ways. But I think what really defines a family are the small moments – the everyday moments, the funny rituals that develop, the in-jokes, and the quiet moments that reveal so much without anyone realising it at the time.

One of the rituals my family had was to get together once a week for a takeaway dinner. Even though Hilde wasn't living with us she'd always come too. It was the highlight of the week for Sam and me. Sometimes, if the weather was good, Dad would pick us up after school and we'd go down to the strand at Williamstown with a bundle of battered fish, potato cakes and chips wrapped in butcher's paper and sit near the beach.

Dad would never wait until we got there to eat. He'd tear open the packet while he was driving, pull out some steaming hot chips and eat them on the way. The smell of those fish and chips used to fill the car and I'd be salivating, wanting to get my hands on my share.

Once we found a table and all sat down, the seagulls started to muster around us, squawking, diving, hoping for a morsel to be thrown their way. Sam has always been fiercely protective of us and it didn't matter who (or what) you were, he always stood up for the family.

One night at Williamstown the seagulls were hassling us more than usual and Sam kept getting up to chase them away. He ran with his arms flailing about, shouting, 'Go away, birds, this is our dinner!' He ran so far that the birds circled past him and flew back and snatched his chips, gobbling them down, not caring at all about my crazy little brother, who was dashing about like a maniac, fighting a losing battle.

Dad, Hilde and I laughed so hard, but when Sam came back to sit down after his third failed attempt to scare the gulls away, he seemed really sad. It was like he'd suddenly realised he couldn't protect us at all. That day he was outwitted by seagulls but from that moment on it was like a weight settled on his shoulders. He was just one seven-year-old boy against the world.

I laughed at Sam that night but I recognised the vulnerability in his eyes. I sat there eating my chips and laughing, hoping the attention would stay on him because I had a secret. Better he be the brunt of the joke than me. I was too embarrassed to tell my family that earlier that day I'd wet my pants at school. I'd been holding on too long. I didn't know what to do, so I took off my undies and put them in the bin. Luckily my skirt wasn't wet, but I spent the rest of the day holding my skirt down, making sure it didn't blow up in the wind and show me naked underneath. I didn't play, I just sat and watched and hoped that no one would find out.

After we'd finished our dinner and the gulls had moved on to harass another family, Hilde decided we should have a wheelbarrow race. I was absolutely horrified. For the game to work, Sam and I needed to be the wheelbarrows and Dad and Hilde needed to be the pushers. I refused to play.

Sam was perched on his arms, with Dad holding his legs poised to race. I grabbed hold of the bench, pulled my knees in tight together and didn't move.

'Come on, Con, don't be a spoilsport. We can't race if you don't join in,' Hilde pleaded.

I shook my head and didn't move.

Hilde came over and started tickling me and I writhed around, giggling involuntarily, 'Stop it, Hilde, stop it.' I was getting upset but I couldn't help laughing. The tickle turned into a wrestle and Hilde outmanoeuvred me, prising me away from the bench, and before I knew it I was on the grass. She grabbed my legs, and we were off and away.

Sam and Dad raced ahead. Sam always wins races, no matter what it is – running, egg and spoon, wheelbarrow – he always wins. Just when I thought I was going to get out of this with my dignity intact a gust of wind blew my skirt over my head. Hilde dropped my legs and I collapsed onto the grass, grasping for my skirt, trying to save any remaining dignity I had left.

'Connie's wearing no knickers!' Hilde pointed and laughed. They tried to hold the laughter in but it burst out uncontrollably and they laughed uproariously. I sat on the ground, red-faced, and burst into tears.

All these years later, I remember that night. I remember feeling small and sad and completely separate from my family. I was the clever one. I was the organised one. But now I was also the bare-bottomed one. I didn't like being the joke. I didn't like it one bit.

—

Maybe the reason I was so upset was because my hold on my position as the smart one in the family was feeling shaky. The truth of the matter was that Sam wasn't bad in the classroom, it was just that I was that little bit better. I'd earned my 'smart' title. I couldn't compete with him on most things, but knowing I was good at something was really important to me and there wasn't enough of a gap between us for me to relax. I couldn't stop studying, stop trying, stop busting a gut to be the smartest. If I lost that title then who would I be?

When I was in Grade Six and Sam was in Grade Five, I had one of those 'once in a lifetime' teachers – Mrs Giddens. She challenged me. She put words on the spelling tests that I struggled with, just for me, just so I wouldn't get ahead of myself and start thinking I was too smart for the rest of the kids in my class. She appreciated my intellect, and challenged me to take it to the next level. Mrs Giddens made me realise that I could be whoever I wanted to be. She understood that I wanted to be a success, and encouraged me to explore how I could make that happen.

She set projects for me and I worked hard and put everything into them. They were always interesting, always challenging.

And then she set a project on . . . transport. Why would I want to research and write about planes, trains and automobiles? I was appalled.

I went home to tell Dad, half expecting him to tell me not to worry about it, just to do it quick and get on with the real stuff. But he didn't. He said, 'Con, something I have found while writing my books is that anything is interesting if you look at it long and hard enough. Do your research, work as hard on this as you would on any assignment, and you will find out that it's interesting.' I thought he'd be on my side, but he had a lesson to teach me.

So I begrudgingly started my research. I was surprised to discover that motorcycles were invented before cars, and that the production line that Ford pioneered is the building block of all manufacturing today.

Later that afternoon, I wandered into Dad's room, where he was sitting at his desk, writing his latest book with his favourite type of pen – the kind that Sam and I bought for him every Father's and Mother's Day. 'Dad, what do you think was invented first, the car or the motorbike?' I asked.

'I don't know, Con, maybe the motorbike, since it could have been developed from the bicycle,' he replied, glancing up from his notepad.

'Yep. You're right. I would have thought the car would be invented first, you know, from horse-drawn carriages.'

'I guess transport isn't such a boring topic after all, Con.' He laughed, picked up his pen and resumed his writing.

That's what I mean about small, quiet moments. I look back now and think this is one of the most precious gifts Dad ever gave me as a parent. He showed me to get on with it, and that if I was going to be disenchanted and disappointed, that was my choice, because there is always something good to be found in any situation. You just have to look hard enough. Well, most of the time!

I completed that project on a huge piece of cardboard with a fancy, lettered heading, coloured in perfectly. Of course I got a good mark, and mine was chosen to be one of the posters to be put on display in the corridor. When my classmates called me a teacher's pet, I was proud of the label – what was wrong with that?

But then something happened that made my crown slip.

There was an announcement at the weekly assembly. Our school had been chosen to send some children as representatives to the Asian-Pacific Children's Convention, which was to be held in Japan later in the year. I started to tremble with excitement. Maybe politics is where I would display my greatness, maybe this could be the beginning of my burgeoning political career. I could be a politician, a minister of parliament, or even the prime minister – Australia's first female prime minister. Yep, that could be me. I had to apply. Surely I would be chosen.

My confidence faltered when I overheard Sam discussing his application with Dad in the kitchen when I got home. As I loitered outside the door, I could hear the excitement in Sam's voice at the prospect of travelling overseas. Then I realised that he had an advantage over me. He was learning Japanese at school while I was learning Latin. Slowly but surely doubt crept in.

—

Sam: I was busy thinking ten-year-old thoughts when they made a very special announcement at assembly. Our school had been allocated ten places at the Asian-Pacific Children's Convention for ten- to eleven-year-olds, to be held in Fukuoka, Japan! While I had no idea that this was mostly due to the fact that Black Rock Primary was one of the only primary schools in the state to offer Japanese, I did know that we could apply as long as we fitted into the age bracket. After a brief few moments of panic I established my eligibility and set about dreaming of a trip overseas. The world beckoned, beseeching me to explore it. I hungered for something more. I could be some kind of pioneer, maybe? Someone who went to Youth Conferences and engaged in wholesome and meaningful stuff like holding hands, lighting candles, singing songs and releasing balloons and doves into the sky in the name of unity. Becoming a Youth Ambassador and representing my country on an international stage? Gee whiz and holy moly. Maybe I could become one of those people who counted.

Dad helped me with the application form, which I printed in my neatest writing, and when notice of my interview came, I quizzed him about it over the dinner table.

'You must show an interest in their culture.' Dad advised. 'It's very different from ours. Geisha girls, temples, sumo wrestling and such. Learn about it and find what you're interested in.'

Off to the *Britannica* it was then. There's something lovely about an old-fashioned Google search, and I drifted through the thin pages with wonder.

I knew that Craig was my number-one threat. He was a ginger-nut genius. Even his face was enquiring. The teacher would ask for his help when maths got tricky and it was widely accepted that he'd spend all of his hours outside school buried in scholastic endeavour – just another savage untruth floating around the yard, I realise now. I had him on social skills but he creamed me in smarts. With my wonky maths I had somehow surmised that the likelihood of them choosing two boys from my class was next to none. If I could edge Craig out I might be in with a chance. I envied Craig. Every day he came to school with a large Hershey chocolate bar and he was so bloody clever. He would surely be chosen. He deserved it more, really.

I sweated my way through the interview – my very first audition. While I chided myself afterwards for my lack of articulateness, I could at least take comfort in the fact that I had given it my best shot. I waxed about how interested I was in Japanese culture, but it all felt a bit false. I didn't quite believe myself. Was I actually interested in their ancient culture or did I just want to channel Huck Finn and go places? I concluded that although they would probably have seen through me, I was still sort of almost maybe in with a semi-fighting chance. Hopefully Craig had stuffed up his interview. Not really, but kind of.

An interminable wait followed. Finally, the time for the winners to be announced arrived. I stared, terrified at the principal at assembly as he read out the list of ten names. My heart was about to pop. Would I be gifted the golden ticket? Craig's name was read out. I nodded to myself. I expected that. I tried to look at him but I couldn't yet. I steeled myself as they kept reading out names that weren't mine. Just. Don't. Cry. Then it came through, 'Sam Johnson – 5D.'

I knew that my life changed significantly in that moment,
but it wasn't until I turned 36 that I realised just how much.

—

The principal stood at the front of the assembly, explaining that there were so many more applications than there were places, and they were all good, but, by necessity, only a few had been chosen. My heart sunk, how could Sam get chosen? Why not me? I worked so much harder than him at school. He just winged it – never put any *real* effort in.

I could feel a lump in my throat and I fought back tears. I wanted to scream, 'Where is the justice?' My political career was over before it even began. I looked down, unable to clap, unable to enjoy this success for my little brother. I concentrated hard on the floorboards of the assembly hall, tracing the wood grain with my finger. If I looked up people would see how upset I was, how awful I was not to be happy for my brother. They would realise that Sam had taken my crown.

Now who would I be?

CHAPTER 4

THE GIRL WHO HAS CANCER AND THE BROTHER OF THE GIRL WHO HAS CANCER

Sam: I exhausted the first of three rolls of film I'd been allocated for my ten-day trip to Japan before we'd hit 20,000 feet. I'd somehow scored a window seat for my first trip into the sky and it absolutely blew my noodle as we went up through the clouds. I was seated over the wing and all the flaps on the wings terrified and excited me. This was even better than my bike!

I stayed with a host family and saw temples, sumo-training facilities, judo, tea ceremonies and sure enough, 10,000 kids from across each and every South East Asian nation (even including the Federated States of Micronesia!) did indeed hold hands, sing songs, light candles and release balloons into the sky, all in the name of unity. Watching 10,000 white balloons, one for each kid, was pretty special and I didn't mind that there were no doves. Not one bit.

I was walking with my host family along a street when we passed a massive park. I looked in to see a whole big bunch of kids unicycling around the place on a couple of basketball courts. I had seen a unicycle in a circus, or a book, or somewhere, but I didn't realise they were commonly available, or that anyone could ride them. It looked fun. It was 1988 and, as it turned out, there was a thriving unicycling scene in Japan. I wanted to go and try, but we were on our way somewhere and I only paused to watch for a few seconds before walking on.

Before the Children's Convention in Japan, I'd always planned on becoming a tennis champion like Ivan Lendl. He was number one in the world, and I'd seen his penis when I was seven (which isn't nearly as creepy as it sounds). Let me explain: Dad worked out pretty quickly that novels don't pay, so after Mum died, with three young kids to feed, he started writing commissioned histories. He effectively became a sports historian and when I was seven he tackled a history of the Australian Open Tennis Championship, which led to him walking me through the bowels of Melbourne Park during the Australian Open. We walked into the change rooms just as Ivan Lendl, number one in the world, turned around to throw his used socks in a waste bin and virtually flung his massive cock into my face, leaving me almost literally gobsmacked. While I'd love to say that it was Ivan Lendl's penis that inspired me to aim to become the world's greatest tennis player, the truth is a lot more pedestrian.

I had shown enough skill having a casual hit around on the street with Dad for him to book me in for a lesson at the local tennis club. On the day of my first lesson, I held my newly bestowed wooden racquet shakily as we approached the club. Yellow balls flew through the air – it was a hive of activity and the atmosphere thrilled me. I was very nervous to meet my coach, but he was supportive and it felt just great to be out there, running free, but with enough fun challenges – like keeping the ball in the court – to keep me occupied. And what boy doesn't like hitting stuff? In the car on the way home I knew I'd found something special, something that I might be good at.

For me, tennis wasn't just a dream. It was an ambition. I knew it wouldn't just magically happen, because Dad wasn't one of those parents who told their kids they could do anything if only they believed enough. If you told him you wanted to win Wimbledon, he'd break it down and, if anything, undersell its achievability.

'Sure,' he would explain, 'you can hold the trophy up, but a lot's got to go right to get you there. You could do everything right in the world, use all the talent you have and it still might not happen.' He explained what a 'grinder' was – someone who devotes their whole life to something, who does their utmost, and still achieves average results. If I was willing to accept that it would take a lifetime of sacrifice and hard work, and that I might never achieve the heights I dreamed of, he would support me the whole way. As long as I was happy to end up a grinder.

Dad was a realist. And he was never about being number one; doing your best was always good enough. He knew I knew every shot in the book. He knew I had the skill. He knew I had the application and the work ethic – he knew because he'd fostered it all in me. My game was bloody good. I held a tennis scholarship and achieved an ATP Junior ranking of sixth in my state. I won some decent tournaments and came close in the bigger ones. But big question marks lay over my 'temperament'.

Still, if I wasn't on my bike, I was smacking a tennis ball against a brick wall. It wasn't about mucking around either. The wall was an opponent and for all the thought I put into it every shot may as well have been match point. That's where I made my volleys what they were; against those walls. Despite having a massive problem with my attention span, I could devote hours to something if it was physical or menial. That's why I was the proud owner of such a large and tremendous vegie patch. It's why I was able to quite happily push my volleys to the limit against a wall for four or five hours, and back it up day after day after day. I just really liked trying hard at it because tennis was one of the few things I'd found that made me feel good.

One normal weekday, I stood on our small patch of grass out the front practising my shots, waiting for Dad to come and pick me up to take me to tennis. I had joined a larger club a few suburbs from home and while I could ride the distance on my bike, it wouldn't leave me with enough in the tank to go a hundred per cent when I hit the court, so Dad always drove me. But this day Dad was late.

The minutes overlapped and I started tiring of swing shots – where was he? This wasn't like him. Maybe he rang and I didn't hear the phone? I checked my watch. I wouldn't make my lesson. I started swiping my racquet low to the grass, clipping it into the air.

I looked up for the umpteenth time to see if Dad was coming and there he was, slowly entering the drive, with Connie in the front seat. I waved, but was barely acknowledged. Something was very wrong. Connie looked cold and lonely and was hugging her knees and Dad's face was more grey than normal and he had a very serious expression on his face. I was confused. What could have happened?

Dad turned to Con and I lip-read him saying, 'Wait here.' He got out of the car and headed towards the front door. He didn't look at me. He was walking differently – he looked older. I glanced back at Con but she was buried in herself. I decided to follow Dad inside to find out exactly what was going on. I banked left into the living room and looked down to see him curled up on our off-lime two-seater sofa. At first I thought he must be very tired, but then I saw his shoulders heaving. Then I heard the sobbing. Then it turned to weeping. I can remember the sound so clearly even now. It was the sound of utmost pain.

I said the first thing that came to mind: 'What's going on?'

Dad barely looked up at me. 'Your sister's got a tumour in her leg,' he said.

It sounded pretty serious. I didn't want to press Dad any further while he was so upset, even though I really wanted to ask what a tumour was. I didn't know Dad cried. It was the worst sound I had ever heard.

—

I didn't know what a tumour was either and I didn't want to look stupid, so I didn't ask. I shared the bag of lollies with Dad as he drove us home and tried to keep my leg from moving.

We didn't talk much. Dr Liefman told us we had to go to the hospital but Dad needed to stop home first to pick up a few things and take Sam to tennis. None of us talked much in the car but Sam and I weren't worried. As far as we were concerned, I just had a sore leg.

Once we'd dropped Sam off, Dad drove me to the children's hospital. I was admitted and assigned to a room with five other kids. They did more X-rays and I had a heap of doctors talking to me, asking me questions. They took Dad out of the room so they could talk to him too.

After a while Dad had to leave for a bit to pick up Sam. All the other kids in my room had either their mum or dad with them and it made me sad wondering what it would be like to have a mum. I felt very sorry for myself about my leg already, and looking around at all the other kids with their parents made me feel even worse.

I tried to make sense of what was happening to me by working out what everyone else was doing there. Diagonally opposite my bed there was a girl with just a few strands of long blonde hair left. She was in a wheelchair. Her name was Natasha and she told me her tumour was in her spine and she had been on chemo for three months. She said the doctors told her she would never walk again, but she was full of fire, and insisted angrily that she would walk, and run for that matter – she had her basketball to get back to. She wasn't going to let the doctors tell her how her story would end. Her mum was with her, and so were her six little brothers and sisters. They made a racket and I'd get used to her mum always yelling at one of the kids to be quiet, stop mucking up or to be nice to each other. Natasha seemed like the sensible older sister, who took control and looked after them when she wasn't too sick.

Next to me was a boy about my age, Mark Fletcher, who had a huge smile and big white teeth. His teeth were straight, except for one eye tooth which was a bit crooked and gave his smile a noticeably different sort of charm. He was tall and lanky, with a full head of brown hair. He stood out because he just didn't seem as sick as the other kids in the ward, in beds or roaming the corridors. And of course, he had so much hair. He knew all the staff by name and made in-jokes with them every time they came to do a blood test or check his blood pressure. I knew right away he wasn't a newbie. I was curious. His mum was there with him and his little brother. His little brother seemed to know the staff as well as Mark did and over the next few days I eavesdropped, mainly through boredom, and worked out from their conversations that he and his brother were both sick, they both had haemophilia, a blood condition, and had been in and out of the hospital since they were born. I can't imagine what that would be like. Just thinking about it makes me shudder.

There was a girl in the bed opposite me, who was also about my age. She didn't look like there was anything wrong with her, but then I guess I didn't look like there was anything wrong with me either. Her mum sat beside her bed. She was well dressed, had nice neat hair and make-up. She seemed like a mum out of a magazine and she talked to her daughter, stroking her hair occasionally. 'That's what it must be like to have a mum,' I thought.

The girl looked over at me and caught me staring. 'I'm Jacqui, what's your name?' she offered.

It turned out that Jacqui had come in that day too. She'd been playing netball when all of a sudden her hip got so sore that she couldn't walk anymore. She was 12, like me, and in Year 7. She asked me where my mum was and I brushed over the question and changed the subject quickly. We got talking and her mum went off to get a cuppa, leaving us to chat. It felt good to have someone to talk to, someone who was just as scared to be in hospital as I was. She had a tumour too and was staying in hospital until they worked out what to do, just like me.

—

The next day I found myself bored and watching the clock, hoping I didn't have to stay in hospital too much longer. It was so noisy and I found it impossible to sleep with so many people in the room. But worst of all it was just *so* boring. Dad had said that he would bring Sam in after school so I was just waiting for the day to pass, waiting for Sam to get there. Who would have thought I would ever be so keen to see my little brother?

The nurses came and went, always asking questions about how I was feeling, and whether I had been to the toilet. Gross! Why did they need to know if I'd had a pee? I mean, really.

Tick. Tock.

Tick. Tock.

A lady called Pat came to see me at one point. She was a teacher. They had a school at the hospital, but she said I wouldn't have to go until I'd been in hospital for one week. 'Am I going to be here that long?' I wondered.

I spent the rest of the day doing homework while I waited for Dad and Sam. For English I had to write the front page of a newspaper, and for Geography I had to draw a map of Europe. That kept me busy for a while at least and stopped me from going totally crazy from boredom. I talked to Jacqui a little more, but she had her mum, and then her dad and little sister came to visit. I began to wonder what was taking Dad so long. I started watching the clock again.

Three-thirty rolled around and I thought, 'Great! It won't be long till they get here now.'

At 4.30 pm I thought, 'Where are they? Shouldn't they be here by now?'

And by 5 pm I started to wonder whether they were coming at all.

At 5.30 I heard Dad's footsteps and Sam's voice coming down the corridor. I could have cried I was so relieved. It had been a long day and I wasn't used to being on my own. Whenever Dad left me alone I always had Sam with me, so it was always me and Sam. Never just me. Never.

Dad was carrying a plastic bag full of clothes for me and Sam had a tennis ball in his hand, which he would periodically bounce and catch, bounce and catch. Dad kissed me and gave me a big hug and I felt all the love in the world flooding from him to me. He embraced me and I felt safe.

'You've been a very brave girl, Con,' he said. 'I know it isn't easy being in hospital by yourself.'

I didn't understand why Sam couldn't miss school or Dad couldn't miss work, so I said so. I told Dad I didn't feel brave at all. I was hoping for another hug.

Dad sat down to hug me again and then explained in that careful, thoughtful way he had that I was going to be in hospital for a while so Sam had to keep going to school and he had to keep working to pay our bills. He'd called Hilde and she was on her way to Melbourne from Sydney where she lived now. Once Hilde arrived it would be easier. She'd be able to stay at the hospital or run around after Sam so that Dad could be with me more. After telling me how much he loved me, he asked, 'Would you like an ice-cream?'

He left Sam and me alone while he went to buy me something from the hospital snack bar. Mixed lollies yesterday in the car, and an ice-cream today? Dad didn't usually let us eat junk food, so the fact that he was not just allowing it but encouraging it made me think that something pretty bad must be happening. Was I sicker than I realised? Why would I be in hospital for a long time just because of a sore leg – a tumour or whatever they were calling it?

'Hey, Sis,' Sam whispered, looking behind him to make sure that Dad was gone. 'I don't know what's going on, do you? Last night I was waiting at tennis for hours! It was dark and everyone had gone, even the coach, and I just had to wait there until Dad came, and when he got there he was crying again.'

Sam looked across at me to make sure I was listening, and getting it. 'Con, he never cries!' he said, palms facing up, shrugging. 'Whatever is happening, I don't think it's good. Really. Have you ever seen him cry? I haven't. Never. What does it mean anyway, to have a tumour? Do you know what it is?'

I had to tell Sam that I didn't know what a tumour was either and then he started talking about making a welcome-home sign for Hilde. I wanted to know if she was coming by herself or bringing her husband, Ceri, and their little boy with her. Jonathon was nearly six months old and Sam still called him 'the baby', like we used to when Hilde was pregnant, like he still wasn't used to Jonathon being born and alive and having a name. I wanted to see Ceri as well. He was always so much fun – he did backflips and handstands, and took us to the movies and bought us cool stuff.

'Have you checked the place out? Been on a bit of an exploring mission yet?' Sam asked.

Of course! That was what Sam and I could do, we could explore things. I grabbed my crutches and off we went. There were four other rooms like mine, with six beds in each, and on the other side of the corridor there were rooms with just one bed in them. Most of those single rooms had the blinds drawn and lots of people around. I didn't think I wanted to be in one of those. Towards the end of the corridor on the right was a massive kitchen. It was all stainless steel, with huge steel benches, big taps and big sinks. The fridges had glass doors on them, not like our fridges at home, more like what you'd find in a shop or restaurant. We checked out the fridge, but there was only milk and yoghurt and a big stack of jelly cups in there. The freezer had heaps of little tubs of ice-cream, hundreds of them. I remember wondering if they were for the kids or the staff.

Sam cheekily grabbed a jelly cup and popped it in his pocket as we left. Then, at the very end of the corridor on the left, we hit the jackpot. A playroom! There were games everywhere, and toys, and tables with craft stuff, and best of all a TV – with a Nintendo! We didn't have a TV at home, let alone computer games. We couldn't believe our luck!

Like most boys his age, Sam was completely Nintendo-obsessed. Earlier that year he had saved up his paper-round money with the intention of buying one, and he'd asked Dad to buy a TV so he could use it. Dad refused and banned him from buying a Nintendo, even though it was his own money. Sam was furious. He didn't understand – he thought that we didn't have a TV and a Nintendo because we couldn't afford them, not because Dad didn't want us rotting our brains away in front of them.

—

Sam: All through primary school I was a busy little fella. At age nine I scored a plum gig delivering the daily papers and quickly proved myself adept enough to handle two rounds, in addition to filling in for any adult who may have had too many the night before and couldn't make the early start. So I was up at the crack six days a week. I've never been a morning person, but the lure of a wage proved very tempting.

I'm not sure why, but I became completely fixated with money as a youngster – perhaps it was because Dad never had much of it. I understood that money could help solve problems and my grand plan was to earn enough so that Dad could write novels all day long and not partake in the soullessness of writing commissioned histories, which we knew killed him. Somehow, even at that age, I knew that money meant power. A power that my family didn't seem to have. Now I just see money as toxic, but back then it certainly seemed the answer to everything.

Every payday I would reward myself with a Cherry Ripe (or sometimes a Bounty), and bank the rest. I was unstoppable – soon I added the local weekly paper to my repertoire, then I took up pamphlets, and before I knew it a Sunday paper started up. I was banking over $40 a week! It wasn't long before the dollars started stacking up. As far as I was concerned, I ran an empire. Christmas time was especially lucrative; most of the customers on my route left out a little festive gratuity, and sometimes presents too.

Connie still likes to remind me of what a tycoon I was. One night, we were all eating around the dinner table when I excused myself to pee. When I returned, I ploughed back into my dinner, but it wasn't long before Connie and Dad started snorting with laughter, barely holding it together. Clearly something was up and I wanted in. Turns out, Connie had added her peas (which she hated) a couple of carrots and two brussels sprouts to my plate while I was indisposed and I'd eaten all of her vegies for her, none the wiser. They, of course, found this hysterical, and I felt stupid. I stormed off, and as I huffed away I tried to get them back with the one thing I could think of . . .

'I'm going to count my money!' I said.

This sent them right over the edge. They laughed as if nothing had ever been funnier.

I went straight to my moneybox and started counting. First I divided my coins into groups. Then piles. Then I started tallying. It made me feel better. The whole family still gives me shit about it – the time Sam went off to count his money!

—

As far as we were concerned, just because we couldn't play computer games at home didn't mean we couldn't play them in hospital. Sam switched on the console and plonked himself down in a beanbag in front of the TV. Unsurprisingly, it turned out I was as uncoordinated playing computer games as I was with sports, so my attempts were over pretty quickly while Sam's game went on forever. I didn't mind, it was fun watching him play.

When Dad came to find us, we sat and ate our ice-creams, and then he told Sam to stay there while the two of us had a talk back in my room.

Dad explained that I was going to have an operation on my leg the next day. 'The doctors need to find out what sort of tumour you have so they can work out what sort of medicine to give you to make you better. Do you understand, Con?' he asked.

'Yeah, are you going to be here? Will you be here when I wake up?'

'Of course I'll be here.' He explained that his friend Joan would be looking after Sam so that he could stay all day. We spoke about how I wouldn't be able to eat anything else that night and how I'd have to wear one of those dreadful hospital gowns – the type that meant you might accidentally flash your bottom – and how once I'd recovered from the operation I could go home.

I listened to his every word, about how it would hurt after the operation but that they'd give me some medicine to help make it not so bad, and when Dad stopped talking I asked sheepishly, 'What is a tumour, anyway?'

'Oh, Con, it's just a lump, like a growth of unhealthy cells. They'll take a little sample from the growth tomorrow and look at it under a microscope and see what sort of growth it is. Then they'll work out how to treat it. They might just cut it out, or you might have to have some stronger medicine as well. We'll have to wait and see.'

Later, when Dad and Sam left the hospital, I watched them walk down the corridor, getting smaller and smaller the further away they got, and Sam kept turning back and waving, and jumping – acting so goofy he made me smile.

———

I ended up being in hospital for a week and I was so excited the day I got to go home. I was going to miss Jacqui but I was over the moon to get out of there. If I hadn't been on crutches I would have raced out of the building.

When I got to our front door, Hilde was there with Ceri and Jonathon, and all my friends from school.

Surprise!

They had made me a welcome-home banner, with my favourite lollies stuck all over it. I laughed, and hugged Hilde. Ceri rubbed my head, scruffing up my hair and baby Jonathon reached out his little hands towards me, smiling and babbling. It felt good to be home.

Once the adults went to the kitchen to talk about adult things, it was just me and the girls from school. All my closest friends were there and there was a lot to catch up on.

'Have you heard? Scott Robinson asked Julia out, not Julia Mahoney, Julia Jones! Can you believe it? I mean she is so uncool, I can't believe a hunk like Scott would ask her out!'

'And John finally dumped Suzie the floozy, about time.' Everyone talked over each other, gossip and rumours aplenty.

Kelly joined in, 'My mum says you have cancer. She said I shouldn't hang out with you anymore because it'll hurt my feelings when you die!'

The babble stopped and a dramatic silence fell over the room.

Cancer?

Dying?

Everyone was quiet. Nobody knew what to say, me especially. 'That's not true. Why did you say that, Kelly?' was all I could manage.

At that moment Hilde poked her head around the doorway. 'Everything alright, girls?' she asked. 'It's very quiet in here.' Then she took one look at my devastated face and realised something was very wrong.

'Kelly says I've got cancer and that I'm going to die and that she isn't going to be my friend anymore! Why would she say that? I have a tumour, that's what Dad says, and I'm not going to die, am I?'

Silence.

'Am I, Hilde?'

Why isn't she answering? I thought.

Hilde moved to my side. 'You do have a tumour. Some tumours are cancerous and some aren't. We don't know which sort you have. But you are not going to die. Even if it is cancer, you're not going to die. The doctors have lots of good medicines to help kids with tumours get better, whether it's cancerous or not. But it might not even be cancer. We won't know until the results come back.'

Hilde was calm. She wrapped her arm around me, comforting me. 'Now, Kelly, did you say that you didn't want to be friends with Connie anymore?'

'That's not what I meant,' Kelly stammered, trying not to cry. 'It's just that . . . it's just . . . I mean, Mum just said . . . she said, you know, that it would hurt my feelings when Connie, I mean, sorry, I mean *if* Connie dies. So she said . . . um . . . that, maybe, I shouldn't hang out with her anymore, that's all. Of course we'll still be friends, you know.' Kelly had shrunk before our eyes – shoulders slumped, head down, eyes down. She looked even more embarrassed than me!

Hearing Hilde's explanation made me feel so angry. Angry with Dad for not telling me that tumours could be cancerous and that I might have cancer. And angry with myself for not knowing and feeling too silly to ask. I felt like I had a concrete block in my tummy and a storm in my head.

How can I have cancer?

I thought only old people got cancer.

Can kids even get cancer?

Don't people die of cancer all the time?

There was so much I didn't know. So much I didn't understand.

The party wasn't really the same after that and a little while later Hilde asked me to go for a walk with her. We wandered down to the park and sat on the swings, gently swinging back and forth. Hilde explained that because I was sick she was going to move back in with us for a little while. Her plan was to go back to Sydney to pack up their stuff and get organised, and then she and Ceri, and little baby Jonathon would all be moving in with me, Dad and Sam.

I had weird mixed feelings about this. On one hand I was thrilled – Hilde was always a bit like a mum and a sister rolled into one, and I hated that she was living so far away. I loved the idea of her being close by again. But at the same time I felt sick with worry – things must be really bad with my leg if she was giving up her life in Sydney to move here.

'Hilde, is it that bad?' I asked, looking over at her. 'Am I going to die?'

'No, you're not going to die,' she said adamantly, looking me square in the eyes.

But even then I knew that wasn't true.

We were all going to die one day.

—

The next few days were a waiting game. There was nothing else to do while we waited for the biopsy results. Finally, Dad got the call, and it wasn't good news.

Dad explained to me that my tumour was cancerous, and that I was going to have to have chemotherapy to make me better. He told me that chemotherapy is a strong drug that would make me very sick and make my hair fall out. I would have to have more operations to have the tumour removed, and I might have to have my leg amputated. The good news was that lots of people with my type of cancer do get better. If I took my medicine and had the operations, I wouldn't die.

When I look back on it now I think, how can a 12-year-old process such information? Dad always talked to us like we were adults, but getting my head around all that was tough.

In the house we were living in at this time, Sam and I had a magic wardrobe between our bedrooms. We could sneak past all the clothes and through into each other's room. We loved it because Dad didn't know if we were staying up late together. That night, after Dad left my room, shutting the door behind him, I sat there and watched the cupboard door open. Sam poked his head out and whispered, 'You still up?'

He came and sat next to me on my bed and we chatted.

'Dad and Hilde seem pretty stressed out,' Sam said. 'Dad told me that I have to be nice to you, that I have to be gentle, and no fighting. It must be pretty bad.'

We both decided it was, especially because Dad had bought me some Kentucky Fried Chicken on the way home from the hospital.

I told Sam I was scared. He lay down next to me and we talked until we both fell asleep.

CHAPTER 5

CHEMO SUCKS

Chemo sucks. Basically what happens is you are pumped full of drugs that kill cancer cells. Sounds great, right? The problem is those same drugs also kill hair cells and white blood cells, because they target and kill any fast-growing cells, even healthy ones. The needles hurt, the chemo burned as it flowed into my veins, and it made me so sick. It is toxic and my body tried to get rid of the poison by throwing up. I couldn't stop vomiting.

I had two different cycles of chemotherapy, and each cycle went for three weeks. First, they gave me a drug called cyclo-phosphamide (cyclo), then doxorubicin, a drug they called the 'red devil' because it made people so sick it must be evil and it was bright red, like cordial. The cyclo cycle meant five days in hospital on a drip and then home to recover. The red devil meant three days in hospital, then home to rest. While I was in hospital I vomited every five or ten minutes. I couldn't eat, I couldn't get out of bed. I could hardly move. They gave me a drug called Largactyl to help me sleep through the sickness at night and it zonked me out so badly that I vomited all over myself and wet the bed. They were constantly washing me and putting new sheets on the bed, but it was the only hope I had of getting any sleep.

By day five I was vomiting less, maybe once every half hour. By day six it was every hour, then by day seven the vomiting stopped. Seven to ten days after each treatment my white blood cell count dropped and it made me very susceptible to infection. Every cough or sniffle had Dad taking my temperature, because if I got a fever I could die as I had no white blood cells to fight any infection. We had never had a thermometer in our house before, Dad always just felt our foreheads to see if we were sick, but now he was diving for the thermometer at any hint of a problem.

During days 14 to 21 of the cycle I began to get my strength back a bit. I could eat and was hardly vomiting at all. If I felt strong enough during this period, I could go back to school. I could almost be a normal kid.

The chemo started killing the tumour cells immediately. Within about a week I could walk again without crutches. The pain in my leg had gone. It made everyone think the chemo must be working. That had to be a good thing.

We moved house again not long after I started chemo. We had been renting the house with the magic wardrobe, and I heard Dad telling Hilde that the owner kicked us out because Dad didn't mow the lawn and the house looked messy from the street. Dad didn't have time to mow – he was too busy working and looking after me. That had been our first rental and then we moved to a new house closer to our school. It had a dishwasher and a breakfast bar but no magic wardrobe. The lounge and dining room were all one massive room with big glass windows along one side so it was really light and spacious, and it kind of felt like you were in the garden – but without the rain and the mozzies. I loved that house. Housing prices in Victoria had soared a few years back, so the upshot of it all was Dad couldn't make renovating worthwhile anymore. But he was cool, he just went on as normal, and perhaps he was even a little relieved that he didn't have to renovate. Now all he had to worry about was writing, and us kids. At the time, Hilde was pregnant with her first baby at the age of eighteen, and Sam and I were getting to high school age and turning into teenagers, so he had more than enough to worry about without having to renovate at the same time.

In the previous few houses I'd always had the biggest bedroom, and Sam had to reluctantly accept the smaller one. He said I was spoilt and that I always got my own way. When we moved into the new house, though, it was his turn to choose the bedroom he wanted. Dad's bedroom was at the front of the house and our two bedrooms were at the back. One of them was huge, with floor-to-ceiling windows along one wall, looking out into the garden, and built-in wardrobes along the wall opposite. It was beautiful, and as soon as I saw it I wanted it. The other bedroom was small, poky even, with hardly enough room for a single bed, no cupboards and a small window looking out onto a fence. I realised that all those times I got to have the good room were now coming back to bite me – now I was going to end up with a small stuffy little room looking at a fence! But, as always, Sam surprised me.

'Con, you can have the big room, 'cos you're sick and everything. I'll take the small room,' he said.

I don't know if I would have been so kind if the tables were turned. But that's Sam. He's always had a huge heart.

———

Sam: Matty Davis was the first friend I remember having. He was an odd little unit, like me. With him being pigeon-toed and me sporting a decent lisp, I suppose we made quite the pair. His dad had a beard and was obsessed with these new things called computers. Matty had inherited his dad's obsession and spent much of his time trying to convert me into this new cult. The whole operation was run out of the bearded one's back sunroom and everything revolved around this screen with lots of green code type stuff and it had a thing they called a keyboard, which controlled the screen and a cassette player that was the actual game – loading took half an hour but the return was clear. There were bricks, a ball and a floating bat thingy which I couldn't get enough of. Remember when you had to wait for special things?

Matty had his own way of thinking, which generally didn't make much sense to me. One day we were playing a typical game of backyard cricket; I was bowling, he was batting and his old red heeler was a fieldsman. I bowled my best ball at him and he smacked it into the bushes. I went to fetch the ball, having watched where it went, but there was no sign of it.

'Look in the branches. It might not have fallen to the ground.'

I searched high and low. I factored in every possible ricochet and was still left confounded.

'I know! We'll find another ball . . .'

'We don't have another ball.'

'The dog'll have one in the kennel.'

Matty went headfirst into the kennel and his bum wiggled around purposefully. He emerged with a punctured, matted old tennis ball. 'You bowl the exact same ball, I'll hit the exact same shot, only this time we'll properly look at where it goes and it'll lead us to the other ball!'

I was pretty doubtful. 'The balls don't weigh the same. I can't get the same speed with a lighter ball.'

This presented no issue for Matty, who quickly burrowed into his dad's shed to emerge moments later with a roll of electrical tape and splashes of smug. He strapped the mangled tennis ball in bright yellow and tossed it to me.

'How's that?'

I weighed it. 'That's about the same.'

'Alright then!'

His pigeon-toed gait took him back to the crease in complete confidence. While I didn't share his unshakeable belief in his new theory's efficacy, I did know that I'd be short-changing him if I didn't at least try to bowl the exact same delivery. I surprised myself with the facsimile I produced and was further surprised by the seemingly fully replicated on-drive. It was one of those slow motion moments. We tracked the ball through flight, watched it hit, then scurried to test the accuracy of our re-creation. Two grubby little kids parted the bushes to reveal . . . the two balls touching each other!

'They're kissing!' said Matty.

We laughed our heads off.

—

It was hot. I was still wearing my school uniform, even though it was way after dark. I was sitting at my desk looking out into the darkness of the backyard, procrastinating. I should have been working on my Geography assignment on houses in Mesopotamia, but I was resting my head in my hand, leafing through the pages of my textbook without even looking down at them. I stared out into the blackness. I couldn't believe I had cancer.

I shifted in my chair and pulled my hand away from my head. Multiple long hairs were stuck to my palm.

It was happening.

I stared at my hand in disbelief, repulsed by the sight of all that hair. I tentatively put my hand to my head again, and gently combed my fingers through. Clumps. Stringy, disgusting clumps. I jumped up and rushed down the passage into Dad's room without knocking.

He was sitting at his desk, with the typewriter pushed to one side, writing in a notebook. A beer sat on the corner of the desk, and without looking up he took a sip, before saying, 'Kids, how many times do I have to ask you to knock?'

I didn't know what to say, so I just stood there, stunned. He swivelled around and saw my face and my hands held up to show the hair in them. Dad swept me into his arms saying, 'Oh, Con, it's started.'

Everyone had told me this was going to happen, the nurses and the doctors had tried to prepare me, but it didn't make it any easier to deal with. My eyes welled up, my chest heaved and I couldn't stop the flow of tears. I sobbed uncontrollably, tears soaking the sleeve of Dad's shirt. 'Dad, I can't go to school tomorrow. I can't go to school ever again.'

He held me in a comforting hug, and started stroking my hair with that instinctive soothing touch of a parent, then apologised awkwardly and started stroking my arm instead. 'Con, you don't have to go to school tomorrow. We'll go to the hairdresser, and look at wigs. You can stay home as long as you need.'

He said all the right things, and held me like I needed to be held. I wanted him to make this go away. I wanted him to make this stop. I wanted him to tell me it was all some awful mistake, that I didn't actually have cancer, and that my life would go back to normal.

I know that Dad would've liked that as much as me. But he couldn't do it.

—

The next morning Dad took me straight to the hairdresser to have my long hair cropped short, so it wouldn't be as hard to lose it, or as noticeable. I sat in the chair with the cloak draped around me watching in horror as the lady cut off big chunks of my beautiful long hair.

'Well, I guess I won't be getting that perm for my birthday then, Dad,' I said, trying to make light of the situation.

'When your hair grows back, I will get you a perm. As soon as it grows back you can have whatever style you want.'

I knew he meant it and I wished that it made me feel better. I'd been asking for a perm for months. Initially Dad said no, but then I talked to Joan about it and told her how much I wanted one, and she'd talked him around and convinced him that I was old enough to have my hair styled any way I liked. She pointed out that at least I wasn't asking for a tattoo. Just when he finally agreed to it, this happened. Joan didn't live with Dad but they'd been friends a long time.

The ladies in the hairdresser told Dad that he didn't need to pay, and that I could come back for another haircut whenever I wanted. It seemed like everywhere I went, every time I met someone new, they felt sorry for me. They got this look on their faces and even if they didn't say the words I knew what they were thinking – 'You poor thing!'. The fact that everyone felt sorry for me, or for Dad and Sam, made me realise that what I was going through was really serious. This was something people feared, and they knew it could happen to anyone at any time. I could see, behind the sympathy, a part of them breathing an inner sigh of relief, thankful that it wasn't them, or their own daughter, going through this.

I left the hairdresser feeling worse. How was I going to go to school without hair? Everyone would tease me. They teased Jessica because she had red hair. They teased John because he had a stutter. They teased Stuart because he was short and they teased Travis because his ears stuck out. Kirsty was teased for not showering enough. Max was teased because his mum was fat and Matt copped it because his mum was tall and skinny and wore tight miniskirts. If they got teased for that stuff, what was going to happen to me?

No hair.

Scars.

Crutches.

Cancer.

—

When I wasn't in hospital but wasn't well enough for school, Joan would come over and take care of me. She taught me how to sew, and thanks to her and my Home Economics teacher I knew how to make windcheaters, bags and summer dresses. I'd proudly take up Sam's school pants and sew on buttons when they fell off our uniforms or Dad's shirts. I loved sewing. With a needle and thread I could fix things. I may not be able to fix myself or cure cancer, but I could fix a shirt for Dad, or a school dress for me.

One day I found out that kids with a life-threatening illness get to make a wish. Lots of my friends had made wishes. They'd wished for TV systems, stereos, tickets to sports games and rock concerts, holidays with their families to the Gold Coast, new bikes, Sega or Nintendo computer game consoles – all sorts of things. I'd been secretly hoping that I'd get to make a wish as well, and then a lady came to see me during one of my visits to the hospital and she explained that I could. I was thrilled because I knew exactly what I wanted. A sewing machine! With a sewing machine I'd be able to make my own clothes – no more op-shop clothes for me! Dad always encouraged creativity and hard work, so I knew he'd buy any fabric I asked for. I'd have the best wardrobe in the whole school, and all the pieces would be one of a kind. My mind was made up before the wish lady had even finished speaking, 'I would like a sewing machine.'

I could see she was taken aback, and she asked if she could speak to my mum. I wasn't sure why, but I explained that Mum had died a long time ago. Then she asked if my grandma had a sewing machine, or if my sister had a sewing machine? What about my dad – did he have a girlfriend? Does she want a sewing machine? I wasn't sure why she was asking and when I told Dad about it later he explained that it was an odd wish for a child, so she was probably wondering if someone had asked me to get a sewing machine for them. We both laughed. Maybe it was a little odd, but it was what I wanted.

The woman had gone on to ask what else I would like if a sewing machine wasn't possible. What else could I think of that would be nice to have . . . 'Maybe a bike?' she prompted. I told her that Sam and I shared our bike so I'd never had a new bike and that, yeah, that would be kind of cool, but I really would prefer a sewing machine.

A few months later, I was told to invite a few friends around to my place to celebrate me receiving my wish. Dad was there with Joan and Hilde, Sam was there, and a few of my friends from school came around. Two people from Make-a-Wish arrived and they started to explain that children make all sorts of wishes but there had never before been a wish for a sewing machine. They told us that not every wish can be made to come true because they rely on donations from corporations. I tuned out because I realised I wouldn't be getting my wish, that a sewing machine was too expensive and I was crazy to ever think that I could get one. They asked me to leave the room so they could get the wish ready. I hobbled out on my crutches, curious. If it wasn't a sewing machine, what could it be?

Before long, they called me back into the room and there was a rectangular-shaped parcel on the bench with a big red bow on it. It was the right shape. It was the right size, I ripped the wrapping off quickly and it was . . . a sewing machine!

I was so happy, and Dad was so happy for me, and proud of me for asking for something so sensible. He told me we could go to the fabric shop the next day and get some fabric and cottons so that I could get started straight away. I couldn't stop smiling.

But there was more! I was told to go into the dining room but I didn't want to go, I wanted to check out my sewing machine. I couldn't be rude, though, so I did what was asked and there, in the middle of the room, was another huge parcel wrapped in brown paper, with another huge red bow on it. It stood in the middle of the room on its own. I pulled the wrapping off to reveal a sparkling red ladies racing bike with ten gears, a pack-rack and a basket! It was the most beautiful bike I had ever seen in my life, and it was mine. I was confused.

'But . . . why? They can't both be for me?'

'Oh yes they can,' one of the Make-a-Wish people replied, 'they are both for you. We were so impressed with you for making such a sensible wish, that we thought we'd try to get you both the things you wanted. We didn't know how we were going to get a sewing machine, and we approached every manufacturer until Janome came forward and said they would donate one, then we thought you deserved a little something else too. That's when we started looking for someone to donate a bike. They are both for you, darling. You deserve it.'

I couldn't believe my luck. What a great day, not only did I get my wish granted, but Dad also told me that I would be getting another present in a few months' time. A little brother or sister. Joan was pregnant and we would soon have another little bubby to play with. A few months later my half-brother David arrived just as Dad had promised.

—

By the time my second session of chemo came around I still had some hair. It was cropped short – like an army buzz cut – but, still, it was more than what most of the kids on the chemo ward had. Their heads shone like billiard balls, silky smooth. And no one wore a wig either. I couldn't understand how they could all bare their heads like that, especially the girls. I was going to wear my wig everywhere I went once I'd lost all of my hair. I didn't want my baldness to be like a beacon that screamed out to the world, 'I have cancer.'

Jacqui started chemo the same day as me, and it turned out that we even had the same tumour, a Ewing's sarcoma. Hers was in her left hip, mine in my left fibula, which is the skinny bone between the ankle and knee joints. The tibia is the thicker bone, the one that bears all the weight, and the fibula just helps with rotating the ankle. The doctor said that if you could choose a bone to get a tumour in it would be the fibula because you don't really need it and they can cut the whole bone out if they have to. That's what they were planning to do to me, but first they had to give me a heap of chemo to kill as many of the cancer cells as possible before the surgery.

When I was diagnosed, Dad went to the state library and read everything he could find on Ewing's sarcomas. He told me a few things, like about how it is a bone tumour that only kids get. That it happens mainly to young teenagers, and that the chemo is pretty effective, but that it was a fairly new thing. Apparently ten years earlier not many people survived my cancer. Like the doctor, he told me the best place to get it was in the ribs or the fibula, because those bones can be cut out after chemotherapy. The hip was the worst place to get it because the chemo and radiation wasn't as effective on tumours in the pelvis. I didn't tell Jacqui that. Dad also said it was good news that I only had one tumour, because sometimes the cancer spreads, and more tumours grow in other parts of the body, like in the lungs, and once that happens the chemo doesn't work as well. So it turns out I was lucky.

Having Jacqui going through chemo with me helped. I had someone to talk to who knew what it felt like. Unlike me, Jacqui was really sporty and even though the pain in her hip had gone, her mum wouldn't let her play netball again. She was really annoyed because she'd already missed four games and the final was only two weeks away. I told her I didn't really like sport so I wasn't missing it like she was.

We talked about our friends' reactions to us getting sick. She told me her friends were like mine, they didn't really know what to say and she felt awkward around them. Some of her friends had gone all weird and thought they could catch cancer off her or something.

'Mum's spoiling me, though,' Jacqui told me with a smile. She showed me her fingernails, wiggling her fingers at me. 'Look, bright pink nail polish, and she got me some lipstick as well. I get to choose what channel the TV is on and I get to hire videos and watch them whenever I like. It's cool. But I'd rather be healthy and normal, and back at school. I don't miss the homework, but I miss my sports and my friends. And I feel like a freak. Have you got a wig yet?'

It was good to have Jacqui there. No one else knew what I was going through. I felt different from everyone at school and everyone in my family – this cancer thing just made me feel so isolated.

Hilde's husband, Ceri, must have understood because when I started losing my hair he whispered to me, 'Don't worry, Con, when your hair falls out, I'll shave my head too, and we can be baldies together.' He grinned at me cheekily, and I didn't tell anyone else about our little conspiracy.

The last of my hair fell out after my second round of chemo and my head was as smooth as every other kid's head on the cancer ward. Now was the time. Ceri had thick blond hair, like Patrick Swayze, and I couldn't believe he was willing to give it up just to make me feel better. But he did. First we hacked it off with scissors, then clipped it into a buzz cut, then we finished it off with a razor. He was going to be just as bald as me, and he promised he wouldn't grow his hair back until mine grew back. We were like brothers in arms, baldies together, ready to conquer the world. Now, if I stood out, I wouldn't be the only one.

CHAPTER 6

NOTHING MAKES SENSE

After about eight months of chemo I had the operation on my leg. They took out my fibula – the whole bone, from the ankle to the knee. I didn't feel so lucky afterwards because it hurt so much. Ten days later they told me I should be walking again but I struggled. The physios kept trying to stretch my leg out, they told me it had atrophied, which basically meant the muscles had shrunk and I couldn't straighten my leg, so obviously I couldn't walk on it. I hated physio. Eventually I managed to get around okay with my crutches so it was time to go back to school.

I wore a wig to school, and even though everyone knew it was a wig I didn't really care. I had to try to keep up the normality a bit even if I was only kidding myself. I couldn't manage my school bag and my crutches at the same time, so Sam would meet me after each class and carry my bag to the next class for me. Sometimes he walked with me, and other times he just ran ahead and dropped it off, so that he could get to his class on time.

At the end of third period on that first day back, Sam picked up my bag from French class and ran ahead to leave it at the Maths classroom for me. A big group of Year 7s were gathered in the hall, waiting for their next class to begin. I struggled past them on my crutches, straggling behind the rest of my group because I was so much slower. Richard Kane, the most popular boy in the year, was leaning on the wall, with a group of kids surrounding him, hanging on his every word. He saw me and I heard him say, 'Hey, watch this. This'll be fun.'

He stepped forward to block my way, confident and full of bravado. He puffed out his chest like a bird in mating season, and said, 'Where are you going, cancer kid?'

I tried to pass him. I felt the eyes of the whole group on me, piercing me and making me leak from a thousand places. I felt weak, vulnerable and at his mercy.

In one sweeping motion Richard pulled the wig off my head, held it in the air triumphantly and shouted, 'So it is a wig then, cancer kid!'

I felt the anger build up inside me and once it began it was unstoppable. I knew I shouldn't respond, but I couldn't help myself. I dropped one crutch and with my free hand I grabbed Richard by the hair. It hurts a lot more to have your hair pulled when it's real than when it's a wig. I pulled him to the wall, half leaning on him, half pushing him, and violently thumped his head into the wall. I couldn't hear anything. I couldn't see anything but his red face, fearful and shocked. I swung my crutch around and started walloping him with it. I could see that he was scared, but I showed no mercy. Rage was driving me and I was acting on instinct, any rational or reasonable thought escaped me. He would not get away with this.

'Connie! Connie! Stop!' someone was shouting in the background. I turned to see my friend Jess looking at me, pleading for me to stop. 'You've made your point, let's go.' She offered me my other crutch and my wig, and we walked off together.

As we walked away I heard a lone clap, then others joined in and all of a sudden the whole group was clapping.

'Good on you, Connie!'

'You showed him.'

'Little Connie beat up Richard Kane. Who can believe that?'

But I didn't feel like this was a victory. I just felt sad.

I didn't go to Maths. Instead I went to the principal's office and dobbed myself in. A few teachers gathered around to hear the story and the principal took me into her office. She asked what happened, wanted every detail. I expected to be expelled or suspended at the very least.

'Now, Connie, if the other student complains, I will have to address this issue. But, just between you and me, he probably deserved to be put in his place, and as long as I hear nothing from the other party, you will hear no more about this from me.'

I walked out of the office, relieved. From that day on I wore a bandana to school, because I didn't ever want to be humiliated like that again.

—

Sam: My friend Matty had a weakness. When in deep distress he cried like a seal. He'd suck back big banks of air and follow it up with an alarmingly seal-like honk, attracting laughter and derision from all around. Jamie Roberts was rough. He was constantly rocking a black eye, bruise or graze and was famous for sticking his fingers down his throat and vomiting everywhere just to get out of class. It didn't take long for Jamie to cotton on to Matty's chink and one lunchtime I watched him reduce Matty to tears just so he could laugh, point and mock. The experience haunted me. I'd said and done nothing.

Of course it was straight to the Oracle for me.

That night over the dinner table I quizzed my dad. 'What is tough?'

'What do you mean?'

'What does tough *mean*?'

Dad took his time, picking up on the question's gravitas and, after a seemingly huge vacuum of time, said, 'Tough is sticking up for your friends.'

But I hadn't done that. I wasn't tough. Next time I would be proper tough.

Of course, the next time rolled around pretty quick. Tan bark, monkey bars and a student-painted dragon mural bordered our little fracas. Jamie started in and went about picking apart Matty's self-esteem with cyclonic delicacy. The more I wanted to say something, the more terrified I became. I was pretty sure my heart was going to smash right through and out of my chest. Still I did nothing. It wasn't until Matty was right on the verge of breaking that I bit the bullet.

'Stop it, Jamie!'

Jamie seemed surprised by my intervention and offered a typical, 'Or what?'

I had nothing and fell back on what I'd been fed. 'You think you're tough? You don't know what tough is!'

Jamie tried to laugh me off but I wasn't quite done.

'Tough is sticking up for your friends. Leave him alone.'

It actually worked, somehow. He quite literally slunk off with his henchmen, punctuating his retreat with a gob of phlegm that said 'smoker'.

Matty broke into the widest grin. I grinned back. Dad was right. He knew how to win.

—

I hadn't seen Jacqui at the hospital for ages, I didn't know if she was on a different cycle, or if she had finished her chemo. If you get an infection you have to wait until you recover from it before you can start chemo again, so she might have had an infection and had to wait. I'd been meaning to call her for ages, but because I'd left it so long I felt guilty and put it off. But I'd been thinking about her.

It was day ten of my latest chemo cycle and my white blood cells were down so I couldn't go to school. Sam was at school and Hilde and Ceri had taken Jonno to the zoo. Dad had to go out for a while but he was not going to be long. I had the house to myself for the first time in a long time so I decided I'd call Jacqui and tell her about Richard Kane and how things were going.

Jacqui's mum answered. I always felt funny talking to grown-ups on the phone so I said hi and told her who it was.

'Connie, how lovely to hear from you.' She sounded tired. 'How are you? How are you feeling?' She was genuinely interested.

I told her I was pretty good and asked if Jacqui was home.

'Yes, love, she's at home. She's been at home for about six weeks now. She's very sick.'

I could hear Mrs Keogh start to cry.

She said, 'Jacqui is pretty sick, sweetheart. She's in a coma. Do you know what that is?'

I didn't really know, but I could tell it wasn't good.

'It's like she's sleeping. She isn't talking or eating, or doing anything by herself anymore, but the doctors say she can hear us, and I'm sure she'd love to hear your voice.'

I was terrified. 'I don't really know how to talk to someone in a coma. What should I do?' I asked.

'If you don't want to, that's okay, but I know it would cheer her up to hear your voice. It's up to you. Would you like me to hold the phone to her ear so you can have a chat to her?'

'Um . . . yeah. I mean, okay, but what do I say?'

'Just tell her about school, and hospital, and your friends. But don't ask any questions, because she can't answer you.'

I heard the sounds of movement down the phone line and then a distant, 'Okay, Connie, she can hear you now.'

I didn't know what to do so I just started talking. 'Hi, Jac. It's Con. I haven't seen you at the hospital lately. That must be a relief. I hate going to the hospital. I'm not at school today, day ten, low white cells, so I'm home alone at the moment. It seems funny, but I kind of miss going to school. The other kids would think I'm crazy, they'd love to have days off like we get, but it gets kinda boring after a while.'

The phone line was silent. It was weird having a conversation with someone who didn't answer. I didn't know what to say so I just babbled on, talking rubbish.

'Dad's been watching the tennis, he's crazy for it. He even hired a TV and watches it in the middle of the night! Sam wants to stay up late and watch it with him but Dad says it's too late and he can't. Do your parents let you stay up late to watch it?' A question – what was I thinking?

'So Jacqui, how's Erica?' Another question. I tried to cover it by keeping up the chatter. 'Sam's at school today, thank god. He's driving me crazy. Always teasing me about reading *Dolly* magazine. Have you got the latest issue?'

Of course there was silence down the line again, and I couldn't handle it anymore. I started sobbing. 'Jacqui, I wish you could talk to me. I don't want you to be this sick. It sucks, Jac.'

'Hi, Connie, it's me again – are you okay?' Jacqui's mum was back on the line. 'I know it's hard, but I think I saw Jacqui smile while you were talking to her.'

I started crying uncontrollably and she explained how sick Jacqui was and that the doctors said that she probably wouldn't wake up. 'We brought her home so she could be here with the family, because she didn't want to be at the hospital anymore. You know how much she hated it.'

I suddenly realised what Mrs Keogh was telling me. 'I've gotta go, Mrs K. Bye.' I hung up abruptly. I sat on a kitchen stool, with my legs curled up, pulled my jumper over my knees so I was wrapped up in a ball, and sobbed. I couldn't stop. I couldn't move. All I could do was cry. I wanted my dad, or my sister, or even my stinky little brother – anyone to take my pain away. I sat in the same spot for what felt like hours.

'I'm home, Con,' Dad called out as he opened the front door. I heard him fumbling about in his bedroom. 'Con? How are you darling? You okay?' he asked as he walked in to the kitchen to see me curled up in a ball, crying.

He came straight over to me, cuddled me, felt my forehead, checking for a fever, 'Are you sick? Are you in pain? Have you been vomiting? What's wrong?' He was panicking.

Through the sobs, I tried to explain my phone call with Jacqui. He held me and I saw a few tears roll down his face, though he tried to pretend that he wasn't crying too. We sat and talked and he listened and reassured me. Later that day, when I felt less emotional, I asked if he'd stay next to me while I called back to apologise to Mrs Keogh. He stood next to me with his arms around my shoulders, rubbing the top of my arm as I dialled the number.

'Hi, this is Connie, I rang a few hours ago and talked to Jacqui. Is that you, Mrs Keogh?'

It wasn't, it was Mrs Keogh's sister, Jacqui's Aunt Sandy. She told me she'd been there when I called. An awkward silence stretched between us.

'Connie, have you got someone with you?' Sandy asked.

'Yep, Dad's here with me,' I muttered.

'I'm sorry, Connie, but Jacqui passed away this afternoon, not long after you talked to her.'

Dad took the phone from me as my body shook. I couldn't believe that Jacqui was dead.

—

I'd never been to a funeral before. I was still finding it hard to understand that Jacqui was gone. It made my head spin to think that we both had the same tumour. Same leg, hers just higher up in her femur, and maybe that was the only difference between living and not.

Dad was driving. Hilde was in the passenger seat and I was in the back. It was perfect for asking questions because they couldn't watch me and I couldn't see their facial expressions. I needed to talk about the confusing things that were going through my head and this seemed like the best time.

Death was so permanent. More permanent than anything in life. Since Mum had died she'd faded from my memory. I'd lost the sound of her voice. I couldn't remember her hugging me. I didn't even remember what she looked like. We didn't talk much about Mum. Her absence was a real and palpable part of my life. But she was gone, and she'd never come back. Jacqui was gone now too.

'How did Mum die?'

I heard the hum of the tyres on the highway, going at 100 kilometres per hour. I could see the buildings rushing past. But I didn't get an answer.

I watched Hilde turn to look at Dad and Dad turned his head to look at her. I didn't think Dad was going to answer and then he spoke. 'The truth is she committed suicide. Con, do you know what that means?' Dad stated, without a hint of emotion in his voice, but I could see his fingers go white on the steering wheel.

'I've heard you say that, but what does it mean? It sounds like she committed a crime or something?'

'It means she took her own life, that she killed herself.'

This made no sense to me. I thought my mum was sick. How was it even possible to kill yourself? Would she have used a gun? I pictured a dead body lying on the floor surrounded by blood. What I really didn't understand was how she could leave her own kids. How could she leave us alone in this world?

'I don't get it, Dad, didn't she love us? Weren't we good enough for her?'

'Oh, sweetheart, it wasn't that. She was sick, and her sickness caused her pain, and it was too much for her. It wasn't you, or Sam, or Hilde.'

'But how could she be in pain when she had three kids? I just don't get it. Don't kids make their mums happy?'

'It's complicated. Because of her illness, she couldn't be happy enough to want to live. Even if she'd had a hundred kids, she wouldn't have been happy. It still wouldn't have made her healthy or taken away her pain. She loved you, and your brother and sister very much. It was just that love didn't prevent the balance from tipping the wrong way.'

'So is it better for her that she's dead, 'cos at least it doesn't hurt anymore?' I asked.

'I guess so, Con, I guess so.'

—

When we arrived at the church, the car park was full, the street was lined with cars and there was a huge crowd out the front. Everyone was wearing black, except for Jacqui's school friends, who were all in school uniform. Seeing all those uniforms, and realising that Jacqui would never wear her uniform again, made me cry.

Dad and Hilde were right there beside me and they hugged me tight. We went inside and sat at the very back of the church. In front of us was a row full of school girls. We stood for a hymn and I noticed that one of the girls had blood on the back of her dress. Nobody said anything to her.

The service had a lot of religious stuff in it. We were told Jacqui was one of God's children and now she was back in God's arms. It didn't make me feel any better. I didn't want to think about her being in God's arms. I didn't want to think about me being in God's arms.

Jacqui's family were at the front. Her little sister, Erica, sat quietly. Her mum stared straight ahead. Mr Keogh put his arms around his wife.

The coffin was so small. As it was carried out I couldn't look at it. Her mum stood up and then collapsed into her husband's arms. Tears streamed down his face, but he stood tall and held his wife.

It just didn't make sense to me. How could Jacqui be gone? How could Mum be gone? How could anyone just be gone? I didn't get it. On the way home I stared down at the program for the service. How was it possible that a whole life could boil down to one photocopied piece of paper?

CHAPTER 7

THE SILVER LINING

Losing friends sucked. Chemo sucked. Operations sucked. Endless needles sucked. Being sick really sucked. But there were heaps of people at the hospital, and outside it, who worked hard to make kids like me as happy as we could possibly be, given our situation. They were there to distract us from the hellish treatments we had to have, counsel us through it all and take us away from that goddamn hospital to places where we could forget that we were sick for a day, a night, or a week.

One of the major supports for me was the Challenge network. Challenge is a not-for-profit organisation that gives support to children and families living with cancer. Their website says that since 1983, they've 'helped over 25,000 children and families, making a real difference to their quality of life from the moment they are diagnosed, through treatment and beyond'. Their pledge is that throughout a kid's cancer journey, they will never walk alone. Challenge runs camps and brings celebrities into hospitals to visit sick kids. They organise warehouse parties, concerts, visits from TV stars and tickets to all of the coolest, latest stuff, and they'd raised the money for the Nintendo in the playroom on the ward that Sam loved so much.

I can tell you from personal experience that they definitely deliver support and make a huge difference. The kids at school were jealous of all the fun things I was doing, but they didn't get it. I didn't tell them about how awful it was to spew up every few minutes for five days in a row. I didn't tell them that I wet the bed because of the medicine I had to take. I didn't tell them that I would get so sick I couldn't even feed myself. But I did tell them every time I met someone famous.

Sam went to CanTeen Camps (CanTeen is another great charity that supports young cancer sufferers and their families). I think he wanted to go on camps that I wasn't on. He needed the space to experience the effects of cancer as a sibling of a patient. There were a lot of siblings on these camps and, sadly, lots of them had lost, or would lose, their siblings. The cancer experience was very different for Sam than it was for me, so the camps were different too, and I think that linking up with other siblings helped him deal with the impact my cancer had on his life. I wasn't the only one to lose my innocence because of cancer – Sam did too. People underestimate the impact it had on him.

—

Sam: Needless to say, with Connie in hospital regularly and so sick, I ended up with a lot more of that independence I craved so much. I became a competent cook. I probably felt like Dad was at the hospital all the time and Connie probably felt that Dad was home all the time with me. It must have been pretty hard on the old man. Dad always had such a solidity to him until Connie got sick. Sometimes I would see an uncertainty in his eyes, which made me uncertain. It was too hard for me to share his doubts so after a while I decided that Connie wouldn't die and that Dad was wrong to worry about it. Connie was the toughest person I knew. She'd be alright. I didn't ask too many questions, but it became clear in time that a tumour was a type of cancer and that cancer was a horrible disease that could kill you, even if you were only a child. I visited Connie in the hospital once, maybe twice, during the initial stages of her treatment, but I avoided the hospital like the plague after that. I simply couldn't handle the reality of the place. I felt like I was walking through rooms of people waiting to die even though I knew everyone there was actually fighting for life. I always found something important to do if Dad was around and asked me if I wanted to go in and see Con, but he had usually left for the hospital by the time I got home from school, which worked fine for me. That hospital my sister was in was big and scary and smelled like sickness and I didn't want to be in it or see Connie in it with all those wires in her body.

When Connie became sick, I became more marginalised at school. It wasn't enough that I had a lisp and couldn't keep my mouth shut for more than two seconds, now I had the bald sister who had cancer. Some of the kids assumed I had caught it and that they would too if they hung around with me. Connie would get teased a lot. Much as I'd like to say that I was her protector at school, the truth was that we were in different years and there wasn't a lot I could do. I was naturally protective, of course, but there was certainly no caped heroics. If someone made the wrong comment at the wrong time, I could fly off the handle – all of the frustration of not really knowing what was going on just boiled over.

Connie and I became 'charity cases' – Connie attached herself predominantly to the Challenge Cancer Support Network and me to CanTeen. Connie never wanted me on the same camps as her (something to do with me being the most annoying brother in the world!) and while there was definitely some overlap, it became clear pretty quickly that when it came to camps, we were to go our separate ways. Any kid who has been on a cancer camp will tell you what fun it is. Just because kids have cancer doesn't mean they don't want to have fun. I felt like these camps were built just for me and I realise now that they actually were! They were designed to give kids a break from the reality of having a child cancer patient in the family. They aimed to get you away so you could have fun and forget about cancer, and they gave the parents a break at the same time. We did ropes courses, canoeing, abseiling, archery, water sports, discos, arts and crafts – I really was in heaven. And every other kid knew exactly what it was like to go through what I was going through.

'Discussion Group' was the only part of the whole camp that was compulsory. I didn't want to go because it sounded ominous and I didn't feel like talking and I was doing just fine with everything squirrelled away deep down where it was quiet. I was reminded by Penny, a leader whom I loved and hoped to one day marry, that it wasn't so bad and that I should attend if I wanted to enjoy the rest of the camp; besides, I wasn't required to talk. I could just listen if I wanted to. Fine then, I would go, just listen, then get back to having fun.

So I went. We had been split into small groups of about eight or so. We all sat in a circle. We could say anything we wanted. We could talk as little or as much as we liked. Kids who had been to camps before took the lead, sharing their stories, one by one. I was amazed. Everything that they talked about I could find something to directly relate to. I was in a group of siblings, so all of our experiences were alarmingly similar. In a jiffy, Penny turned to me and asked me if I wanted to share. My fears had been alleviated. We were clearly in a safe place where anything goes, so I jumped in. I started talking about how I hated it when I answered the phone because the first thing people would say was 'How is your sister?' and how every time I felt like saying 'I'm fine, thanks for asking', but would instead say, 'I'll let her tell you'. No one ever called to speak to me and I hated picking up the phone then because all they talked about was cancer.

Dad wasn't around anymore and I got lonely. Nobody cared about me, everybody only cared about Connie – all that kind of stuff. Anyway, before too long the old waterworks were on full blast and I didn't feel embarrassed because other kids had cried and no one really got teased on camps. Everyone looked after each other. I stepped out of that little room with the weight of the world lifted off my shoulders. I suddenly felt really good. So light. Everything was going to be okay. These discussion groups were a pretty good idea after all! And now that Penny had seen how emotionally sophisticated I was, it was more likely she would love me back and marry me one day.

—

Sam may have had Penny but I had celebrities! Because of Challenge, Sonia Dada, an American band who were touring Australia, came to the hospital and sang their hit song 'You Don't Treat Me No Good' just for us, in a room away from the ward. Challenge took me to see *Les Miserables*, and afterwards I met the cast and crew. I had a nosebleed in the middle of the show, and the nurse had to treat me in the dark in the audience because I wouldn't leave – the show was too good and I didn't want to miss anything. There was always a nurse with us, wherever we went. Whether it was to a concert, a party or a camp, there was always at least one.

I got to meet the Red Hot Chili Peppers, Ugly Kid Joe, Pauly Shore from *Encino Man*, Steve Vizard from *Fast Forward*, Glenn Robbins from *The Comedy Company*, Molly Meldrum, Johnny Diesel, Les Hill from *Home and Away* and they were all fabulous experiences, but the BEST THING EVER was meeting Boom Crash Opera.

It was a bit embarrassing the first time I met Richard Pleasance, songwriter and bass player from the band, because until that moment I have to admit I hadn't heard of them. Richard gave me a copy of their record *These Here are Crazy Times* and signed it for me. We had a photo together and he went on his way. I went home and listened to the record and absolutely *loved* it. Then, when I went back to school in between treatments, I showed some of my friends the photo and told them about it. Susan went weak at the knees. 'Oh my god, did you meet Dale, the lead singer? He is SO hot!' Julie piped in with, 'That song, "Dancing in the Storm" is the coolest song I've heard in ages, and yes, Dale is hot.' Rachael agreed. It seemed everyone knew who Boom Crash Opera were except me. But once I'd heard that record I started to get a little bit obsessed (and that might be a slight understatement).

The next time Richard came into the hospital he brought three other band members with him: Peter Farnan, songwriter and guitarist; Peter Maslen (Maz), the drummer; and Dale Ryder, lead singer. They came around to every bed, spending a little time with each child and when they got to me I hogged them. I just kept talking. Boldly I asked what was next on the agenda for the band and if they had been affected by cancer. They humoured me, and told me a couple of tales about grandparents who'd been sick. Then (I'm not sure why) I asked them if they smoked. Dale was embarrassed but he was honest and told me that he did. I couldn't believe it. I lectured him about it, asking why he would smoke when he knew that it caused cancer and pointing out that he could end up in a cancer ward himself one day if he kept going. He laughed kindly and said that if I ever saw him smoking a cigarette I was allowed to rip it out of his hand, break it in half and squash it to pieces on the ground.

Before they moved away from my bed they gave me a Boom Crash Opera T-shirt and I asked them to sign it, but I also asked Dale (who I now had an immense crush on) to sign my pillowcase. The other guys in the band teased us, saying I wanted to sleep with him next to me at night, and that I couldn't get enough of him. Dale ignored them and signed my pillowcase. It immediately became my most treasured possession. (Technically, it was hospital property but they were never getting that pillowslip back!)

Even though I loved meeting celebrities, it was the camps that made Challenge so important for me. The camps were awesome. They had summer camp, winter camp, water-skills camp, ski camp, spring camp and more. I went on every camp I was allowed to. When the forms came in the mail I'd get so excited. I'd pull out the list of activities and a form for Dad to fill out and want him to sign it straight away.

Spring camp was my favourite. They held it near a lake and organised for a hovercraft to take us for rides over the land and the water. It was incredible. We'd go horse riding, quad biking, ride little PeeWee 50s around the camp and we'd get to go jet skiing. There'd be so much action packed into one week. Although I loved all the physical activities, they also had the best craft activities ever. We'd do screen printing onto T-shirts, then paint them in, and we'd get to keep them once they were done. We'd do plaster painting, and real basket weaving, with cane. I made cane baskets and did screen printing with Natasha. During woodwork I made Dad a box to keep his pens in. But the best thing about all these camps weren't the activities or the craft, it was being with a group of people who were going through something similar to me. No one was teased for having no hair or being on crutches. If you farted on the bus, or had a crush on one of the other kids at camp then you would cop some cheek, but it was never mean-spirited or made you feel like a freak.

I met some great people at the camps and for a shy, white sheep like me who was just starting to become attracted to boys and slowly learning to be a bit more social, camp was the perfect confidence boost. My illness didn't factor into anything because every person there was dealing with the same things.

I liked meeting boys without having to worry about them calling me 'cancer kid' and ripping my wig off.

Troy Henderson was a country boy who wore an Akubra hat and cowboy boots. He lived on a farm way out west and had to travel for hours to get his chemo. He was very good looking, but not my type. Katherine was into him.

Steve Liechard was a blond-haired pretty boy from the city. I liked Steve's rebel factor, he was a bit of a bad boy, always doing things he shouldn't, and usually not getting caught, but I stayed well away from him because Sophie was mad about him.

Karl Ferrington was tall, a little older than us, and Natasha had the hots for him. She blushed every time he talked so everyone knew how she felt.

Then there was Mark, who I already knew from hospital. Mark was tall and lean, with a full head of hair. Because he had haemophilia, he knew he would never be cured and he'd have to be in and out of hospital for the rest of his life. He was the pick of the bunch for me. He had a bright smile that was gentle and cheeky at the same time, and his eyes shone because he was a happy person. We both loved listening to music and he'd always give me one side of his headphones on his Walkman so I could listen along. He knew I couldn't afford my own Walkman, but to tell the truth I preferred listening with him.

On the last night of that camp there was a disco. Natasha didn't want to go because she couldn't dance in a wheelchair. I convinced her to come and told her I'd spin her chair around even though I was still on crutches. With me and my crutches, her chair and Steve's titanium knee giving way, we really were a mixed bag on the dance floor, but it didn't matter. That's why I loved those camps so much.

That night 'Walk This Way' by Aerosmith and Run DMC came on, and I was singing the words and having a bit of a boogie on my crutches when I saw Natasha was crying. 'I can't walk this way, or any way, and I never will again in my life! I hate this, I want to leave.' I tried to make her feel better and then the next song started, 'Run To You' by Bryan Adams. You just don't realise how many references there are to walking and running in songs. They are everywhere. We both didn't know whether to laugh or cry but then one of the leaders grabbed Natasha by the hands, and pulled her along behind him while he walked backwards, then stepped forward, propelling her backwards. They were face to face the whole time. It was so cool, then he spun her around, under his outstretched arm, like in ballroom dancing when the boy spins the girl by the hands. Natasha was smiling so hard, her tears were forgotten.

Finally there was time for one slow dance before the disco ended. 'It Must Have Been Love' by Roxette came on and all the couples teamed up: Steve with Sophie, Natasha with Karl, Katherine with Troy. Mark came up to me and I ditched the crutches and limped onto the dance floor, knowing I could lean on him. I rested my head on his chest and we moved our feet clumsily from side to side, holding hands. It was perfect.

If I could choose I definitely would choose never to have had cancer, but those people and those camps are memories I am very glad to have. I think they changed me in a good way. But it was going to be hard to say goodbye to them all when I was better and had to go back to the 'real' world. I wasn't sure how I could do that, I wasn't quite the same person I had been.

CHAPTER 8

NO SUCH THING AS NORMAL

I thought that life would go back to normal after I finished treatment and started going to school regularly again, but it wasn't quite that simple. I had these strange mixed feelings about everything. I loved that I didn't have to go to the hospital anymore, and I sure didn't miss the chemo, the vomiting, all the needles, the pain, being away from my family and all the other awful stuff. But I missed my friends, especially Mark, and the nurses too, and I just didn't feel the same as I had before cancer came along. I'd missed so much school and it felt like everything had changed while I'd been sick. Suddenly half my friends had boyfriends, and some of them were starting to wear make-up and were worrying about fashion. I didn't fit in anymore and I longed to be with my hospital friends again – they just seemed to get me.

Chemo is a powerful thing. It kills cancer, but it also kills hair cells and white blood cells, and stops menstruation and puberty. When I was first diagnosed, a lady had come to see me – a social worker. She had tight black ringlets and a low-cut top that showed off her bust. She asked me if I wanted to talk about the cancer or chemo, or if I wanted to talk about 'girly' things, like periods, breasts and boyfriends. In the midst of everything else and having only just learnt what a tumour was and how much my life was going to change, I couldn't believe she thought I'd want to talk about 'girly' things. Didn't I have bigger things to worry about?

I'd listened as the doctors told Dad that I wouldn't have a period, develop breasts, or have any signs of puberty while I was on chemo. I had heard them tell him that the treatment might mean I could never have children of my own. I heard so many things, but didn't really take much notice of any of it, the only things I was interested in was when the chemo would finish, when the cancer would be gone and when I could go back to being a normal kid.

When I'd finished treatment I didn't go back to being a 'normal' kid but I did finally want to know about those 'girly' things. I'd always talked to Dad about everything, but not this time. And there was no way I was going to talk to Sam! I needed a woman and so Hilde was my first port of call.

I told her about the girl at Jacqui's funeral with blood on the back of her dress and how I was worried about getting my period and how I didn't know what to do when I did. Hilde explained everything – what a period was, what pads and tampons were, what changes happen to your body and your thoughts, how you get interested in boys all of a sudden – that type of thing. I thought of Mark and my friends with boyfriends and when Hilde finished I wasn't so freaked out. But I still wasn't ready for what happened next.

—

Three weeks after my last chemo session, Dad took me to the mall to get my ears pierced. We were both keen to do something to celebrate the end of treatment, and my hair was nowhere near long enough to get that perm he'd promised me, so pierced ears it was! We were on the escalator heading up to the jeweller when I suddenly felt hot and wet between my legs. I didn't know what it was, but I thought I might have wet my pants. I was so embarrassed. I told Dad I needed to go to the toilet straight away, and he waited outside while I went in.

My period had arrived in the middle of Southland Shopping Centre. I panicked. It hadn't soaked through my jeans, so I cleaned myself up as best I could and stuffed a heap of toilet paper in my undies in the hope that that would work for a while. I walked out and whispered to Dad that I needed a chemist and some money because I'd just got my first period. I couldn't look at him as I spoke.

Dad adopted his usual no-nonsense approach. 'Okay, Con, not a problem. We'll find a chemist.'

Dad waited outside while I went up to the counter. Two pretty cashiers were chatting away. I stood there for what seemed like ages and they didn't even look at me. Finally one of them rolled her eyes as she noticed me and said, 'How can I help you?'

I told her what I wanted and she waved a hand towards the far corner of the shop and went back to her conversation.

I found the section and was completely overwhelmed by the selection. There were pads, panty liners, minis and maxis for light, moderate and heavy flows, and there were a heap of different brands – it was all just too much.

I went back out to Dad, trying very hard not to cry, and told him I didn't know what to buy. He walked in and went up to the counter with me trailing behind. This time the shop assistant stopped talking straight away.

'Hello, sir. How can I help you today?' she asked with a smile.

My dad lowered his voice. 'This is my daughter. She's just finished treatment for cancer, and she has started to menstruate.' He was so polite and matter-of-fact, but kept his voice low. 'She doesn't have a mum, and I don't know what to buy for her.'

The shop assistant looked shocked and her smile faltered but she walked out from behind the counter, and took me to the section. She smiled as she handed me a bright blue packet. 'These ones might be good for you. I used them when I started too.'

I was so embarrassed. I'd read in a Judy Blume book from the school library, that you needed a belt to wear with pads.

'Thanks . . . um . . . but what about the belt thingy?' I asked.

'This is all you need,' she said. 'You just open it up and stick it into your underpants.'

I kept my eyes down as we paid. I didn't want to get my ears pierced then. I just wanted to go home and see Hilde.

—

After I'd finished a year and a half of chemo and there was no sign of recurrent illness, Dad decided it was time to move house again. We had spent three years at Sandringham Secondary College, the longest Sam and I had ever spent at one school, because Dad decided it was best to stay in one place while I was sick. Before that we had been to five different primary schools in six years.

Before I got sick, I used to get really excited about moving. I'd think about the new friends Sam and I would make, our new teachers and classes, the new house with new bedrooms, the new area we would explore. It felt to me like every new world was full of possibilities. And, of course, I always had Sam. Wherever we moved I still had him to play marbles and Monopoly with, to go bike riding and exploring with, to write and perform plays with, to build and race obstacle courses with. And even though we fought a lot, we always had each other's back; if anybody dared to tease or fight with one of us, the other one was there in a flash. I could beat Sam up, but nobody else was allowed to touch him, or they would have to deal with me. He would happily tease me, but if anyone at school dared mock me, he was there fending them off, putting them in their place and reminding them not to upset his sister again.

After I finished chemo I lost the passion for moving. I was happy. I had put down roots. I didn't want everything to change again. I had my friends at school – even if I felt a bit removed from them – and my friends at the hospital, who I still got to see on camps. I had never felt like I belonged as part of a group before, and now that I did, I didn't want to leave. I didn't say all this out loud but I hoped that Dad would change his mind.

He didn't.

I started at my new school, Mornington High, with what can only be described as a head covered in peach fuzz. It was kind of like baby hair – only a few millimetres long and all soft and wispy. Plus, I was still on and off crutches because every time I got off them for a while I'd twist my ankle and end up back on them. So I wasn't only the new girl; this time I was the new girl on crutches with funny hair and no breasts (because the chemo had halted my development in that area as well). I looked like a boy. It wasn't exactly the best start.

After a few months I made friends with a girl called Alissa. She was only a little older than me, but she seemed much, much older. She had long strawberry blonde hair, wore make-up and always had the latest clothes, whereas I wouldn't have known what to do with make-up and just wore whatever clothes I'd made myself. We'd sit together on the bus to and from school, and we chose our electives so that we would be in all the same classes. After school I'd rush home from the bus stop, knowing that she would ring me as soon as she got home so we could gossip about the day's happenings. Alissa was hooked on *Neighbours* and we still didn't have a TV so she would give me blow-by-blow descriptions of what had happened the night before. She thought it was weird we didn't have a television and that we were really poor. I didn't like it when she seemed to pity me, but other than that it was like we were sisters. We went everywhere together, finished each other's sentences, and pooled our pocket money, so what I had was hers and what she had was mine.

Sometimes we went down to Main Street after school instead of going straight home. We'd hang out at the chicken shop munching on roast potatoes – the nicest, cheapest, snack in the shop. All the boys hung out there too, including a boy called Quentin, who I kind of liked. It was also where the older guys hung out. They'd finished school and worked at the supermarket, so they had money and shouted us roast potatoes from time to time. Alissa thought a guy called Clarky was hot, and she wanted to be with him. He was 18, we were 14. She encouraged me to like Clarky's mate, Pete Smith, or Smithy. Smithy was cute, but I only had eyes for Quentin.

I was desperate to look more like Alissa, so for my birthday I asked for nothing but new clothes. It was the mid-nineties, and hip hop had finally made it to Mornington, so everyone was in super bright Cross Colours pants and midriff tops. Alissa had this really cool matching tracksuit that she wore whenever we had a casual day, or on the weekends when we went into town. She was bigger in the hips than me, and envied my small frame, but teased me for having breasts like egg yolks. Everyone teased me for having no tits. It was the bane of my life. Boys, girls – it didn't matter. I was a target for teasing. I also had the most awful crooked teeth. It didn't matter to me before, but it mattered now. I was so self-conscious about my teeth that I wouldn't smile. I'd deliberately keep my mouth shut whenever I could. I begged and begged Dad for braces, but he told me we couldn't afford them. He told me I was beautiful just the way I was, and anybody who teased me for having crooked teeth wasn't worth being friends with.

It's hard to admit but it was around this time that I realised my family wasn't normal and didn't do things that other families did. Our house didn't look like other people's homes because Dad didn't place much importance on housework. It was dirty, and people noticed. The first time Alissa came over she asked me why our toilet was so disgusting. I told her it had always been like that. She taught me how to clean a toilet, so I'd clean it every week to avoid the embarrassment again. But it wasn't just the toilet. Alissa only wore her school uniform once before her Mum washed it. I begged Dad to buy me more uniforms so I could do the same, but we didn't have the money, so I'd take off my uniform as soon as I got home and wash it. If it didn't dry overnight I'd iron it, the heat making the moisture sizzle, and dry the whole dress, one iron triangle at a time.

I started to feel ashamed of my dad. I used to love the records in his collection and Sam and I would sing along to Helen Reddy, Dory Previn or Air Supply. Then, one day when Sam put on a record, I fobbed him off. I didn't want to be a part of it. Dad's music wasn't cool. Dad wasn't cool.

It wasn't a huge step to go from shame to hate, and it didn't take long before I started to hate Dad. For not getting me braces. For not getting me more school uniforms, for not letting us have a TV. For not giving us enough pocket money. I didn't want to spend time with him, and he didn't understand what was going on with me. He thought I was going to stuff up my life by not studying as much as I used to, but he didn't understand that my new friends were far more important to me than my school grades.

The days of hanging out with Sam and wanting to spend time with Dad and Hilde were gone.

CHAPTER 9

'SMELLS LIKE TEEN SPIRIT'

It was probably inevitable that my feelings towards my family would change. Isn't that what happens to all teenagers? But looking back, it makes me sad. I can see now that I wasn't fair. My dad was a good dad and he *always* wanted the best for us. I thought Dad shopped at op shops because we were poor, but it was because he didn't want to waste money unnecessarily. We didn't have a TV because he wanted us to have a childhood where we played, imagined and read books – and we did, we absolutely had that kind of childhood. For so long my whole world revolved around Dad, Hilde and Sam – especially Sam.

When we were little we'd spend our days building obstacle courses out of ladders, hula hoops and junk from the garage. We wrote plays, made sets and costumes and performed them for Dad and Hilde. We collected stamps and shells, which I proudly categorised and arranged according to my strict rules of order and organisation. We had pen pals from whom we anxiously awaited the latest correspondence. We built cubby houses out of blankets that spanned the whole room from the top of the piano to the curtain rails. They were private. Dad and Hilde weren't allowed in. We were the Connie and Sam club. We built a treehouse in the big wide tree that stood tall outside my bedroom window in our house in Black Rock. That was private too. We grew vegetables that we ate once they matured. Sam was an especially keen green thumb. We explored the world using a set of *Encyclopaedia Britannica* and the globe that Dad got us for Christmas one year. We played Guess Who, Test Match, Monopoly and Connect Four. Uno was a favourite and occasionally one of us would cheat, resulting in attitude and fisticuffs.

When we were younger, Sam and I were endlessly fascinated by the stories of Dad's boyhood, or his life before we were born, and one of our favourite stories was about Jim the Tip Man. We would beg Dad to tell us about Jim again and again. When Hilde was little, Dad went to Daylesford to play in a tennis championship. While Dad was playing tennis, Mum went for a walk and in her travels she came across a house that took her fancy, and she bought it on the spot. She somehow convinced the owner to accept a hundred dollars (that Dad had won at the races the previous day, and she had swiftly confiscated) as a deposit. When Dad finished his tournament, she said, 'I bought a house here. We'll move to the country, it will be good for your lungs, and good for Hilde to grow up here!' Dad didn't have a choice, and the house was a bargain, but there was a catch. The house came with a caravan on the back of the property, and in that caravan lived Jim. Jim was a little bit crazy and he had an obsession; he spent his days at the tip, searching for things that tick, or might tick if he tinkered with them a bit. He collected old discarded clocks and watches and filled his caravan with them. Then, by night, he would tinker away, fixing all the treasures he had found during the day. From Dad's account it sounded like there wasn't much room for sleeping in that caravan, it was just too full of clocks. Jim didn't shower much and was what some people might call a bum, or a hermit, but to us he was simply intriguing.

We never met Jim the Tip Man – Mum, Dad and Hilde had moved to another house in Daylesford by the time we came along – but we felt like we knew him. One of the many theatre productions Sam and I put on as kids was about Jim. We wrote the play together and rehearsed it. Sam always went over the top when we put on a production; he really got into character, and his portrayal of Jim was exaggerated and theatrical. I, of course, took the more sensible role of the mother in the story. Sam may have been the star of the show, but I wasn't going to let him interfere with the production, sets or costumes.

The set was comprised of all the junky-looking items I could find around the house and garage. A plank of wood, a frypan, a garden hose and, let's not forget, the clock off the kitchen wall. A bowl here, a shoe there, and a caravan painted onto the biggest piece of cardboard I could find in the house, Blu Tacked to the wall behind the pile of junk.

My costume was a mismatch of womanly items: a pair of glasses that came as part of Nanna's inheritance, a scarf and my brown cardie over a yellow shirt with my plaid skirt. There were no high heels in our house, so I wore my sandals and tied my hair up in the most mature-looking bun I could muster. I even used Nanna's walking stick. I didn't see any difference between someone who was thirty-something, and someone who was seventy-something; they were all in the same category – old – so, to me, the walking stick fit perfectly. Sam's costume was a black tracksuit, with a few green garbage bags cut up and taped together into something that resembled a pair of pants and a top. I don't know where we got the idea that just because Jim loved to forage at the tip, that he would wear garbage bags for clothes, but it all added to the mystique and the ambience of the play.

When the big moment came, we mustered Hilde and Dad, and Laura – a friend of Dad's – to come to our production. I had made up little tickets, which I issued to the grown-ups before ushering them to their assigned seats, which I had numbered with labels sticky-taped to the backs of the kitchen chairs. Sam mocked a drum roll on some old pots while they were getting seated, I dimmed the lights and we began.

Although I felt like the play went for an hour or two, in reality it probably only lasted a few minutes, ten at most. Sam acted out Jim's character as a super crazy, fuddy-duddy old man who foraged around the tip looking for old clocks. One day he uncovered an antique clock that someone had unknowingly discarded. Although it didn't work, it was still worth quite a bit, and with a little love and care Jim might just be able to get it ticking again and sell it for a small fortune. Then he wouldn't have to live in a caravan anymore. Predictably, Jim tinkered away, and got it working, and sold it to the Queen for a million dollars. He was able to pay me $10,000 as thanks for living in my yard, and he moved into a mansion, became friends with the King and lived happily ever after.

Our performance was met by claps, whistles and a standing ovation – the only appropriate response to such a great production. When Sam came out and bowed the clapping crescendoed, but when I came out for my bow the clapping subsided. 'Oh, Sam, you were great, a perfect Jim the Tip Man.' 'Sam, you could be an actor.' 'Oh, the star of the show, Sam, nominated for an Oscar after his stunning performance as Jim the Tip Man.'

I know that actors get all the glory, and I didn't expect accolades for my amazing set design, costumes and direction. I expected the star to take all the credit, but my dad never missed a chance to compliment me, 'Con, Sam wouldn't have shone so bright if he hadn't had a cracker producer and set designer behind him.' He smiled at me proudly, and I knew that he appreciated my hard work. After that, Sam wasn't just a star tennis player, a speedy swimmer and a great footballer and golfer – he was an actor too. Maybe I was a little jealous (okay, a lot). But people like him need people like me to shine.

Up until we moved to Mornington I liked my family. I may have wanted a pool or a trampoline, or a shiny new bike with Spokey Dokeys and streamers and a basket like other kids in the neighbourhood, but I had something better . . . I was never bored. Dad always said, 'Only boring people get bored.' There was no way my family was going to be categorised as boring. And up until the age of 14 I believed I was the glue that held everything together. I was mature, responsible and I had proven it time and again. But then Dad asked me a question that changed everything.

Sam and I had both settled in at Mornington High but it wasn't great. Sam was getting teased a lot. I wasn't hanging out with him anymore. I was spending my time with Alissa and more and more keeping secrets from my family about where we went and the older boys we hung out with.

One day Dad told me he'd been saving up to send Sam and me to a private school. There was a problem, though; he had only saved enough to send one of us. I took the fact that he was talking about this and asking my opinion as a clear indication that I was an adult now. I was mature and sensible, and able to approach such a big question appropriately. I felt the weight of his expectation on my shoulders and stated the only outcome that was reasonable. Of course I should go. I wanted to do Medicine and become a prestigious, groundbreaking doctor, someone on a team who discovers a cure for cancer. I tried not to sound too up myself as I explained it to Dad, but Sam wanted to be a tennis player; he didn't need to go to a private school to achieve that.

I thought Dad would agree, but he didn't. He explained that he thought I was capable and intelligent and that I would succeed regardless of where I went to school. Sam, on the other hand, had trouble staying focused and Dad thought he would really benefit from the extra support a private school would give.

We both knew Sam was doing it tough at Mornington and getting bullied so I couldn't argue without seeming harsh. He would never be someone to fall in with the crowd, he had his own way of seeing things, his own way of doing things. He wasn't into girls. It was his bike, tennis or football.

I wanted to scream and stamp my foot. I wanted to say it wasn't fair. I'd been the one who had cancer, life had already been unfair to me. I deserved this. But I didn't say or do anything. I remained the good girl I'd always been.

'You're right, Dad, Sam needs it more than me. Of course he should go.'

Dad was extremely proud of me for making such a mature decision. Yet again I'd proved that I was the glue that held the family together. I was the white sheep. But my coat was starting to darken. I had lied.

—

Sam: Dad booked both me and Con into an exclusive private school that specialised in the arts when we were little tots. He knew he couldn't afford to educate us privately for all our school years, so he booked us into the best school he could find from Year 10 onwards in the hope that it would provide us with last minute opportunities before we embarked on adulthood.

By the time Year 10 came around Dad had $2,000 saved – enough for one kid, for one term. He simply couldn't afford for both me and Con to attend. The reasons why differ according to who you ask, but I was selected to attend, despite my inferior academic record. I couldn't help but feel that if Connie hadn't been derailed by her childhood cancer, she would definitely have been the one chosen. Not much could stop Connie, but that cancer took a massive toll on her. Her academic development suffered as she focused on more immediate concerns, like her own mortality, for example. Her development as a woman was stymied by chemo and she was told to never hope for children of her own. She endured traumas throughout her treatment that

I couldn't begin to understand. She lost dear friends. How many funerals should a child have to attend before you say enough is enough? I dodged all the bullets. And I got to go to a swanky new school too. It's like I got all the luck.

Dad thought it best if I go to this new school 'with a language under my belt', and urged me to write to the family in Japan that hosted me as part of the Asian-Pacific Children's Peace Convention years earlier, to ask if they would take me in for three months before I hit Year 10, with the aim of me picking up a language in that time. Up until that point I'd only spent my almost-considerable earnings, first as a paperboy then as a gardener, on a single Aboriginal dot painting and one chocolate bar per week, so I had enough saved to cover the return airfares.

While Connie was busy doubting Dad's abilities as a father, I was desperately trying to prove that I could do without him, making good on the sense of independence that he'd fostered in me. Connie got driven everywhere; I used my bike and public transport. Connie sometimes expected a certain level of material support; I never asked him for anything, and prided myself on it. Despite the fact that my grades could never match Connie's, perhaps it was my initiative and purposefulness that played a part in Dad deciding to arm me for private school. One thing was for sure, Connie deserved the position more, but it fell to me.

Snail mail informed me weeks later that my former host family were happy to put me up again if I could get there, so we made the appropriate arrangements and before I knew it I was flying solo to that faraway land again, this time to learn a language I wasn't sure I needed.

My host family actually remembered me stopping to check out the unicyclists in the park that day years earlier and had enrolled me in classes at the 'Fukuoka Unicycle Club' before I'd even arrived. I had only shown a passing interest in the one-wheelers careering about the place when I was eleven, but they remembered, followed through and before I knew it I'd become a fully fledged unicycle nut.

I started with the basics. Head up, back straight, arms out. Within days I was riding backwards, and before long, I was pirouetting spectacularly on a 'giraffe' (a five-and-a-half-foot-high Miyata, which, at the time, was the world's best unicycle). I came back home with a language under my belt and a fancy Miyata, but more than that, I returned with some skills. Enough skills to earn my next term's school fees. I busked.

Dad was always big on accountability. If you failed, it was your fault. If you succeeded, it was your doing. Either way, grind away and blame no one but yourself. If I wanted to continue with the opportunity that he had provided me with, then I would have to show some mettle and earn some scratch. These school fees would not and could not be met solely by him. I was lucky enough to be chosen for this school and if I wanted it to endure, then I would have to do my bit and help him raise the tuition fees. The new school boasted a world-class gymnasium – I buddied up with a dude who could back-flip until the cows jumped over the moon and before I knew what 'producing' was, I snared him for my new street act on the promise that he could share the spoils with me. I had to raise $240 per week for my fees and with the help of this perpetual flip-flopper (he flipped as hard as I unicycled), then I'd be twice the act and half a chance.

We were shit, I'll be honest, but we were kids trying and effort is usually rewarded, at least in my experience. We busked every Saturday and Sunday at Southbank and while I usually didn't meet my targets, I did manage to go a way towards justifying being chosen for the school in the first place.

The new school was another world. I'd never really hung with privileged types before and there were certainly some adjustment issues, but I had been to a fair few schools by that point, so it wasn't too bad. Only a few weeks in, a group of guys I was hanging off recommended that I audition for the school play, 'The Pink Panther Strikes Again'. It sounded a bit lame but I was in the market for new friends so I signed up. I was given the role of the Mad Scientist and after a few fun-filled weeks of rehearsal it came time to make my debut as an actor.

The first time I stood on that stage and got a laugh, I was hooked. I came home pretty amped. The whole experience was just wonderful. I kind of felt like I'd found something. My interest in tennis had waned and I was looking for something new. This seemed the way to go.

That first night after my first ever turn I lay in bed restlessly, unable to sleep. I didn't know at the time that it is common to take a while to settle after a performance. I just knew that the buzz was better than winning tennis tournaments. I was listening to Dad's Willie Nelson LP in bed (the side with 'Blue Skies' on it), just trying to calm down when I heard the phone ring. It was nearing midnight, and very uncommon for the phone to ring at that hour.

Dad knocked on my door and entered in his undies, half-asleep. 'There's someone on the phone for you. Rhonda someone?'

I didn't know any Rhonda. I went to the phone curious, to say the least. 'Hello?'

'Hello, Sam, my name is Rhonda. I'm calling to tell you that you did a fantastic job tonight.'

'Who are you, sorry?'

'My name is Rhonda. I'm Zoe's mum.'

It clicked. She was the mum of one of my cast-mates and new friends! That must be how she got the number.

'I'm sorry to call you so late, but I wanted to tell you that I thought your performance tonight was outstanding. I'm a television producer, and I'm producing a commercial for Dishlex dishwashers and I wondered if you might like to audition for me?'

'Don't you have to be good-looking to be on telly?'

She laughed. 'We'll see. Are you interested?'

'Sure. Sounds great.'

There was no chance of sleep now. I was being head-hunted! I really didn't know what to make of it. I convinced myself that my teeth would be too crooked and I would never get the part, but it was worth a shot, right? After all, Dad taught me to try.

I'll never forget the script. It was a 15-second spot to play just before the weather on the news, which Dishlex were sponsoring.

I told Mum that a Dishlex was the greatest labour-saver ever invented. She's saving 500 hours washing-up every year. Of course, the fact that I'm saving time drying up . . . (pause before the punch) . . . didn't even enter my mind! (insert cheeky grin).

I won the role and was paid enough to cover my entire fees for the next school term! After I finished the shoot, which only took a couple of hours, Rhonda said she'd drive me home and plopped me in a very nice Mercedes convertible. I'd never been in a car that fancy before.

'We're going to make a couple of stops on the way.'

'Okay.'

She drove me to West Melbourne and explained to me what an agent was, before pointing to a building. I was to speak with a lady called Lorraine about representation. I marvelled at all the head shots on the walls as I walked upstairs. I entered a room and there she was, Lorraine West, a showbiz veteran, sipping on a white wine and sucking back a ciggie.

'You must be Sam?'

'Yes. Nice to meet you. You must be Lorraine.'

'Take a seat.'

I sat down opposite her, nervous as anything.

She took a drag and sized me up. 'So you wanna be an actor?'

'Sure, I'll try it.'

She took another drag. 'You know, you remind me of another young actor who walked through this same door a few years ago. Ben Mendelsohn.'

'From *The Big Steal*!'

I knew exactly who Ben was. I had watched *The Big Steal* with him and Claudia Karvan and Steve Bisley and Damon Herriman *five times in a row* at the cinema, leaving only to dart to the toilet and back. I watched it again and again, all day and into the night. It was my most favourite film. And she was comparing me to the star in that? Shut the front door!

We wrapped up and I got back into the fancy convertible.

'How did you go?'

'Good, I think.'

Rhonda had an *actual* phone in her car and after a couple of minutes, it rang. It was Lorraine, letting Rhonda know that she was happy to 'take me on'. Just like that, I had myself an agent.

Rhonda had one more stop before dropping me home. I caught a glimpse of the sign on the way in – M.E.A.A (Media, Entertainment and Arts Alliance). She marched me to the front desk. 'I need a card for young Samuel here.'

'Ah, we can't just give him a card.'

'After all I've done for you, you'll give him a fucking card, and you'll give him a fucking card now.'

I didn't know it at the time but she was muscling the union for a membership so I could work. I filled in a form and walked out with 'a card', not having paid any 'dues' and not knowing what it all meant. She sped me down the Nepean Highway and home. I had just earned a couple of grand in an afternoon and now I had an agent *and* a magic card too!

Within months I was out-earning my dad and the school fees were sorted. I never had to busk again. It seemed Dad was right all along about the opportunities these kinds of schools offered.

A couple of years later Rhonda got sick with cancer and Zoe lost her mum. I was one of the last in a long line of people that she'd 'discovered' and I'm forever grateful to her for helping me find a life for myself. Without her gifting me with a treasured spot in a like-minded community, I'm not sure I'd have a life to speak of, to be honest.

CHAPTER 10

EXILE ON JOHNSON STREET

Like every teenager before me, and undoubtedly every teenager after me, I felt like the pain I had to endure during adolescence was so much greater than anyone else's. My period cramps were worse, my pimples were uglier, and my first-love heartache was more excruciating. I was surely the first sister who knew the jealousy of feeling like her brother was being favoured. But I did know from all the pep talks at school that I wasn't the first girl who felt pressured into doing things she didn't want to do. I was 14 and spending more and more time with an older crowd, trying to fit in.

It felt like everyone was smoking cigarettes, drinking alcohol, experimenting with drugs and having sex — and considering the people I was hanging out with, that wasn't a hard assumption to make. I thought that I would end up with no friends if I didn't follow along with the crowd and I didn't know how to stand up and say 'no'. Suddenly I was put in situations that I just didn't know how to get out of, and I didn't feel like I could talk to anyone about it. How could Dad understand? How could Hilde understand? Sam was still a kid. He hadn't hit that stage yet, where everything changes. I felt like I was on my own for the first time in my life. My ever-present little brother, who had always been so protective of me, couldn't help me this time. I wouldn't let him.

No one could understand the pressure I felt to conform, to be accepted, to not be different – and it made me angry. As far as I was concerned Dad and I were at war. His calm, quiet way of talking to me didn't cut it anymore. I felt like he was patronising me. (I know now that he wasn't but teen anger can be blinding.) He didn't understand me and he didn't want to. I thought he only loved the idea of who he wanted me to be, not who I really was. There was going to be a winner and a loser in this battle. I decided that I was not going to lose.

Dad knew things weren't good – how could he not! – and he tried to make them better. I think he suspected something had happened that I didn't want to talk about. One night he gently approached me and asked what my favourite thing in the world was. Of course, being 14, music was pretty high on the list. He asked me what I'd buy if I could have anything in the world. I told him that I would get a stereo, with some tapes and CDs to listen to, and that I would go to the Boom Crash Opera concert at the local pub.

Desperate to repair our bond and to understand why I was so angry and unhappy, Dad said he would take me to the concert and he'd make sure that even though I was underage I would get in. He told me that I wouldn't be able to drink, but that I could go with him and listen to the music. I was beside myself. I couldn't believe that he would do that for me and I was over the moon . . . for maybe a minute. Then I started to think that he had an ulterior motive, that he was doing this to trap me, to show me that I was on the wrong track, that my life was out of control and that I was making nothing but bad decisions. I convinced myself that Dad was lulling me into a false sense of security before he came down on me for wanting to go to a pub at my age. I have no idea why I couldn't believe he'd be trying to make me happy. Maybe at the time I didn't think I deserved to be.

The next day when I got home, Dad and Hilde were both there looking very excited. They told me to go look in my room for a surprise. On my bed was a huge, brand new stereo still in its box. This gift wasn't from the op shop, it was the real thing, with a double tape deck, radio and CD player. I should have screamed with joy and rushed over to open it, but instead I was intent on ruining the moment.

'Why did you buy this? Do you think you can buy my love?' I started. 'Well, you can't, and I don't want the stupid stereo anyway.'

I let him have it. My anger about the private school, about uniforms, about not having a TV, about being different, all bubbled to the surface. I told him I knew I was a disappointment, and that I didn't want to live up to his expectations. I told him he didn't understand me and he never would. I was cruel and vicious and I felt a momentary stab of guilt as I watched his face drop and his shoulders droop as he turned and walked out of the room.

Hilde was shocked. She started to tell me that Dad only wanted me to be happy, and that he'd given me the stereo to show that he was interested in what I was interested in – he thought that we could listen to music together and talk about it.

'Why do you think he's taking you to see Boom Crash Opera? How many dads do you know who would take their 14-year-old kid to a pub to see their favourite band?' she reasoned.

I wouldn't listen to her. 'I don't want him to take me to Boom Crash Opera and I don't want his stupid stereo. I hate him.'

'He loves you, Con, he loves us all. You know that, right?' Hilde said, but I wasn't listening, and eventually she left me alone in my room to stew.

Why was I doing this? It was like someone I didn't even know had taken over my body and was making me do all these awful things. I felt hot, angry and was about to start crying when Dad came back in. He sat on the bed beside me, and said softly, 'Con, I want you to know something. I don't want you to say anything, I just want to talk and for you to listen, and you can talk at the end if you want to. Okay?'

I nodded.

'I love you, and I love your sister and your brothers too. I love you more than anything, and I am here to protect you. I want you to know that you can talk to me. I can't be with you every minute of every day to keep you safe; that would drive us both mad. You need to have the freedom to grow up, but if anyone hurts you, or does something that upsets you, or that you know is wrong, you can come to me. It is my job to protect you, and if anyone does anything to hurt you, or anything that makes you uncomfortable, I can help you deal with it. Alright?'

I nodded. But there was no way I could tell Dad how I felt or what was happening. That I was feeling pressured to do things I didn't want to do. Dad kept talking but I had stopped listening. I just wanted the conversation to end.

I ended up going to the Boom Crash Opera gig with Dad, and I accepted the stereo, but I was petrified that I was letting him down. I was sure that if he truly knew me and the person I'd become, he wouldn't love me anymore. It was unbearable for all of us and eventually something had to give – so I moved out and moved in with Hilde.

Hilde was no longer with Ceri and she and Jonno now lived down the road from Dad in the 'Green House', as Jonno called it. Dad struck a deal with Hilde – he'd pay my rent and bills until I was 14 years and 9 months old, at which point I was legally allowed to get a job to support myself. In my eyes it was the perfect solution. I'd get the independence I needed and Dad would get peace of mind knowing that Hilde would keep an eye on me. I could help with Jonno, who was now two years old, so everyone was a winner. In theory. But reality was another matter.

We didn't stay in the Green House long. Hilde, Jonno and I moved to the city and I changed schools, from Mornington High to Princes Hill. As soon as I turned 14 and 9 months I got a job as a checkout chick. My white-sheep traits immediately kicked back in and I took the job very seriously. I wanted to be the fastest at entering the prices and bagging goods. I memorised prices and punched them into the cash register faster than anyone else. I was proud of my speed and accuracy. I learnt where everything was so I could direct customers and I smiled at everyone, even if they didn't smile back. Hilde had told me never to stand around doing nothing, so if there were no customers to serve I'd grab a broom and start sweeping, or get the Spray n' Wipe and clean down the counters. I took more pride in working to pay my way than I did in my school work, which would have been alarming for Dad, but I carefully hid that from him.

Working a couple of nights a week wasn't enough to make ends meet, so I went around to every business in the area looking for a weekend job and scored one at the local bakery/deli. I worked from 6 am to 2 pm Saturdays and Sundays. I learnt all the different types of bread and deli meats and it wasn't long before I was allowed to use the meat slicer and serve in the deli as well as the bakery. I felt important. I was proving I was mature and responsible, and a good reliable employee.

Despite working so hard, money was tight. I was getting $60 a week from my bakery job and earning $44.09 per week at the supermarket. But it all disappeared so quickly. I was paying $60 for rent, $14 for public transport and $15 for bills, which left me with just $15.09 for groceries and spending money. I invariably ran out of money and often risked a $60 fine by taking the tram to school without a ticket.

I floated through these times without any clear purpose or sense of where I belonged in the world. I had no idea who I was anymore. I was too scared to fit in with my old school friends. I was still going to Challenge camps but many of my cancer friends had either died or moved on – leaving their cancer behind and getting on with their lives. I forced responsibilities onto myself and wondered why no one understood me. I was surrounded by people but I felt so alone. And I was pushing away the people who loved me the most.

The one thing that kept me going through this difficult time was music. I couldn't afford to go to gigs (and I was underage anyway) but going to sound-checks only cost me the price of a train ticket to get there. I'd watch Boom Crash Opera do their afternoon sound-checks before a night-time gig – I could listen to them practise and have a chat with the band afterwards. This was a little slice of paradise for me, I just loved it. I'd drag along anyone who would come or go by myself if I had to. One day I went to a sound-check at Transformers in Moorabbin and I wasn't the only underage fan there. There was a group of girls there and they were as mad about Boom Crash as I was. One of them stood out to me. She seemed quiet, sitting at the back of the group just watching the goings-on. At first I wasn't sure if she was there because she liked the band or if she had just come along with her friends. She was a quiet little mystery and I was drawn to her. I got a strange feeling, like I was looking in a mirror except one that reflected what was inside me, looking back at me boldly. No shame, no preconceptions, just honesty, plain and simple. Her friends came up to me to ask how I knew the band, which musician I liked the best, what my favourite Boom Crash album, single and film clip was. We started talking and I found out the quiet one's name was Em, not Emma, just Em. I had a feeling that we were going to be friends.

By this point I wasn't seeing much of Sam, and nothing of Dad, but Hilde would keep me updated on what they were up to. Sam was now acting and building himself a great career, while still managing to keep up with school. He had been in a few ads and he was up for a role on *Home and Away*. When I compared myself to Sam, I told myself I was proud I was working hard for my wage. Who'd want to be some elite actor being overpaid and over appreciated? But I was kidding myself. We were two kids with very different lives now.

When I started at my new school someone told me that there was a guy in our year level with AIDS from a blood transfusion, and that I should stay away from him. It turned out they were talking about Mark Fletcher, my friend from my first night in hospital and many camps. I didn't even know Mark and I were now at the same school. It was good to reconnect with him. I needed a friend and it sounded like he did too.

I always knew that Mark had haemophilia and relied on blood transfusions, and I knew that a lot of haemophiliacs had got HIV from transfusions, but I'd never known that Mark was one of the unlucky ones. Part of me didn't want to believe it. I remembered the things my friends had said about me when I was first diagnosed – thinking they could catch cancer, or that I was going to die and so people should stop hanging out with me. I didn't know if it was true or not that Mark had AIDS but I decided I wasn't going to talk about it unless he brought it up first, and I certainly wasn't going to avoid him.

Because Mark's illness was ongoing, he still spent a lot of time at the hospital. I enjoyed hanging out with him but I felt guilty that I was fixed while he was still sick and had to live half his life in that damned ward. Why did I get better? Why did some of my friends die? Why did Mark have to spend so much of his life at the hospital just to stay alive? I was spending more and more time with Mark and there was no way to forget or ignore my survivor's guilt.

Because I was working so much and Mark had to stay in hospital a great deal, I started cutting class and taking the tram down to the hospital to visit him during school hours. I convinced myself that as long as I wasn't doing drugs and was still working and paying my bills, then I was doing okay and that cutting class wasn't such a bad thing. Once I started wagging it didn't seem such a big deal and then all of a sudden I was cutting school because I wanted to sleep in, or because I hadn't done my homework. I spent more and more time away from school and my grades started slipping badly. Eventually Hilde found out and told Dad.

Dad and Hilde begged me to stay on at school, to not waste my life. 'Did I want to be a checkout chick forever?' they asked. 'What about your dream of studying Medicine?' But everything they said went in one ear and out the other. I had order in my life, I was paying my own way and I was proud of that. True, when I couldn't afford it, Dad paid for my orthodontic payment plan some months (for the braces I had finally made sure I got), but I ignored that fact. I was independent and loving it. How many other 15-year-olds could say that?

I hadn't seen Sam for months. He had a role in *Home and Away* and I was getting sick of people enquiring about him only because he was famous. The first thing they'd say when they saw me was 'How's Sam?' I felt like replying, 'I'm fine, thanks for asking!' Fame is fickle, and it pissed me off, so I stopped talking about Sam and stopped telling people that I had a brother. I also started to resent Hilde, just like I had Dad. I thought she didn't appreciate the help I gave her looking out for Jonno, so I decided to move out of Hilde's place. It was a self-imposed exile from my family. I wanted nothing to do with

Hilde, Dad or Sam. I wished I had a mum and wondered how things would have been if I did. I wondered if I would still be at home if she was alive.

After I moved out of Hilde's place I left school altogether and got a shit-kicker job in a restaurant. But it didn't take me long to work out that Dad and Hilde were right, working fulltime in a menial job didn't earn me enough to have a decent life. Each week was a struggle to pay the bills and buy enough food. I had no disposable income to spend on things like going out, hiring a video or buying a CD. I was 15 and life was way too hard. I hated myself and my life.

Mark was sick and getting sicker. I was pretty much only seeing him at the hospital by this point because he was there so much. Here I was, pretending I was a grown-up, paying my own way and watching someone I cared about slowly wasting away with no support network to fall back on. Mark and I were both too old for the world of children, but despite our best efforts we didn't quite fit into the world of adults either. And now that he was facing death we were trying to work out whether we were in love. We were really close friends and I loved him, that was for sure, but I had no clue if I was in love. If he hadn't been so sick we would have been seeing bands together and being regular teenagers. Everything was heightened because Mark was dying. He loved me no matter how much I messed things up. He told me he adored me, and when he gave me a ring and asked me to marry him I said yes. I still had a stupid teenage crush on the lead singer of Boom Crash Opera, but Mark was sick and he needed me. It must be love, I figured.

I wanted to tell Dad and Hilde my big news but it had been so long since I'd talked to them that I didn't know what I would say. Mark tried to convince me to call them. He wanted me to find my peace with Dad and Hilde. He wanted me to be happy and he understood better than I did the happiness family can bring.

Around this time I started to listen to a local Melbourne band, Manic Suede, and I lived for their weekly gigs. I didn't have to be a grown-up on those nights. I could dance, sing along and just have fun. I didn't have to work, or sit in a hospital room watching someone I loved edge closer to death. I went to every gig I could even if it meant I would be tired the next day at work. I'd tell Mark about the gigs when he couldn't come (which was most of the time). Then, one day, a few of the band members came into the supermarket. We chatted for a while and after that they'd look out for me at their shows. They'd drive me home after gigs to make sure I was safe, and tell guys to keep away from me, as if they were my older brothers. It made me miss Sam. And I wanted him to hear this band with me. I wanted him to experience their music and see how happy it made me.

Finally I gathered my courage and called him and he came over to my apartment in Johnson Street. Sam had his Walkman with him, and played me some of his favourite tunes, I played him some of mine too, on the stereo Dad had bought me. We hung out.

'I forgot how funny you are, Con. Why can't we be friends again and hang out like this?' he said. 'It's cool.'

There'd never been any *real* problem with us. My issues were with myself, with Dad, and then Hilde – never really with Sam. So we started going to see Manic Suede together and formed a new bond as not-quite adults. There was no more competition, no need for one-upmanship, just two friends, a brother and a sister, going to see a band together.

Sam started coming over more and more. On the back of my bedroom door, I had a rope with pegs tied into it, and I'd hung my collection of baseball caps and scarves off them. It was all the headwear I'd collected to cover my baldness. It was a long time since I'd needed any of it, but my collection meant a lot to me. Most of the items were given to me by someone important to me, some who had moved on, and others who had passed on. Sam eyed my collection. Bold and brash he openly asked for one of my baseball caps. He didn't expect me to say no. I thought back to the spoon incident. When Sam asked for something, he got it, and he wanted that cap. He laughed and cajoled saying, 'Oh come on, Con, you don't wear them anymore anyway. At least I'd use it. It wouldn't be hanging on the back of a door wishing it had a life, wishing it could go on a tram, or to a pub, or down the Vic Markets.' He had a point, but I was not the same pushover I'd been and I was steadfast in my refusal. He wasn't getting his mitts on my hat.

—

As the weeks went by Sam and Mark were both in my ear to get over my grudges and talk to Dad and Hilde. I didn't listen to either of them but then one of the guys in Manic Suede, my adopted big brother, heard me and Sam talking and told me to call my dad. He said something that finally got through to me: he said I didn't need to make friends with Dad, I didn't need to tell him I loved him or say sorry, all I had to do was call him and have a chat. I didn't need to change the world with just one phone call, all I had to do was say 'hi'.

The next day I went to a public phone and dialled his number.

'Hi, Dad. It's Connie.'

'Do you need me to pay for your braces, Con?' he asked.

'No . . . that's not why I'm ringing. I just wanted to say hi,' I managed.

'Well, it's great to hear from you. What have you been up to? How are things? How's your new house in Fitzroy? Sam told me it's a great little place and that your housemate is really nice.'

I didn't realise he was so up to date. I didn't know he cared that much. I started to cry.

Dad didn't make a big deal out of me crying. He just asked about work, my house, my friends. He'd heard about Em through Sam, and my favourite band. He asked about Mark, he remembered him from the hospital and thought it was great that we were close friends. I didn't tell Dad that Mark and I were engaged. I didn't know how.

I wanted to tell him that I had decided to go back to school, to finish Year 12, but for some reason I didn't think he'd encourage me, so I said nothing.

I realised I didn't know how to be a daughter anymore.

That one phone call didn't change the world, but it was a start. A weight lifted off my shoulders. I wished I could have reached down the phone line and given Dad a great big hug. All that time he'd just been waiting patiently for me to come home.

CHAPTER 11

NOT ANOTHER GOODBYE

Besides music, one of the highlights at this point of my life was the Challenge camps. I just loved them, and they gave me a break from the relentlessness of the independent life I continued to inflict on myself. There were new kids coming to the camps all the time, and each camp I went on I'd see fewer of my old gang, either because they had died, or because they had resettled into their normal lives and didn't want to go to camp anymore. Mark went to the camps that I went to and we had so much fun. We'd walk around like normal teenagers, listening to his Walkman with one earphone each, singing along. We held hands. We kissed. We were free.

My friendship with Em had become really important too. We had so much in common. We both loved Boom Crash Opera, that was obvious, but it didn't take long to discover that there was more to our friendship than just that. Em drifted away from her old group of friends and we'd hang out together more and more. She was still at school and occasionally I helped her with her assignments, which made me kind of jealous. Part of me wished I'd stayed at school, that I'd made better decisions. Em understood me. She understood why I'd been angry with the world and had so much hatred in my heart. We were different enough to find each other interesting, but we were similar enough to finish each other's sentences. We just fit. She kept things light and she made me laugh a lot. I was enjoying my life again, despite having no money and no future.

Now that I had stopped hating everyone I tried several times to go back to school. I went to my old high school and begged them to take me back, but I was too far behind now so I enrolled to do high school by correspondence, but that didn't work out. I went to TAFE and enrolled in Year 12 for mature-age students. Time and time again I failed and then I just got tired of trying. It wore me down. I started to wonder if I had ever been the smart one. How did I fall from grace and crash down so hard? How did I go from being top of my class, to not being able to complete an assignment? I'd completely lost confidence in my ability to do well at school.

Dad and I were spending more time together. He didn't hold my poor behaviour against me. He wasn't angry, he just talked to me about things that interested me. He knew I was crazy about Manic Suede so one night he asked if he could come along to a gig with me. Sam came too. The three of us hit the dance floor together and played pool between sets – it was great fun. The guys in the band were intrigued and told me they thought my dad was a really cool cat. They all loved that he'd come to see his daughter's favourite band with her. After the last set they had a beer with Dad and I overheard one of the guys say to Dad that he must be very proud of me, because I worked so hard, and tried so hard. I wasn't part of the conversation but I had tears in my eyes as I overheard Dad say, yes, he *was* very proud of me.

That was just the confidence boost I needed. I was 20 years old and I finally felt that just maybe I could get back into school and finish it. It wasn't really about making everyone else proud of me, though, I just wanted to be proud of myself. From my first night in hospital when I was diagnosed, I had wanted to be a doctor. I wanted to be an oncologist, and research children's cancers. With my early academic achievement, I had never doubted this future. Medicine was my destiny. But it had all gone wrong. I might have learnt the lessons the hard way, but I knew for sure that I was not destined to work in a supermarket or a restaurant for the rest of my life. I was going to try again, and this time I would succeed. I would finish Year 12, then aim for medical school. I was determined to get back on track.

Around this time Challenge was organising a massive gala ball for Halloween as a fundraiser and one of the attractions was a dance routine choreographed by the Sydney Dance Company and performed by some patients and their siblings and friends. My friend Natasha – who had proven the doctors wrong, ditched the wheelchair and was walking again – was in it, I was in it, Mark was in it, and there was space for a few more, so I was ecstatic that Em could join in too. The dance was to Michael Jackson's 'Will You Be There'. It was really moving, and we all took great pride in our roles – Mark, Em and I practised every chance we got until we knew the routine by heart.

Just as I started to spend more time with Dad and Hilde, and started to get my life on track again, Sam was starting to achieve real stardom. It seemed to me that Sam always had the magic touch. Whatever he put his hand to he was good at, and he was such a nice person that people wanted to see him succeed. First he did his paper round and saved up so much money that he was able to invest in Australian Aboriginal art, and through this he found himself in the papers, on the radio and even on the TV; then he'd won himself that place in the Asian Pacific Children's Convention; and then he was going to be an international tennis player, and was good enough to be playing, and sometimes beating some of the top players in Australia in his age group.

I wasn't surprised that when he turned his attention to acting he really flourished. His looks and his voice are distinctive and he was landing every role he auditioned for. He'd been on so many ads and shows, that he could barely walk down the street without getting recognised. Sadly, the more acclaim he received the less he seemed to enjoy it. Suddenly I could see he was finding the fame really hard to cope with – he didn't seem to trust anyone, he pushed his friends away, and eventually he pushed me and the rest of the family away too. The easygoing brother I'd always known had disappeared and he was in a pretty dark place. I recognised the anger but he was hard to reach. It seemed that one of us was always struggling; just as I had turned things around he started going off the rails.

Hilde was always close to Sam, and had been there for him in the same way she'd always tried to be there for me, even when I pushed her away. Hilde never stopped trying to help me, and once I decided I was going back to school she found ways to make that easier for me too. She encouraged Dad to employ me in one of their bookshops, so I didn't have to work in the crappy jobs I'd been doing for so long. Dad and Hilde had opened a second-hand bookshop in Melbourne a few years earlier and then a second. It had been a natural progression for Dad to go from collector to shop owner – and he was good at it. Dad gave me shifts and actively encouraged me to study while I was working. Getting paid to study – it doesn't get much better than that, does it?

Then Dad said I could live above one of his bookshops in exchange for working weekends, that way I didn't have to pay rent and all my bills would be covered as well. Dad wasn't in a position to support me financially while I went back to school, and I wouldn't have accepted his help even if he was, but this was an arrangement my pride could cope with. I still felt that I was working hard, and living my independent life, but he was helping relieve the financial pressure and giving me the space to study.

This time I was determined to make it work. I was humiliated that I'd been a drop-out but I put that behind me and used it to spur me on. I didn't want to be a drop-out again, I couldn't handle the disgrace. I knew I had to get back into the habit and study hard every day. I had to learn to prioritise and work on the most pressing stuff first, then get to the rest. I wouldn't let myself slip. Every day had to be a good day.

It was hard but I was keeping up, meeting deadlines and still finding time for music and friends. My results were good. The only bad thing was that Mark was very unwell. He went up and down, we'd think he was fine and then he'd get sick again. Very sick. Every time we'd all rush to the hospital and say our goodbyes. I begged him to get better so we could do the dance together at the Halloween ball. I doubted he could hear me, but I'd hold his hand and whisper in his ear, 'You have to get better, Mark. We can't do the dance without you.' He was thin and tired, his skin was grey and his lips unbearably dry. After days of sitting beside him with no response, thinking every breath would be his last, I felt him squeeze my hand ever so slightly. He recovered, but each time this happened he was a little weaker. I think he was determined to dance at the ball.

The night of the ball finally rolled around, and the room was packed – there were over 300 people there! Mark and I were waiting in the wings, ready to go on. It was so quiet you could have heard a pin drop. The lights dimmed and soft music started. It was gentle and graceful and our two key dancers pirouetted into the spotlight. The music built and we stood as still as statues in the background, waiting for the drums to start. I was shaking. The first drum sounded and our feet began to shuffle then our bodies joined in. The full lights flicked on and we danced. I was so proud, so happy to be a part of this moment I thought I would burst. Here we were – a group of kids who had fought cancer or other life-threatening diseases, and the friends and family who had supported us through it, and we'd won. At that moment I had never felt more alive. As the last notes sounded, the audience rose to a standing ovation, there were shouts and whistles – it was a moment of triumph for us all. But it was over far too quickly, especially for Mark.

Not long after the dance Mark fell ill again. I prepared myself for the worst. I held his hand. I told him how much I loved him. That I needed him. I visited him every chance I had. I wanted this to be another false alarm. I needed it to be another false alarm. But it wasn't. No matter how willing his mind was, Mark's body just couldn't keep fighting. One morning I got a phone call telling me that things were really bad. I rushed over to the hospital but by the time I got there he was gone.

An anger fired up inside me, I was more angry than I had ever been. This wasn't right. How could someone like Mark be gone, after fighting his whole life, and others who weren't as kind or as loving still be around? How could his life be over?

Who would ever love the colour green as much as him? Who would be the number one fan of Guns N' Roses? Who would I listen to music with? Who would show me our dance moves when I forgot them? Who would smile handsomely at me when I was being aggro, and tell me he liked how independent I was? Who'd love me like he did? It wasn't fair. Nothing about it was fair. And I was angry.

Em stayed with me and we cried together. I put on Michael Jackson's 'Will You Be There' and went through the dance moves in my head. The last thing I'd said to Mark was, 'You have to wake up. I can't remember the dance, I need you to show me.' Without Mark, I felt like there was no dance, no music, no laughter, no light.

I didn't know that they don't put a headstone on a grave straight away, it goes on later, after the earth has settled. I hated that there was nothing to show for his life so I built a big, wooden cross and painted it bright green, Mark's favourite colour. Before the funeral I looked in every shop I could afford to shop in, searching for a green dress, or skirt, or shirt – something green, something he would love. I finally found a green skirt, and I wore it in his honour. I kept the funeral program. I looked at the two-dimensional photo that didn't truly capture his spirit and wondered how his life could be reduced to a two-page program.

I wasn't sure how I could go back to school, how I could just get on with my life without Mark. How could I act like everything was okay? Nothing was okay. But somehow, life finds a way to go on, and though I felt like screaming, I suppressed it, looked down and kept going. I listened to my Walkman, not looking at the people around me. I constantly wondered how Mark's mum was. How his brother was. I kept in touch for a little while, but we always said the same things, always talked about the same memories, and eventually it was longer and longer between calls until I just called on his birthday and death-day.

I think Dad was worried that I'd go off the rails again and give up. He reminded me that Mark was proud of me and that he'd wanted me to finish school and get into Medicine as well, so I had to keep at it. He was right, but somehow it still felt wrong.

Grief is strange because it never goes away but eventually it hurts less to be out in the world. As time went on I could think of Mark and smile, instead of cry. I was going to make sure I lived well, for myself and for him.

CHAPTER 12

IF AT FIRST YOU DON'T SUCCEED

Returning to school was one of the hardest things I'd ever done in my life. It would have been easy for me to give up again after Mark died, but I didn't. I was determined to leave my checkout-chick days behind and claw my way back to a different life, so I committed to the TAFE course and gave it everything I had. If I could, I wanted to get into Medicine and research and work on helping to find a cure for haemophilia.

I'd always achieved full marks on tests at school before I got sick – it was something I'd expected of myself and almost took for granted. But going off the rails changed all that. I'd learnt that I had to earn every point and knew it wasn't going to be an automatic thing anymore. And when I did succeed, my victories tasted that much sweeter because I knew I'd given it my all.

My final marks for English, Biology, Chemistry and Literature were all well above 95, but I let myself down a bit with Maths, and ended up with a Tertiary Entrance Rank of 92.9. I was over the moon, but couldn't help being disappointed that I was three points below what I needed for the Rural Medicine program, which had an entrance score of 96 or higher. I didn't let that disappointment get on top of me, though, and enrolled in a Bachelor of Science majoring in Biochemistry at university, which I intended to use as a stepping stone to get into Medicine the next year. Dad and Hilde were proud and so were Sam and Em. I knew Mark would have been proud of me. Most importantly, I was proud of myself. And it felt good.

For the first time in a long time I also felt hopeful. I was working in the bookshop on Saturdays and Sundays to pay for my board and going to uni during the week. Living above Dad's bookshop was suiting me perfectly. It was in a cool area – right on Glenferrie Road in Hawthorn and only five minutes from uni – and there was no way I could have afforded a place on my own. It was a fairly rundown building but it had lots of character. It didn't have a lounge room, just three bedrooms upstairs and then a kitchen, laundry and toilet at the back of the shop downstairs. If I had a big night and slept in I had to get dressed and walk past all the customers in the bookshop just to get to the toilet.

The three bedrooms were connected by a long narrow hallway, made even narrower by the bookcases that lined the walls, which stored all the spare stock for the shop. Each bedroom also had its own set of bookcases and there were probably 10,000 books stored upstairs. A friend of mine, Naomi, lived in the tiny room at the back end of the building. It was just big enough for a single bed and a chair. Dad lived in the middle bedroom, which was a reasonable size, and he had a telly on a bookcase at the end of his bed. (Finally he had a

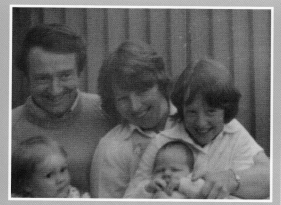

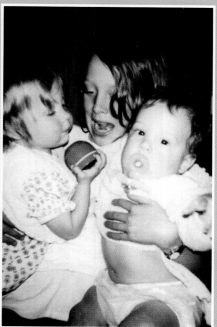

ABOVE: This is the only photo we have of our whole family. Me, Dad, Mum, Sam and Hilde.

RIGHT: Big sister Hilde wrangling me and Sam.

BELOW: Me, Aunty Marg, Dad, Sam, Hilde, Uncle George and Cousin Jamie in the backyard of one of Dad's renovation purchases.

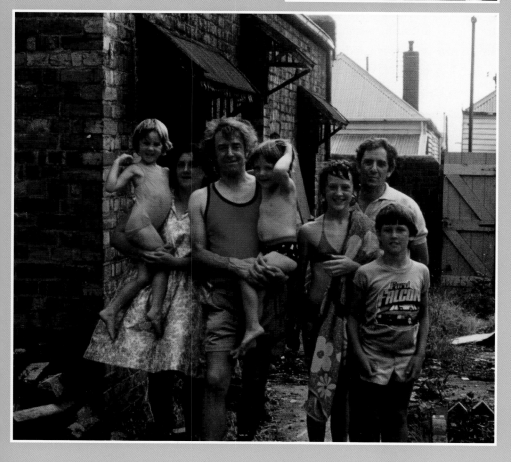

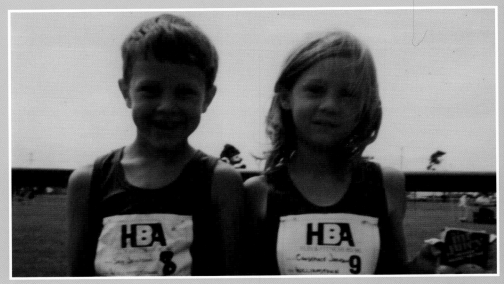

ABOVE: Me and Sam at Little Athletics.

RIGHT: Anyone for table tennis?

BOTTOM LEFT: Me and Sam just after I finished chemo.

BOTTOM RIGHT: Always the performer: here is Sam juggling at Black Rock Primary.

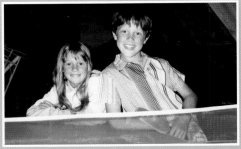

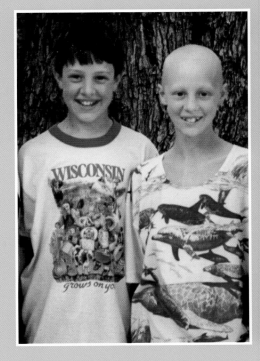

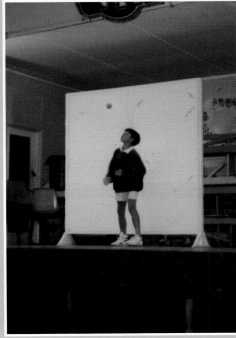

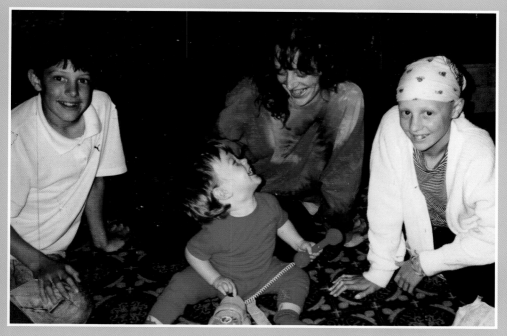

ABOVE: Sam, baby Jonno, Hilde and me.

BOTTOM LEFT: Me and Dad playing 'Whac-a-Mole' during one of my hospital visits.

BOTTOM RIGHT: Me with Diesel (aka Mark Lizotte), but my heart still belonged to Dale Ryder from Boom Crash Opera.

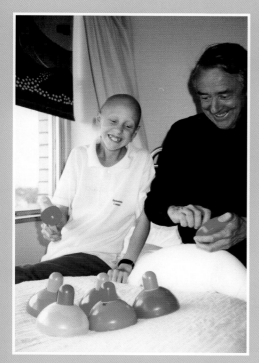

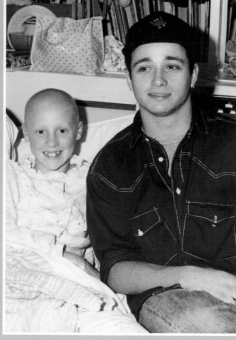

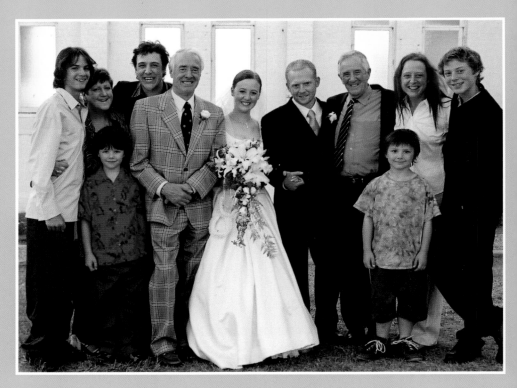

ABOVE: My and Mike's wedding day in our church at Harden in October 2004. Left to right: Dave, Aunty Marg, Sully, Sam, Dad, me, Mike, Uncle George, Aussy, Hilde and Jonno.

BELOW LEFT: Dad and Sam, a favourite picture of mine.

BELOW RIGHT: Dad and baby Hamilton. He was such a good grandpa.

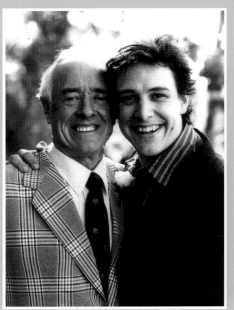

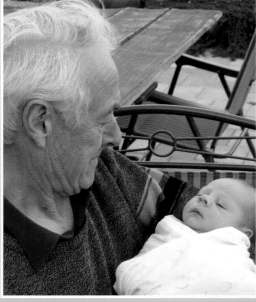

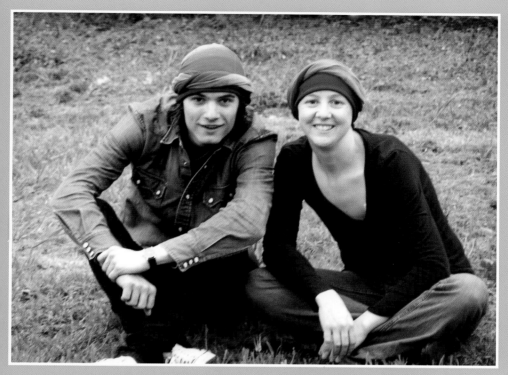

ABOVE: Dave wearing a bandanna in a show of solidarity during chemo in 2010.

BELOW: Family time before my mastectomy operation: Mike, Hamilton, Chris (Nanna), Willoughby and me.

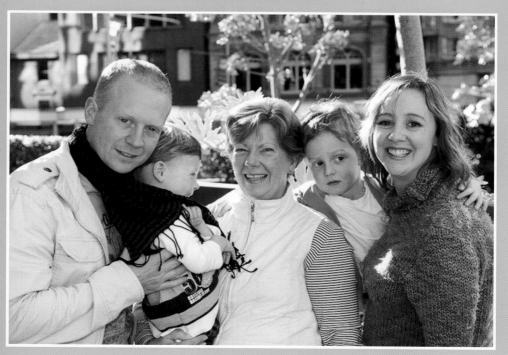

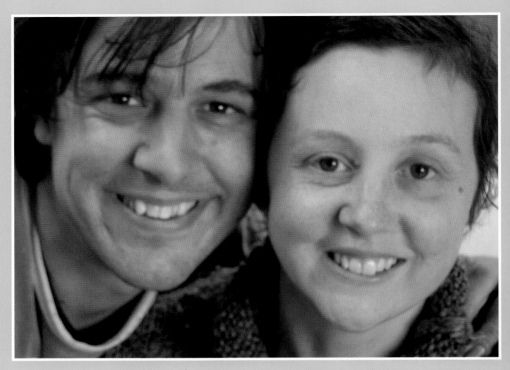

ABOVE: We've had our ups and downs but when I've needed him Sam's been there.

BELOW: We both had to learn 'The Facebook' to get Love Your Sister happening. This was our first post together.

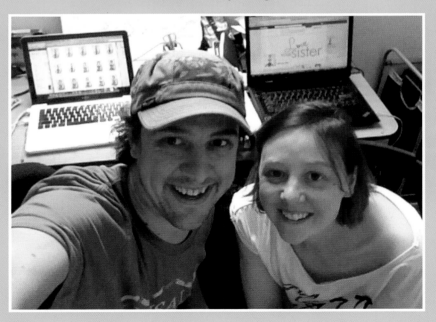

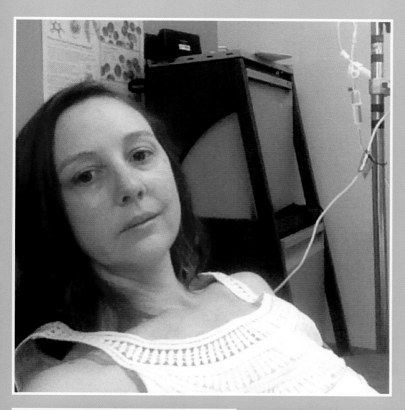

ABOVE: Having chemo just before the Love Your Sister launch in February 2013.

Molly Meldrum is a big supporter of Love Your Sister. Here he is (LEFT) with me during my first chemo when I was 12. On launch day (BELOW) he presented me with an authentic 'Molly' pink Akubra.

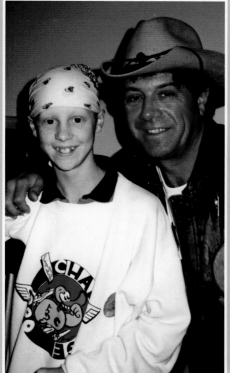

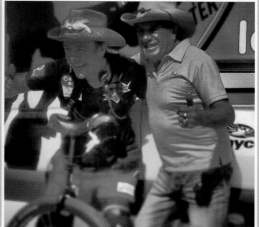

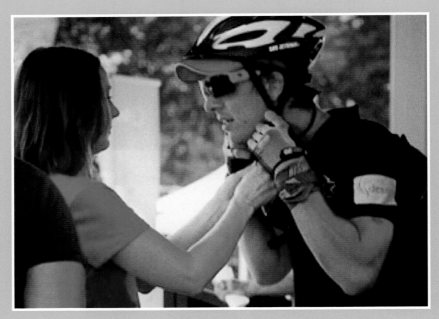

ABOVE: A final gesture of love before Sam rode away for the whole year.

BELOW: Sam riding off from Federation Square, high-fives all round.
The support blew us both away.

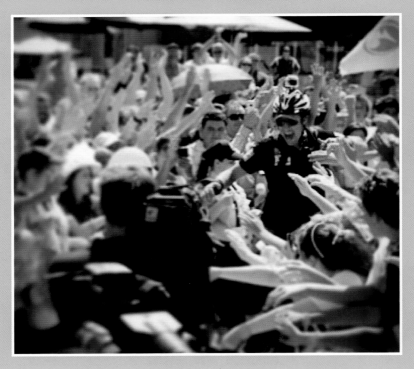

TV!) I was the lucky one – I had the huge room at the front of the building, with a balcony looking out over Glenferrie Road. I loved that balcony and spent hours out there, watching the goings-on of the street below. The trams rolled past at regular intervals, dinging their bells all the way, cars banked up behind the trams and I'd watch as people got cranky and impatient, keen to keep moving. Over the road there was a video library, a clothing store, a picture framing shop and a noodle restaurant.

Noodles were my favourite meal. They were cheap, filled you up and came with a heap of vegies. I often went to the Noodle Box for dinner with Naomi. We'd get our noodles and eat them on my balcony, looking down on the street while we ate. We could see right into the window of the Noodle Box, and had a good view of the blokes who worked there. Naomi liked one guy especially. She thought he was hot. He was good looking in a traditional sense, I guess, but he didn't get my attention. There was a really nice red-haired guy who always served us – he was more interesting to me. He always smiled kindly when we went in and after a very short time he'd memorised my order: kway teow with extra broc, carrots, 'shrooms and shoots. He'd always pile in extra vegies. Naomi called him and the boy she liked the 'Noodle Boys'.

One day I was walking through uni and I felt a tap on my bottom as I turned to walk up the stairs. I was horrified. Who would have the nerve to touch me on the butt? I spun around with, I am sure, a disgusted look on my face, only to see the red-haired Noodle Boy standing there awkwardly holding a book, half brazen, half guilty.

'What are you doing here?' It was one of those strange moments when you see someone in a different context and it takes a second or two to place them.

'Well,' he answered, 'what are YOU doing here? You're the Bookshop Girl.'

I was so taken aback that I forgot to reprimand him for tapping me on the butt. 'So what are you studying?' I asked.

'IT and Business. What about you?'

'Biochem. So you just work part-time at the Noodle Box while you're studying?'

'Yep. Same as you, Bookshop Girl.'

'Shut up, Noodle Boy!' I hit him playfully on the arm, suddenly remembering that he'd just tapped me on the butt. 'And what makes you think that you can just slap me on the bottom out of nowhere? You're lucky I didn't punch you!' I said cheekily, to let him know that I was just fooling around.

'It wasn't me, it was the book!'

We talked for a while about what we were studying and he offered to give me a hand with a programming assignment I was having trouble with. He said we could get together some time. Maybe over the weekend?

I walked off, trying to act casual. I wanted to look back to see if he was looking at me, but I stopped myself. I felt like jumping up and down and squealing. I got to the top of the stairs and couldn't help it, I looked back. He was still standing at the bottom of the stairs, watching me walk away. He grinned and waved clumsily. He was pretty cute!

I realised that I had just agreed to a date with this guy and I didn't even know his name. How embarrassing! I couldn't keep calling him Noodle Boy. Then I realised that he didn't know my name either.

—

I was surprised by my reaction to this guy. I'd only recently decided that I didn't want a boyfriend. I just wanted to focus on my studies and forget about men altogether. Over the previous few months it had seemed like everybody I met was only after sex, nothing else. I was sick of feeling like I was being used so I'd decided to stop dating altogether.

Having these feelings for Noodle Boy made me feel vulnerable and foolish. I told Naomi about what happened, and she could immediately tell I was into him. We talked about it and she agreed with my decision to play it cool and keep my distance for a while. That lasted until the next Saturday when Naomi and I went in to get some dinner.

Red-haired boy's face lit up and he said, 'It's the Bookshop Girls.'

'And here are the Noodle Boys,' we joked back.

Naomi's Noodle Boy served her, and mine served me. It was awkward, but he seemed happy to see me and I was definitely happy to see him. We talked around other customers and eventually I asked if he was serious when he offered to help me with my assignment. It turned out he was.

'Yeah, I can have a look at it. When is it due?'

'Tuesday. So I don't have long.'

He said he was working until 11 pm for the next two nights. He surprised me when he offered to help me after work. I was delighted and a little bit excited as well.

He told me he just had to see if he could get out of something he had planned and that he'd call me. I looked out the window and pointed to our phone number printed on the bright yellow sign of the bookshop across the road. I didn't normally answer it after hours, but I was going to that night!

About an hour after I got home the phone rang and I picked it up while looking down at his shop. I could see him waving up at me.

'Hey, Bookshop Girl, how you going?'

I laughed. He still didn't know my name. This was getting awkward. 'Hi, Noodle Boy,' I said.

'I was supposed to go out tonight, but I pulled out, so I can come over and help you with your assignment if you want?' He sounded nervous.

I was stoked and offered to pour him a drink to make up for missing his night out. I hung up and realised I hadn't asked his name. D'oh!

—

I tried to study while I waited for Noodle Boy to arrive but I couldn't concentrate. Finally, at 11 pm I went downstairs and sat at the counter, in the dark, looking out at the street through the book display in the front window. There were people walking past, some drunk and silly, staggering and loud. A couple walked up hand in hand and stopped to look at the books on display.

'Look at this one, honey. It's that book I was telling you about, *The Long Walk to Freedom* by Nelson Mandela. It's only nine dollars. We should come back when they're open and get it.'

I smiled to myself. I love people who love books.

Eventually, the lights went out at the Noodle Box and all the staff milled about out the front for a few minutes, chatting. There was only one girl who worked there. I watched Noodle Boy kiss her on the cheek as they said goodbye. I wondered briefly if they were more than just friends or colleagues. I was a bit jealous.

I unlocked the door and held it open for him. I showed him around the shop and out the back – the makeshift kitchen with the laundry and bathroom. We had two dogs and they jumped all over him. Upstairs I explained that we didn't have a lounge room, so I had to invite him into my bedroom. I pointed at Naomi's door and Dad's door and told him who lived in each room.

'I feel awkward, but I don't know your name,' I finally admitted. 'I'm CJ.'

He laughed, relieved. 'Yeah, it's funny. I'm glad you asked, CJ, my name is Mike.'

I offered Mike a vodka, which he accepted, so I poured a very weak one for myself as well – I still had homework to do. We worked on the assignment for a little while but then we started talking and we took it in turns playing songs to each other from my CD collection. He liked most of my music, and teased me a little for the Spice Girls in my collection. I kept topping up our drinks and they were getting stronger and stronger as the night wore on. We talked for hours, about life, how we wanted to live, what we were working towards. We talked about the environment and politics. We talked about uni and why we were studying and what we wanted to be when we 'grew up'. We talked about our families and our friends, our best friends, our favourite bands and pubs around Melbourne. Before we knew it, it was three in the morning. I had to start work at 10 am, he had to start at

1 pm. It didn't seem strange that we decided he should stay the night but I told him I wasn't going to sleep with him.

I turned out the light and told Mike I was taking off my jeans because it wasn't comfortable to sleep in them but not to get any ideas. Mike followed my lead and took his jeans off too. It was dark, but there was a streetlight just outside my window, so I could still see him a little bit. He reached over and put an arm around me, in a half hug, and I gently kissed him on the lips. He kissed me back.

'I am not sleeping with you,' I reminded him.

'No, of course not, CJ. I'm not sleeping with you either, we only just met.'

—

I woke to a soft knocking at my door. 'Con, are you there?' It was Dad. 'I'm going to the bakery. Do you want anything for breakfast?'

'Could you please grab me a couple of croissants?' I called out.

Mike's face was ashen and his eyes looked like they'd pop right out of his head. 'Oh shit, I have to get out of here. I can't believe your dad's here,' he whispered.

I managed to convince him to stay for a croissant before he had to go to get ready for work, and I had to open the shop.

Dad came back and knocked before walking in. 'How are you, Con? Oh! Hi, how you going, mate? I'm Joe, Connie's dad.'

Mike stammered as he introduced himself. I love my dad, he was so cool, he bought me a nice bakery breakfast, was nice to a guy he found in my room and didn't freak out at all, just introduced himself and then left to get on with his day. (What a difference a year or two made to my attitude!)

'He seems pretty cool,' Mike said once Dad had gone. 'When I lived at home I never could have brought a girl home and have her sleep in my bedroom. My mum and dad would freak right out.'

We talked for a bit more and then Mike left, telling me he'd come over with lunch for me. I spent the first two hours of my shift in a daze, going over everything we'd talked about, re-feeling every emotion and unable to sit still because of the buzz that ran through me whenever I thought of Mike. Before I knew it he was back with lunch from the deli. He didn't know what I liked, besides noodles, so he'd brought a selection of everything. I couldn't help but like this guy and it seemed he liked me too. Things were really looking up!

Over the next three weeks, Mike stayed at my place nearly every night, and if we weren't there we were at his place. One night we were at mine, lying in bed watching *Ally McBeal*. I had a really cheap and nasty futon, totally matching my fiscal position. During an ad break I started to tidy the bedroom a little bit. Mike had a bag of stuff, and I made some space on one of the bookcases for him to put his things. I was just pottering around and I picked up a pair of his undies. I couldn't believe what I was seeing. They had little roaring tiger faces all over them in purple and orange. They were truly awful.

'Mike, what are these?' I swung them above my head like a lasso. His face went bright red, from the neck up, like a thermometer reading a fever. I felt a bit mean but I couldn't stop myself because they were just so hideously hilarious. I put them on my head and ran around the room laughing hysterically and he got up to chase me before tackling me onto the bed.

CRACK!

The bed collapsed. It took me a moment to realise that we had broken the bed. Nobody was going to believe that we broke the bed laughing – nobody!

—

After we broke the bed Mike offered to bring his over. That meant he would have no bed at his place. He had effectively moved in. This was really going somewhere! But I still wasn't sure if Mike felt as strongly as I did.

I'm a fiery type, and the most inane things can set me off. My temper is the characteristic I most hate about myself. I regularly lose it, drop my lolly, lose my shit over little things that other people just brush aside as unimportant.

Things like:

When I go to the movies, I don't understand why people sit close to me when there are hundreds of seats elsewhere in the theatre where they could have plenty of room. I move away, flabbergasted.

When I catch the tram, and am stuck next to a sweaty man with bad body odour who is holding the overhead straps, exposing his stench to me and the world. I take offence, and find it hard not to say something.

When someone parks in the driveway at the back of our shop. I get pissed off, even though I don't have a car and can't park there anyway. It's the principle of the matter.

I know this about myself. But I wasn't sure how Mike would react when he learnt about this side of me. It didn't take long for me to find out.

I had been hauling washing to the laundromat since I was

14 – that's eight years of weekly haulage – because I had never been able to afford a washing machine. I had, however, bought myself a little trolley with a basket on top and a basket below, that made the weekly haul a lot easier. Now that I had Mike's washing too, I had to go to the laundromat more than once a week and it was starting to wear thin. I was choosing to do the washing and though I consider myself a feminist, I still wanted to do his washing because I wanted to be a good partner and I thought that was what good partners did.

But one night, after literally airing our dirty laundry to every passerby I was sick of it. I needed to blow off steam and Mike copped it as I ranted about being poor and not having a washing machine.

Mike's shoulders dropped. 'Oh, honey, I wanted to surprise you, but I guess I should tell you now, since you're so upset.'

That wasn't the response I'd expected at all. I immediately regretted having just blown my top.

'I bought us a washing machine,' he went on. 'I got it last week from Andrew, my friend who works in the electrical and white goods trade. It's getting delivered on Monday. I wanted to surprise you. I know you hate going to the laundromat, so I bought us a washing machine.'

It hit me then. I knew that Mike was a good guy. He didn't expect me to do his washing, or look after him. He just wanted me to be happy. He had seen the worst of me and he was staying put. I adored him.

CHAPTER 13

LIGHTNING DOES STRIKE TWICE

It surprised me how well Mike and I got along because we were so very different. But it's true what they say about opposites. Mike grew up in a Salvation Army family. I didn't realise that the Salvo's were a religion, I had only ever thought of them as a group who did good things for people in need. Meeting Mike's family gave me an insight into why Mike is the way he is. He is measured, calm and personable. Everyone who meets him likes him, and he doesn't stuff up. He never does the wrong thing. He is always polite, always appropriate. He was a complete contrast to my family, who are all so haphazard, emotive and impulsive.

I was so nervous the first time I met Mike's family. I was worried they'd think I wasn't good enough for their son. I needn't have worried. They opened their front door and both his mum and dad were standing there with big smiles plastered on their faces. They were so happy to see Mike and I got the credit for bringing him home to his family.

I was happy. I had a partner who made me feel like it was okay to be me. No pretending. We were happy together. I was 22 years old, working at Cabrini Hospital as a pathology clerk and blood collector, and with Mike in Dad's bookshops to cover our rent, all while still studying. But something wasn't right. I started feeling sick all the time. Not in a totally debilitating way, but I knew that something was up. I talked to a friend and she told me to get a pregnancy test done. I told her I was on the pill and that after all the chemo I'd had it was very unlikely I'd fall pregnant even if I wasn't.

Mike came with me to the doctor. I'd been seeing my doctor for a long time by this point. He was a gentle soul and knew all about my history with cancer. He took a sample, dipped a tester into it and typed into his computer screen while we waited: *pregnancy test*. His fingers paused over the keyboard and he adjusted his screen so we could both read it. He asked, 'What would you do if it was . . . ?' then before we had time to answer, he typed: *positive*.

Mike looked at me. I looked at Mike. I wanted to jump out of my seat and scream. I was overjoyed. I couldn't believe my luck. I was actually pregnant, after spending the previous eight or so years believing I couldn't have children of my own. It was bliss.

We left the surgery and I was practically skipping to the car. Mike was silent. Then reality hit me and I stopped mid-stride. 'Mike, you need to tell me what you think. I need an honest answer so I can decide what to do with this baby.'

In the time between realising that he might not be as happy as me and the moment when he responded, I had already planned to be a single mum, because abortion wasn't an option for me. I didn't want to trap Mike in a life he didn't want, but this was a gift. I had always wanted to have children and now I was able to. If I had to do it without him, I would.

Mike looked at me earnestly, walked towards me with his arms open, and folded me into him. 'I think we are going to have to go to a car yard and trade in the Celica for a family wagon.'

Wow!

———

Hilde had had her first child at 19, and Dad had always mourned the fact that I probably couldn't have children, so I knew he would be ecstatic at the news, and he was; when we told him he was so happy he cried.

But I was really worried what Mike's mum, Chris, would say. She is a lovely lady, a really nice person, a good Samaritan, but I knew she didn't believe in sex before marriage. I'm sure she knew the truth about Mike and me, but at that moment there was no proof we were living in sin. A baby changed all that. I was absolutely petrified, and I knew that Mike wasn't going to tell his parents any time soon so I called her. I chatted on about nothing much, nervous and definitely not my usual self until Chris finally said, 'Oh, for goodness sake, Constance, what is going on?' She said it with a light, but slightly strict tone and so I took a deep breath and bit the bullet.

'We're pregnant, we are going to have a baby,' I blurted out.

There was a pause.

'You haven't known each other for long. Are you happy?' she asked.

'Yes,' I said truthfully.

'And is Michael happy?'

'Yes.'

'Then that is great, great news!'

We chatted some more about the due date, the test dates and all that rigmarole and when I got off the phone I was able to tell Mike that his mum was okay, and happy for us, but that she wanted us to set a date for the wedding soon. I couldn't help laughing I was so happy. Everything was changing so quickly but it felt good.

—

One night, about three weeks later, I woke up bleeding. Not a lot but enough to worry me. Maybe it was too good to be true, maybe I couldn't really have a baby. Mike took me to the closest hospital. A young intern asked me a barrage of questions, and did a quick feel of my belly. She didn't order any scans and then said, 'You have a tummy bug.'

It was the middle of the night. I was tired and so was Mike. Even though I didn't quite believe what I was being told, I was happy to learn that it was nothing serious, so I accepted the answer and went home. But the tummy bug diagnosis didn't hold for long. The next day I was still bleeding and something was wrong, very wrong. Whatever this was, it wasn't a tummy bug.

Mike drove me back to the hospital's emergency department. This time it was a young male intern and he told me I was miscarrying. There was nothing that could be done.

I instantly felt deep despair. I called Dad. He cried and cried and told me how sad he was for me. I called Sam. He cried and cried. He told me how wrong it was, that I would make such a great mum and that it wasn't fair that this baby didn't make it. I called Hilde. She cried with me and then decided that we should all meet. This was something that our family needed to be together for. She told me I needed to grieve, but I also needed to be with them.

We all met up at a pool hall in Kew. It's this huge, dark hall up a flight of stairs with rows and rows of pool tables. The only lights are the lights over the tables, which shine down onto the green felt. There's a bar and the room is always smoky with music blaring out from a jukebox. We found a secluded little corner where we could all congregate. Dad sat there nursing a beer. His shoulders were slumped and he turned the glass around and around on the spot, in a quiet and contemplative daze. Tears rolled down his cheeks whenever he looked at me.

He told me of the time when a girlfriend of his, a lady I remember well, whom he saw on and off for years during our childhood, got pregnant with his baby. She decided to terminate the pregnancy and didn't tell Dad until after it was done. He never forgot that baby, and never quite got over the loss. He told me that he didn't know my pain, and that he would never understand how it feels for a mother to lose a child, but that he was sad for me. He said he thought I would be a great mum one day, and the fact that I got pregnant in the first place meant that it could happen again.

I hoped he was right.

It was such a quick dream. After growing up thinking that I couldn't have kids, it felt like a sliver of light shone on me for a moment, and then it was gone. I sat there with Mike and my family around me and I couldn't smile, I just sat there crying as the waves of sadness rolled over me. Everyone bought me drinks and I swallowed them all down, hoping the alcohol would dull the pain. I smoked a cigarette or two. Why not smoke and drink? I didn't have a baby to protect anymore.

A few days later I still felt pregnant. I was confused and asked the nurses at work to do another pregnancy test. It was positive. Mike took me to see my doctor and I told him about the blood test at work and gave him the results. He did another urine test and confirmed that I was still pregnant.

Panic seized me. 'But they told me I'd had a miscarriage! I went out and drank and smoked. What if I've done something to harm the baby?'

My doctor reassured me that one night out was not going to do anything drastic. He told me to stay off the booze and smokes from then on. He also wanted to do a scan so he sent me straight to the radiology centre, with its white walls and cheap art prints.

They told me on the spot that it wasn't good news and sent me straight back to my doctor with the report and the scans.

I watched my doctor's face carefully as he read the report and I tried not to cry. He sighed and then explained I was showing all the signs of being pregnant but the baby was actually a genetic mutation with far too many genes – it was actually a tumour. What I had was called a hydatidiform mole pregnancy, and it happened in around one in 1200 pregnancies. There are two types of molar pregnancies, benign and malignant. I needed to have a Dilation and Curettage (D&C), and have the tumour tested to see if it was cancerous.

I was left swimming in a cloud of confusion and grief.

How could I be pregnant, but not be having a baby?

How could our baby be a tumour?

Did I have cancer again?

Had this happened because of the treatment I'd had when I was a kid?

Would I be able to have another baby in the future?

What would happen if it was cancer? I could not and would not go through that treatment again. I would rather die.

—

Mike was concerned about me. It was like a switch inside him flicked off and he stopped worrying about not being pregnant – he wouldn't even talk about that – all he worried about was me.

And all I cared about was that I wasn't having a baby. My baby was gone.

Back at the hospital, my appointments with nurses and doctors passed in a fog. I was just so sad. Through all the chaos and confusion I heard a doctor say, 'I don't know why you are so upset. It isn't a baby, it's just a mass of cells and it's unhealthy. We need to get rid of it for your health.' I was incapable of anger, I just cried more.

I had the D&C and they sent the sample off for testing. They explained that it would be tested there at the hospital. The hope was that it was benign. I couldn't really contemplate it being malignant – the thought of more treatment just horrified me.

Dad was there. Hilde was there. Sam was there. Mike was there. But nobody understood my loss. Nobody understood my grief. I was surrounded by the people I loved but I felt so alone. They were all trying to be positive, they all hoped that it would be benign. But I was still grieving the loss of what I had thought was my miracle baby. We didn't need to trade the car in now. I could throw away the baby books and my lists of possible names. I had already bought a tiny white and grey jumpsuit – something neutral, so it could be worn by a boy or a girl. I could throw it away, along with my dreams and hopes for the new life that was no longer inside me.

A week passed, no results. Another week. More anxious waiting.

Finally the results came in and the surgery called, asking me to come in. The tumour was benign. I was happy, but it didn't take away the pain. The first thing I asked my doctor was when could we start trying for another baby.

He explained that I shouldn't get pregnant again for at least two years. That I had to go on strong birth control, because if I did get pregnant the tumour could come back. And if the baby and the tumour were competing for nutrients and space in the womb, the tumour would win and the baby would die.

In my head I knew that I couldn't risk it, but all I wanted was to try for another baby. Nothing else mattered to me. Work didn't matter. Uni didn't matter. I just wanted to have a baby. I was bordering on insanity the way I was obsessing, but Mike stayed sensible. He took me to every appointment (or should I say dragged me along!), making sure that I received my injections and the care I needed. He just wanted me safe and healthy.

I couldn't understand why Mike wasn't paralysed by grief like I was. I couldn't comprehend how he could just go to work, how he could study, how he could get on the train every day and continue with life like nothing had happened. For me, life had stopped making sense and it made me angry that the world kept turning, that day turned into night and the trams kept rushing past. My world had ground to a halt and I hurt. How could the sun keep shining?

Eventually I had to go back to work. We had bills to pay, and medical treatment isn't cheap. I couldn't leave it all to Mike. But I didn't have the heart to finish my studies that semester and so I just stopped going. I stupidly didn't even withdraw officially, even though I knew that I would have a fail on my record, permanently. I rejoined the throngs of people on the train going to and from work. I started to go out with my friends and family again and the numbness dissipated slowly. I thought it was getting better. And then the phone rang.

'Hi. May I speak with Constance Johnson, please?'

'Speaking. Who is this?'

'It's Mary calling from the Women's Hospital. I need to speak to you about your molar pregnancy.'

'I was treated at Monash. I don't get it.'

'It's standard procedure for all molar pregnancies to be sent to the Women's Hospital after they have been tested locally, for further tests and research. You signed a form permitting this to occur.'

I didn't remember signing any such form, or being told anything about this, but that's not surprising. I wasn't in a very receptive state at the time.

'We've tested your tumour, and we need to inform you that it is a double hydatidiform mole. Do you know what that means?'

I didn't, but I could guess. 'I got told that it wasn't cancerous, that I didn't need to have any chemo, that it was benign . . . Are you telling me it's cancerous?'

'I'm afraid so, Constance. I'm very sorry, but you will need to go back to the hospital immediately to talk to the doctors about treatment. Do you have support with you?'

I sat and listened as this woman explained that she'd contact the hospital and my GP, that they'd receive copies of the test results and would manage my treatment from then on. I sat there trying to make sense of it all. First I was diagnosed with a tummy bug, then with a miscarriage, then with a benign molar pregnancy. And then, months later, when I was starting to get it all together again, THIS! I could feel anger brewing, and something else. Disbelief.

CHAPTER 14

HOW DO YOU LIKE THEM APPLES?

For me, some of the most difficult things to deal with in life are the unknown ones. Often when I've asked a doctor for hard and fast information, something that I could hold onto and that (hopefully) might give me comfort, they've come back with vague responses. 'Every cancer is different,' they'd say, 'and every patient responds differently.'

This may be true – I mean, everyone *is* different and everyone *does* experience their cancers in different ways – but sometimes you just want a straight answer. Sometimes you just want your doctor to whip out their textbooks and tell you exactly what it is you want (or don't want) to hear. Something definitive. Something real.

But this cancer was different – I was told from the start that it wasn't life-threatening, it was just something I had to endure, have treatment for and then move on from. That was the plan, but the reality proved much harder. This cancer had come about due to a pregnancy gone wrong, and for that reason alone, it was more of an emotional punch than anything. It hurt, and that hurt wouldn't let up. I had a physical pain in my heart and I felt it every time I saw a pregnant woman, a newborn baby, or a little toddler tottering around. There were constant reminders of my loss everywhere. Not only had I lost my baby, but I had cancer again as a result. 'How do you like them apples?'

Not so much!

I worried about what sort of life mine would be once I recovered. Would my future be completely devoid of children? I had been given the hope that I would one day be able to have kids of my own – fate had dangled this big golden carrot in my face, had let me smell it, taste it and touch it, and then cruelly yanked it away. And, for the final blow, just so I would never forget what I couldn't have, fate had given me another cancer instead.

Mike was worried about me. Dad was worried about me. Hilde and Sam and David and Jonno were worried about me. But I was only worried about one thing, and it wasn't my cancer: *Poke me. Prod me. Take my blood. Give me drugs that make me sick. Just please don't tell me I can't have kids.*

The cancer was excised surgically, and everything was fine for six months. I took my contraception faithfully, as the doctor prescribed, but still the cancer came back. And that meant chemo. Again. This time it was mild and short-lived – just a few months, and my hair didn't even fall out. Medically speaking, it was really no big deal. Mentally, it was devastating.

I allowed myself to get swallowed up in grief. I hated the self-pitying, wallowing, pathetic creature I had become and

I knew I had to pull myself out of it, but it took me a long time to figure out how. Eventually I managed to come out the other side and to shake off the darkness. Not because I was strong. Not because of positive thinking or because I fought valiantly. Quite simply, I got through it all because I endured. I turned up to the hospital and I took my medicine. Through endurance I somehow conquered.

I was 23 years old and I was a survivor. Again.

—

When I'd started at uni I felt full of possibility. I was enjoying my studies and I finally found a job that I was proud of and happy to tell strangers about.

'Hi, I'm Peter and I'm studying to be an architect.'

'Hi, Peter, I'm Constance, and I'm studying Biochem. I work as a pathology clerk, and I also do phlebotomy.' (That's a fancy word for collecting blood.)

'Oh, so you're a vampire, then?'

'Yes. By night, usually.'

For the first time in my life I had stopped worrying that I wasn't good enough. I felt I belonged. I was happy.

That second cancer had changed things again. Dropping out of uni, and the emotion of losing a baby, getting sick again, dealing with doctors' appointments and chemo swept me away from my happy life for a while. But I knew that I wanted to get that life back.

As planes crashed into the twin towers on screens all around the world, Mike sat in the Department of Defence headquarters in Melbourne, waiting for a job interview. He'd finished university and applied for a position in a graduate program. He got the job, and so we moved to Canberra for his first six-month posting.

We went there thinking it would be temporary, that we'd go back to Melbourne or somewhere else in Australia or the wider world after he had finished his grad program. Neither Mike nor I expected to fall in love with the place. We certainly didn't expect to settle in Canberra and make it our home for many years to come, but that's what happened.

Before we left Melbourne our friends and families joked about it and pitied us for having to go and live in what they considered to be a city with absolutely no redeeming features. We didn't argue at the time, but we soon discovered that Canberra was full of culture and history, and for the stage we were at in our lives, the (quiet) nightlife suited us just fine. For someone like me who is fairly feisty and prone to angry outbursts, Canberra was perfect. There was no traffic to make me miserable and no frenetic madness in the air to make me homicidal. Peace descended on me in Canberra and within six months of moving there I knew it would be my home for life.

The move brought other changes as well. Before leaving Melbourne, Mike and I had purchased a book collection from a friend. He sold us about 200 books, all high-quality stuff that we knew we could sell over time because of our experience working in Dad and Hilde's bookshops. We set up an online store and catalogued our books. We didn't even have the cash for a bookcase so we stored them on the floor in boxes, with their spines facing up so we could see all the titles. I applied the sense of order that I had perfected as a child and categorised the books into sections, then alphabetised them by author surname. We uploaded the information to our website and then sat back and anxiously awaited orders. Slowly and steadily they started to come in.

This wasn't enough to keep me busy though, so I started looking for other work. There was only one position for a phlebotomist available in the whole city, so I branched out and looked for something different. I knew I wanted to work with people who were sick or needed a helping hand, but I wasn't a qualified nurse, so when I stumbled across an advertisement for Disability Support, my interest was piqued. After a one-night training session, I found employment looking after people with disabilities in their homes, and it was something I was instantly passionate about.

Working with people, not molecules, was the perfect fit for me. I surprised myself because my patience for adults in ordinary everyday situations was often a bit short, to put it lightly, but I discovered I had all the patience in the world for children and adults with disabilities.

To demonstrate my everyday impatience, I will tell you a tale that I am not proud of – in fact, it makes me cringe just to think about it – but here we go. While living above one of Dad's bookshops, I came to have a string of 'dissatisfactions', shall we call them, with the patrons of a local restaurant who took to parking in our private car park or across the driveway entrance. Now, if someone parks you in so you can't get your car out of your own driveway, clearly you are not going to be happy. When you are on your way to work (I used to work evenings at my pathology job), it is even more frustrating. And when it happens again and again and again? Well, even the most patient person would lose it, right? It was happening almost nightly and I would have to leave twenty minutes earlier than I needed to, just to allow enough time to act like a parking cop and get some stranger to move their car out of my driveway.

I had already called the police several times but they were not willing to move cars that were not parked in a clearway. They would come, if time allowed, and give out a fine but it could take several hours for them to arrive, if they came at all. Understandably, minor traffic infringements weren't a top priority for them. I had put up signs and customarily put big wheelie bins out the front so that people would be less inclined to park there, but it didn't work. There were always people desperate to park within 20 metres of the door of the restaurant at which they were eating.

I'd regularly trudge into the restaurant and ask politely for the owner of the car with XYZ numberplate to please move their car so I could get to work. This caused great inconvenience to the patrons, who didn't want their dining experience interrupted. Or I'd be told I had to wait until their takeaway was ready before they would leave. Now, I ask you, if I was to go and park in front of their driveway so they couldn't get their car out when they wanted to leave their house, would they expect me to move my car, or would they accept it when I told them to settle down and not to get their knickers in a knot?

So, as you can probably tell, I was pissed. And my patience wore thinner and thinner as the weeks and months went by. After about a year, I stopped being polite when I went into the restaurant to request that a car be moved. And then, one night, a man pushed me too far.

On this particular evening I was reciting my usual spiel at each table – 'Excuse me, but does anyone here own the car with XYZ rego?' – when a big man with a puffed-up chest like a very tanned pigeon, sitting at a table of about 20 people, sat up straight and grabbed hold of the table anxiously.

'Have I been hit?' he asked, panicked. 'Has there been an accident? Is my car okay?'

I tried to remain calm. 'No, your car is fine,' I said, 'but it's parked across my driveway and I can't get out. Could you please move it so that I can get to my job?'

He didn't even hesitate. 'Pfft! You stupid bitch, I'll move my car when I'm good and ready. I'm eating!'

And that was it. I picked up the nearest thing and threw it at him across the table while shouting, 'Move your f#$@ing car – NOW!'

Unfortunately, it just so happened that the thing nearest to me that I'd picked up was a handful of cutlery, so subconsciously I had thrown knives at this man across a table. It was not my finest moment and, as I have said, not one that I am proud of. I could have really hurt someone. I could have been charged. I was very lucky that Mike was there to smooth things over for me when I ran into the house screaming, followed by a very angry crowd of young men with big biceps, army buzz cuts and muscle tees.

So, it might seem incongruous that I would then choose a job that requires patience and empathy, but for these children I had it in abundance. They taught me a lot about life, love and family, and a bit of patience was the very least I could give in return.

I started studying Community Services Work at TAFE, applying the knowledge I was learning on the job to my studies and vice versa. I gave up the idea of Medicine because I realised this was where I could really help people; this was a way for me to have a positive impact on people's lives. I enjoyed it so much it hardly felt like work at all. It had taken me a little while, but I had found my happy again.

CHAPTER 15

I BOUGHT A CHURCH!

Mike was doing well in his new job in Canberra and we had come to appreciate just how strong our relationship was. Having moved away from our families and friends, we had only each other to rely on. We spent a lot of our spare time building up our book collection and found that we worked really well together. Mike has a great knowledge of books and a nose for sniffing out a valuable rare item, and I kept our cataloguing systems up to date and looked after the finances. Every time we sold a book, we'd buy more and our collection grew until we had about 10,000 books packed into our little rental house in an inner northern suburb of Canberra.

When Mike got home from work he would process the orders, and enter in the details of any new stock. Then I would come along and package up the orders, ready for posting the next day. I packed every book with care and precision, applying the dedication and perfectionism that you'd expect from a white sheep. First bubble wrap, then a customised cardboard box, styled to fit the book perfectly, then brown-paper wrapping and a neatly lettered address.

Mike is a touch-typist extraordinaire, and he took pride in the listings and descriptions, while I took pride in the packaging and protection of the orders. Together we had it all covered, and our little internet business grew steadily.

As our book collection got bigger it got us thinking that maybe it was time to invest in some more space and buy a house so we could let our collection grow even further. Just about the only thing we didn't like about Canberra was the property prices. We couldn't afford a small two-bedroom apartment, not to mention a house big enough for us and our books. We were definitely ready for nesting but we needed space, and lots of it. We looked around at industrial and commercial properties, but nothing was quite right, or else it was perfect but not in the right price bracket. Then one day, I spied an ad for an old church for sale in Harden. I had never heard of Harden, so I looked on the map and discovered that it was only about 125 kilometres north-west of Canberra.

The next day I was working with Jack, a young boy with multiple disabilities, who just loved to be on the move. His favourite thing in the world was buses and we often rode them all day. Cars weren't quite as exciting but he loved a long drive, so I thought we could go out to this Harden place and have a look at the church for sale. Jack was thrilled – we'd drive there, picnic at the park and then drive back.

It was quicker than I expected to get there, so Jack and I had a stickybeak around town before visiting the church. We went to both playgrounds and had a walk around, wandering down the main street. It certainly wasn't the most picturesque country town, but it definitely had everything you could ever need. Finally we pulled up alongside the old church, which was perched above the town on a small hill. From the outside it looked quite dilapidated. The front half was all peeling white paint, while the back half was red brick, but I have a pretty good imagination; I pictured it painted a soft cream colour, with heritage-green trimmings, and stained glass in all of the eighteen arched windows. I immediately saw the potential, and I hadn't even stepped inside.

The real estate agent, Bob, was waiting and he let me in through the heavy front door with a long iron key that must have been the original from the 1890s, when the church was first built. Measuring over 15 centimetres long, it looked like the kind of key that could open a drawbridge on a moat, or a royal castle. It was solid, unbreakable and proud. I wanted that key and all it stood for. I wanted to be able to open that door time and again, and walk into this church, into a room full of books and I wanted to create a warm and welcoming home for Mike and me.

The building was made up of two large rooms: the front room where the services would have been held, and the back room, which would have been used for Sunday school and community gatherings. At the very back of the building was another smaller room with a boiler in the corner. It had leaked over time, and the floor there was rotted through. It was clear that a pony has taken up residence in the church. It had most probably pushed its way through one of the doors at the back and sought refuge from the elements there. I could tell this because the floor was littered with horse manure. Quite a grand little stable, really.

There was no kitchen, no bathroom and no bedrooms. But it had loads of charm. And electricity, space, charm . . . Plus, it was cheap, about a sixth of what we'd pay for something the same size in Canberra. And did I mention the charm? I was besotted, and before I knew what had happened, I'd put in an offer.

Driving home, Jack was happy staring out the window, watching the world go by, hoping to see a bus, and I spent the trip thinking about what I'd just done. Who buys an old church in the country without their partner even seeing it? Umm, ME! What had I done?

Mike had spent the day at a book fair in the Southern Highlands with his parents, and they were all at home when I got back. He had bought heaps of boxes of books at the fair and was eager to show them to me. His parents thought we were a bit crazy, buying so many books and cluttering up our house with stock for our online bookshop when Mike had a perfectly good job in the public service. But they accepted it and were never critical . . . but they didn't know I'd just bought a church!

I tried to get Mike's attention without his parents noticing but that wasn't to be, so I finally came out with it. 'Hey, Mike, you know how I went to see that old church in the country today?'

'Yes,' he replied, still leafing through his new purchases, distracted.

The words spilled out in a rush. 'Well, I might have made an offer on it. Actually, I did make an offer on it . . . but it is huge, and has real potential.'

'Potential, hey?' Mike's dad, Ray, said. 'Famous last words. Sounds like a money pit.'

I was about to retort when Chris, Mike's mum, piped up with, 'I'm sure Connie wouldn't buy a place that didn't suit them. An old church . . . I like the sound of it!'

Thank god for Chris, she always fixed everything.

'Well, I need to see it before we buy it,' Mike stated, reasonably.

So I called Bob the real estate agent and we all set off back up the road to Harden. I spent the whole drive hoping they were going to like the place as much as I did (and praying the pony hadn't come home!).

When we reached the church there was a collective sigh of relief. Mike and his mum liked the look of it. His dad kept mumbling things about money pits but I blocked out his negative comments and started planning where we would put the kitchen, the bathroom and the bedrooms. Chris shared the vision that I had for the place. Mike was partly charmed and partly sceptical but he went with me. It was three against one. Mike's dad stopped mumbling.

Mike and I spent the next few months renovating to get the place ready for our wedding. We'd decided that there was no better place to get married than in our very own church. I think renovators always underestimate the amount of work there is to be done and we were no different. We had to completely rewire and lay new pipes for the plumbing. It seemed as though everything needed to be done from scratch and we did as much of the work as we could ourselves. We took pride in every brick we painted, every wall we rendered and every paver we put into place, but it was exhausting and we only finished the renovations of the hall part, where the bookshop would eventually be, on the morning of our wedding. Our cousin arrived to install the lights just hours before the guests arrived. Luckily for me, I wasn't there to watch that part – I was in Canberra with my bridesmaids, having a full-blown panic attack.

I wanted to marry Mike, I was certain of that, but I wanted everything to be just right and the thought of having all those people there and something going wrong almost defeated me. Despite the best efforts of Em and my other friends, I was paralysed with nerves and I didn't manage to get out the door until about ten minutes before the service was supposed to start. We had to phone ahead and tell the groomsman to start serving the alcohol early, as the bride was going to be about an hour late! Poor Mike, he must have thought I was getting cold feet.

Eventually I arrived and everyone was a little lubricated so the mood was happy. I had no reason to be anxious, everything went just as we planned, and the chandeliers our cousin installed were perfect, hanging high from the beams, six metres up in our church. The chairs were arranged like in a real church, and walking down the aisle I noticed all the smiling faces, but I also noticed that the rendering we did on the walls and the repairs we did to the arched windows were just perfect.

In the lead-up to the wedding I'd spoken to Sam about how important my wedding day was to me. I stressed that I didn't want any dodginess marking the special event and he had taken that on board and vowed that he would stay sober until the ceremony was over. That meant a lot. I'd been worried about Sam but he was doing his own thing and had shut himself off from me. I'd been equally stubborn and hadn't reached out. I thought maybe the wedding day would be a turning point. I really hoped so. I gave Sam the job of coordinating the music. He took his job very seriously and promised that he would make me proud.

Many of my friends hadn't met Sam before the wedding, and now that he had been on *The Secret Life of Us*, he was practically a household name, or face and voice at least, so some of my friends were very excited about meeting him, and others, who had heard me whingeing about his fame, were nervous. They didn't want to make a big deal out of him and annoy me. Sam took it all in his stride and was absolutely free with his time, happy in his nature and charming to all of our guests. He was the Sam I'd known as a kid, not the Sam who had been so badly affected by fame that he'd started distrusting people. It made me happy to see my brother like this.

Dad was just so proud. His speech, though a little embarrassing (which is almost obligatory at a wedding anyway, isn't it?) was touching and insightful. The whole room hung on his every word and they all got a glimpse of the father I loved. So many people came up and talked to me about Dad that night, telling me how gentle and charming he was, how caring and special, how intelligent and accepting. In one speech, Dad conveyed to a whole room of people the sort of father he was.

I'd always believed that getting married didn't change the permanence of a relationship, that you could be just as committed to someone and not get married, but that belief changed after I said my vows. I suddenly felt there was an extra level of commitment that I hadn't recognised before.

I BOUGHT A CHURCH!

I was glad that I had dedicated my life to Mike, and that he had dedicated his to me. It made me feel good. It felt right. We said, 'in sickness and in health', we said, 'until death do us part', but we wouldn't truly appreciate the weight of those words until six years later. Blissfully, we had no idea what lay ahead.

CHAPTER 16

BUILDING A LIFE

After the wedding, Mike and I still had a lot of work to do on the church. We'd renovated the hall, which would later become the bookshop, but the house part out the back left a lot to be desired. What would become the lounge room and bedrooms was one big room and that had to change if we were going to live there and start a family (and that was definitely on my list!). We cleared the garden of the chest-high weeds and put in plants. Slowly but surely we were creating a home and I wanted to share it with my family.

On Christmas Day 2005 we all came together in our little church in Harden for a family celebration. That day was everything I had always thought family Christmases should be. Dad, Hilde and Jonno came with Sully and Aussy (Hilde's kids from her second marriage). Sam came with his partner, Lainie, and our half-brother David came down from Queensland. The whole family was there, all in one place at one time. This hadn't happened before. Not since we were kids.

I made handmade Christmas crackers with Sully and Aussy out of Glad Wrap rolls and wrapping paper. We put little chocolates that we'd made inside and got a pack of crackers so they still went bang when you pulled them apart. I cooked a massive roast lunch and we all sat at a long table at the back of the bookshop to eat.

After lunch we all played board games. Dad and Mike played chess, while Lainie sat on the couch trying to beat her previous high score on Simon (an eighties electronic game). She had never played it, and she was now well and truly hooked. Then of course the Trivial Pursuit came out and Dad and Hilde thrashed us all, showing us up to be not as smart as we liked to think we were. But Pictionary was the highlight. We all rolled around the room laughing at Dad's rendition of half a gee-gee with four flies hovering around the horse's rear end. No one was ever going to guess that the word he was trying to draw was 'forge'.

Everything was perfect . . . until it turned sour as we were saying goodbye. I made the mistake of asking Sam for some money he had borrowed. His mistrust of people bled into the family arena, and I instantly became one of the many people asking him for money, help, or a ticket to stardom. It wasn't good and it would take a while for us to fix it and find our way back to each other.

I didn't dwell on missing Sam. I was busy working in the church building bookcases, designing and renovating the house and tending to the garden. Mike was working fulltime in Canberra in his public service job. We spent a lot of time apart. I would go to Canberra on the weekends to work my disability job, so we were never in the same place at the same time. We were too busy to think about starting a family for a while. But one night, a few months before that family Christmas, we sat down on the couch in our little house at the back of the bookshop, which was now open five days a week and doing a good little trade, and I said, 'I think I'm ready, I want to try again'. If we could actually fall pregnant all those years ago, surely we could do it again. I didn't want to push Mike into such a big decision but, as always, he was right there with me. He was ready too.

I had been on strong contraception since the molar pregnancy and it took some time until things got back to normal but within three months of getting my cycle back, I was late. Could it be that easy? Three months? I didn't dare to hope, but I could think of nothing else. I finally went to the doctor. Yes, I was pregnant. This time, upon having an early scan we discovered that there was a nice little regular round-shaped sac with a little heartbeat in there. We were going to have a baby.

Things were good and I was hopeful that it would all be okay. I wasn't really thinking about anyone else at the time. I was in my Harden bubble. Then, when I was 13 weeks pregnant, I got a phone call from Dad.

'Con, are you sitting down? Is Mike with you?'

A sense of foreboding hung heavily on the phone line and I was scared.

'I don't want you to get too upset and for anything to happen to the baby, but you have to know before you hear it on the radio.'

'For crying out loud, Dad, what is going on? Is everyone alright?'

'It's Lainie,' Dad said. 'She's gone. She's taken her own life.'

I was sitting on the edge of my bed, and I collapsed back and started to sob.

Poor Sam. First Mum, now Lainie. I wanted to be with him. All my anger fell away and I sobbed for him. I sobbed for his loss. For his heartache.

Dad told me that he wanted me to stay in Harden and look after myself. He assured me that he and Hilde would look after Sam, and that all I had to do was stay home and look after the baby growing inside me.

I felt so far away.

I hung up and the pain started shortly after. Then the bleeding started. I rang Mike at work and asked him to come home. By the time he got to Harden I had already been transferred by ambulance to Wagga Hospital. That three-hour drive must have felt like forever for him.

There was nothing we could do but wait and hope. I rang Dad and I could hardly talk between gasping for air between sobs. 'Dad, I'm miscarrying, I'm losing the baby.'

Dad stayed with Sam and he knew that Mike would look after me. He told me to 'just hang in there'.

Just. Hang. In. There.

The baby was listening! Slowly, the bleeding subsided and eventually Mike was able to take me home. I stayed in bed for days and crossed my fingers. No more bleeding. Please, no more bleeding.

The hardest thing was I couldn't be there for Sam. I never even saw him while he was dealing with one of the hardest experiences of his life. I couldn't go to Lainie's service because I couldn't fly, and I didn't want to risk a long drive either. It was safer for me to stay put and I prayed that this baby would hang in there and that Sam would be okay. I had to try to control my anxiety about everything and focus all my energy on carrying this baby.

Days turned into weeks and gradually I started to believe that just maybe I could carry this baby to full term. I was 32 weeks when my waters broke. Mike was at work. I convinced myself that I had just wet my pants, that the baby was putting pressure on my bladder. I called Em and told her what had happened, hoping she'd laugh too. She didn't. She told me she was booking a flight right then and called my next-door neighbour and asked her to drive me to Canberra Hospital straight away. Em knew this was not good.

I was well and truly in labour by the time I got to Canberra and I had to come to terms very quickly with the fact that I was having a premature baby. I was terrified. The doctors and nurses explained that when the baby was born they might need breathing apparatus to keep the child alive. Mike and I already knew we were having a boy and I was in shock as I listened to someone tell me that he would not be born ready to feed, but that he had a very good chance of survival with medical intervention. The medical team managed to delay the birth by about 24 hours, to allow the steroids they were giving me to take effect on his little lungs, and get him ready to try to breathe on his own when he was born. We were very lucky; at 32 weeks he at least had a chance.

It was a difficult labour, and he was the wrong way around, so forceps were needed because he went into distress. Then I saw him, a little purple bundle of skin and bones. They put him straight into a humidicrib and raced him off to the neonatal intensive care unit (NICU). I knew I wouldn't get to hold him when he was born, but it was still a shock to me when they whisked him away. It was all so medical and dramatic. I was really scared.

Our boy was breathing on his own and he didn't end up needing machines to keep him alive. For a premmie, he was quite big and strong. We named him Willoughby and as soon as I was well enough, and they had stabilised him, I was allowed to go and see him in the NICU. I couldn't believe how perfect he was, and was completely overwhelmed by how much love I felt for someone I had only just met. He was perfect in every way and my mind filled with all the promise of his future.

A midwife came along and 'milked' me, explaining that every drop of my milk was precious; it was good for the baby and gave him a better chance. After that, I became obsessed with expressing milk and became a little dairy cow. I measured every millilitre I expressed but was hard on myself for not producing much. I thought I would kill Willoughby by not producing enough milk to put through the nasal gastric tube.

Willoughby showed himself to be a real trooper, and he grew bigger and stronger every day. Within two weeks he was out of intensive care, and four weeks later we were taking him home – a fortnight before his due date.

For my family, struggling to deal with the sadness of Lainie's death and worrying about Sam, Willoughby's homecoming was a much-needed moment of joy. And for me, I was now the mother I'd always wanted to be.

CHAPTER 17

THE JOHNSON FAMILY ROLLERCOASTER

Looking back on my family life, it seems that we were never all happy or healthy at the same time. When I finally looked like I'd put cancer behind me, Sam was battling his own demons. But with Willoughby's birth I was hoping things would settle down, for all of us.

Mike and I had always wanted to have more than one baby, and we wanted to have them close together. Sam and I were born 13 months apart; Hilde's youngest kids, Sully and Aussy, were 11 months apart. The relationship Sam and I had as kids was really special and I could see how close Sully and Aussy were. I hoped for something similar for Willoughby, so Mike and I started trying for another child almost straight away.

Before we even realised just how hard it is with a newborn, we found out that we were expecting our second. I couldn't believe our luck! I felt very fortunate and was very excited for Willoughby that he'd have a little brother or sister so close in age to him. But then anxiety kicked in and I started to worry that I might not be able to love the new baby as much as I loved Willoughby. That I'd favour Willoughby to the detriment of this new baby. I couldn't comprehend how I could find enough space in my heart to love the new baby as much as I loved Willow and became quite anxious about it. I tried not to let it show and concentrated on looking after Willoughby and myself and just hoped it would be okay. Mike was still working in Canberra but he also had to travel a lot so Willoughby and I were our own little team.

I was doing well, had our routine down and my anxiety mostly in check but at 23 weeks I knew something was wrong, I started having contractions. I told myself they were probably Braxton Hicks (contractions that can occur throughout a pregnancy that don't signal labour). Or that I was imagining it. But they got worse and worse, stronger and stronger, and closer and closer together so Chris took me to the hospital. I was examined and told I had an 'incompetent cervix', which explained why Willoughby was born premmie, and now it seemed this little baby wanted to come early too. But 23 weeks was far too early for a baby to be born and have any decent chance of survival. The doctors explained everything but I refused to accept their grim outlook.

Mike was in Perth for work and he couldn't get a flight out. I so wanted him to be there with me as I struggled to take it all in. Chris was there and did a great job of looking after me and Willoughby. The NICU doctors were really good and explained everything to me as they gave me drugs to try to stop the labour. They told me I was in a grey area because before 22 weeks they don't resuscitate and after 24 weeks they do everything they can to keep an infant alive. But between 22 and 24 weeks there was no real legislation so I had to make a decision about whether or not I wanted the team to work on the baby when he was born.

From my work in the disability sector, I have had a glimpse into what it's like to raise a child with disabilities and the impact it has on families. I also know and value so many people who live their lives with a disability. There was no way I could make this decision so I just hoped to God I wouldn't have to. I prayed that my labour would stop. And, luckily for me, it seemed that someone was listening.

Through some stroke of luck, some miracle, or effective medical intervention, the labour did stop. I spent the rest of the pregnancy on my back, not allowed to roll onto my side, but I was allowed to get up to go to the toilet and shower. Mike still had to work so we had a roster of people coming up from Melbourne to help. Hilde, Dad, Em and Chris (Nanna) all took turns looking after Wib, but Nanna was there the most and they forged a strong bond. Em made me a big, bright incubation chart and Mike and I crossed off every day as a huge milestone. The first aim was to get our baby to 28 weeks, then to 30, then to 32 weeks, then 36. We had some more close calls but the doctors managed to stave off seven threatened labours and I managed to 'cook' our baby to near-term. I was sent home at thirty-six weeks with the words that 'if he is born now he will be a normal-term baby' ringing in my ears. Em came to stay with us and we just waited.

At 39 weeks I felt the contractions again, and this time we could let it happen. Willoughby's brother, Hamilton, was born an hour later – just two minutes after the ambulance arrived at the hospital. I was shocked by the speed of the delivery and, although it wasn't easy, he was big, strong and healthy and that was all that mattered. Mike didn't even have time to get home from work before he was born, but Em was there and she talked me through the contractions and held my hand. When Mike walked in an hour and a half later, I was sitting in bed nursing our new baby boy. My fears of not being able to love Hamilton were assuaged the minute I held him, the minute I saw his little hands and feet, his little nose and tiny little frown. My heart had expanded and I found I could love Hamilton just as much as I loved Willoughby, and there was still plenty of room in there for Mike and all of my friends and family. The heart is an amazing thing!

—

Just after Hamilton was born we heard a whisper on the bookshop grapevine that a successful Canberra bookshop was going on the market. We saw this as an opportunity to really make a go of the bookshop thing, and hoped that Mike might be able to leave the public service and stop commuting. We loved the idea of actually being able to pull a fulltime wage and to devote our time to what we love. It was a romantic notion and we were sucked into the idea before we even knew if the rumour was true.

Mike wanted this, but Mike doesn't ask questions unless he knows the answer. Because we didn't know the answer, he was reluctant to do anything. Me, on the other hand, I love risk, I love excitement. I love the thrill of the chase.

So I chased. I picked up the phone, called the bookshop and introduced myself. All I had to say was that I was Joe Johnson's daughter. Dad had been a writer for 20 years, a book collector for 30 years and a book dealer for just as long. Anyone who knew books knew Dad. It turned out the owners were willing to entertain the thought of selling, so we talked numbers, we talked books and we made a time to meet. The deal was exciting and it had the potential to transform our lives, but in the end it didn't go ahead.

Then, as they say in the classics, when one door closes, another one opens and we heard of another shop owner in Canberra who was thinking of selling. Before we knew it we had bought their business. What were we thinking? We had one shop in Harden, a shop in Canberra, and two kids under two. Suffice to say, we had a lot on our plate. We moved into a rental in Canberra and used all the space in the church for the bookshop.

Dad, being the ever-generous soul that he is, realised we could use a little help, and after a little to-ing and fro-ing, he packed up and left Melbourne and came to live with us. He helped us with the shops and the kids, both of which he had extensive experience with. I was thrilled to have his company. He planned to stay for a year, and we made the most of every minute of that time. Dad was a doting grandfather and it melted my heart to see glimpses of what he would have been like when Sam and I were babies. Willoughby quickly became the apple of his eye.

Willoughby would wake in the morning, put on my slippers, then shuffle out to the granny flat where Dad lived and knock on his door. They had a ritual; Willoughby helped Dad toast the crumpets, then they'd sit down together and eat them. They were a tandem team and watching them go through their morning routine was a pure delight. Dad talked to Willoughby throughout the whole process and Willoughby made noises that were starting to sound like words, with an earnest expression and an expectation that Dad could understand him. After breakfast, Dad and Mike would head off to the shops, while I stayed home with the kids. By this point I had given up on working in the shop with two young kids, and we had employed staff to work fulltime at the church. Dad and Mike worked the Canberra shop, heading to Harden once a week to restock and check up on everything.

I ran our house like a well-oiled machine. The kids had a routine and they went to bed the second I saw a sign of them being tired, then I spent their nap times cleaning and getting ready for the next activity. We passed the days with train sets, balls in a sandpit, a vegie garden – which the kids loved to water – painting, trips to the playground, a swing on the back verandah and numerous puzzles and books. There was never a dull moment.

Then, after closing up, Mike and Dad would come home and we'd all have dinner together. Mike and Dad often had a beer together after dinner, and I soon realised that they didn't need me to hold them together, they had become friends in their own right. Dad and Mike shared a powerful intellect and a thirst for knowledge. They made quite a formidable pair. Dad took Mike under his wing and their passionate search for knowledge meant every conversation had spark. Dad had long before mastered the art of conversation, and I never met anybody who didn't enjoy a chat with him.

I loved having Dad around. We talked a lot and just when I thought I knew everything about him he'd surprise me with a comment or an anecdote and I'd think, 'Why didn't I know that?' And he was always there to give me a hand. One day I was painting the exterior of the church. It's a huge building and hence a huge job. Dad was standing at the bottom of the ladder handing me brushes or caulking guns or filling up my paint bucket. He started to tell me something and I couldn't get my head around it at first.

'So, I found your brother,' he said.

'Sam?' I laughed. 'I didn't know he was missing?'

'No, not Sam!'

'Dave? He wasn't missing either last time I checked!'

'No, not Dave! Richard. Your older brother.'

I nearly fell off the ladder. I clambered down and started firing questions at him.

'My older brother? Is this the brother from England? From before you married Mum?'

'One and the same, Con. Yes, that's him.'

Dad had told me the story when I was 19. At the time I'd been getting ready to go to England to do the backpacking thing. I intended to go for two years, work over there and travel around Europe, but I got depressed, spent all my money and came home three months later with my tail firmly between my legs.

Just before I flew off, Dad had sat me down and explained that I had an older brother, Richard, who he'd never told me about. He'd wanted to wait until I was old enough but he never found the right time. I was shocked. For some reason Dad and his pregnant girlfriend couldn't be together. I still don't know all the details but I think it had something to do with her family. Dad had left England shortly after Richard was born. Dad thought I might like to track down my brother while I was in the UK but I was too focused on myself to worry about finding a long lost brother and I hadn't really thought about it since.

'So, how did you find him?' I asked.

'I put it in The Google.'

Dad had only recently discovered the joys of the internet, and I found it endearing that he put 'The' in front of everything to do with searching the web.

He told me he'd entered in everything he knew about Richard, which wasn't much, and went from there. First he tried searching for him under the surname he was born under, his first name and his date of birth. Richard was born on 29 February in a leap year, a memorable date. Nothing came up, so he widened the search by adding the surnames of Richard's mother's parents, Binden and Bore.

What came up was interesting. He found that a book had been published by a Richard Selesnick, that had contained fictional characters named Binden and Bore. Could this be him? Could he be a writer like Dad? It seemed too much of a coincidence for him not to explore it further. He had the same first name, and had named some characters after his grandparents. The next step was to find the author's date of birth. After much work using 'The Google', Dad established that the author, Richard Selesnick, had the same date of birth as his son. Dad had found him.

Richard no longer lived in England but had moved to New York. He had published a few unusual books and Dad immediately ordered all of them. They were rare and expensive, which added to his excitement. He anxiously awaited their arrival, and he wasn't disappointed when they turned up.

The next step was to seek out Richard and see if he wanted to be found. Dad and Em contacted Richard's publisher and left a cryptic message: 'Does the name Joseph Johnson mean anything to you?'

Would Richard know about his father? Would he even know that Dad existed? Had he been brought up in another family with a stepfather, never knowing that he wasn't his biological father? If he did know about Dad, might he hate him? Might he resent him for not being there? There were so many questions. It was exciting and I wanted to know more. I had fantasies about going to New York to meet him, or him coming out to Australia to meet us. To discover another family member when you are a grown adult is an extraordinary thing. I could understand if he wanted nothing to do with us, but hoped that he would know about Dad, embrace the opportunity to get to know him, and become a part of our family.

An email arrived saying, yes, the name Joseph Johnson did mean something to him. He had grown up with his mother, who had then married and they had become Selesnicks. Richard was brought up by his stepfather, but had been told at a young age that he was not his biological father. He knew who Dad was and he wanted to know more.

They began their relationship by correspondence and Dad was thrilled to find out about him and get to know him slowly over the next few months. We all loved the thought of having a new brother, and entertained the possibility of travelling overseas to meet him. But we knew that this must be very confronting for Richard and that we couldn't push ourselves on him. We would leave the ball in his court and leave it up to him if he wanted to get to know us.

Eleven months passed happily and Mike and I were really hoping that Dad would stay. He'd left Hilde to run their bookshops in Melbourne and he seemed to have settled into Canberra and loved being with the kids. But he had a lifetime of friends back in Melbourne and Hilde and Sam were there along with his other grandchildren, so it was hard for Dad to choose between the two cities. It wasn't going to be a decision he'd make lightly.

We all headed off to Melbourne for a family visit to Hilde's in two different cars. It was the first time we'd all been together since that Christmas before Willoughby was born. Sam was there with his new love, Sarah. Dad and Sam had had some troubles, and Sam and I still had some tension between us. We didn't call each other often and I had no clue what he was up to. I loved my brother but I wasn't going to chase after him – he would've hated that. Things hadn't been smooth sailing for the previous few years but there was a lot of love in that room that day, and a lot of forgiveness. Maybe things were coming good for all of us?

Dad was coughing a lot, but we were used to that; he'd had weak lungs for as long as I could remember. At one point, Hilde pulled me aside and asked if Dad had been sick lately. I shrugged off Hilde's concerns, thinking it was just a bit of a cold. I'd seen Dad moving boxes and running after the boys the day before and he'd seemed fine.

The next day Dad started the drive back to Canberra. I was staying in Melbourne with the kids for a bit longer. We waved goodbye to him and I thought nothing more about it. It was lovely to spend time with Hilde and we talked and caught up. We took the kids to the zoo. It was hilarious because Willoughby dropped his drinking cup near the fence of the elephant enclosure. An elephant stuck his trunk through the fence, scooped up the drink bottle and somehow unscrewed the cap, then held the cup up and drank the water. Willoughby and I watched on, wide-eyed. I was amazed and only dimly aware that Hilde was on the phone in the background.

It was Dad. He'd taken himself to hospital because he couldn't stop coughing. I was calm and told Hilde it had to be a chest infection and that they'd give him an antibiotic and he'd be fine. In my mind, there was no way Dad was really sick. It was an idea I couldn't even bring myself to entertain.

CHAPTER 18

THINGS FALL APART

When we got back to Canberra and visited Dad in the hospital, I wasn't prepared to see him looking so bad. His face was grey and he was slumped in bed when I walked in with the double-decker pram. His eyes lit up and he sat up straighter as soon as he saw the boys. I didn't know if he was genuinely feeling better at the sight of them, or if he just didn't want them to see him in this state. I popped Willoughby up on the bed with Dad, and he fumbled around, trying to pull at the oxygen tube around Dad's ears that threaded to nasal prongs. Dad explained to Willoughby that it was helping him breathe and making him better. Then Dad asked Willoughby if he wanted to go for a walk. I walked behind them with Hammy in the pram, giving the two friends time together. They were silhouetted against the window at the end of the ward corridor, an elderly gent with a two-year-old by his side. Willoughby took the handle of the oxygen trolley off Dad, and he wheeled it at his own pace like it was the most important job in the world. Dad walked slowly next to him. They held hands and talked as they walked.

Dad was tired when we got back to his room, but he had enjoyed strolling with his 'little man' by his side. Quietly, Dad told me that if he was to make it home, with oxygen he might get another 18 months or two years. He had pneumonia and it was clear that his lungs were irreparably damaged. I was shocked. He was too young, too vibrant and too healthy to be thinking that. He really believed that he could die and that the best possible outcome was to live another two years dragging an oxygen bottle around behind him. He must have seen the look on my face because he joked that at least he had a little helper to wheel the bottle around for him. I watched him ruffle Willoughby's hair and tried not to cry.

I couldn't take it in and so I called Hilde while Dad kept up his chat with Willow. I told Hilde what Dad had said and she told me she was flying up immediately. Dad worked out what was going on and grabbed the phone off me. He told Hilde that he was fine and that she needed to stay in Melbourne to look after the shops. He promised her that he would call if things got too bad. Hilde reluctantly agreed to stay in Melbourne. Dad hung up and I pulled out some photos of the kids from my bag. They were of them watering the vegie patch in the nudie. The light filtered through the leaves like the fingers of God reaching down from the sky. There was also a picture of the zucchinis that Dad had planted with Willoughby from seed only a few months earlier.

Willoughby grabbed the photos and showed them to his grandpa. Dad made encouraging noises about the vegie patch and asked simple questions that he knew Willoughby could answer. They cuddled up on the bed while I held Hammy up to show him the Telstra tower on Black Mountain that was visible from Dad's window. Hamilton was more interested in the cars coming and going in the car park below. I still refused to accept that Dad was seriously ill.

I'd booked tickets to take the boys to a show for kids at the Canberra Theatre so told Dad I had to head off. I had tears in my eyes as I left because Dad told me as I walked out of his room that I was every bit as good a mother as he ever imagined I would be. My chest swelled with pride as I left the hospital. His praise meant the world to me. I couldn't wait to get him home again.

I was slightly worried about Dad, but I firmly believed that he would be fine, and that he was just seeing the glass as half empty. The next morning I was woken by a phone call.

It was Dad. There was no hello, no niceties, just, 'I need you to put something in The Google, right now. What does it mean when your fingernails turn black?'

My heart sank as I jumped into action. I fumbled at the computer trying to get online. Why does it always seem to take so bloody long? 'I'll look it up and call you back, Dad. Don't panic. Call the nurse and get some help. I'll come straight in.'

'Don't come in, Con, just look it up and call me back. The nurse is here. I have to go.' He hung up.

I ran around packing some nappies, food and bottles into a bag while the internet connected, then I woke the kids and was just getting them strapped into the car when my mobile rang. It was Hilde.

Again, no hello, no niceties, straight to the point. 'Dad

told me to come straight away with the folder,' she said. '*The folder. Shit, Con, he's dying.*'

—

When we got to Dad's room there was an alarm going off, and heaps of people crowded around him. I felt like I had dropped into a scene in a medical emergency show. I heard snippets of conversations: 'oxygen low . . . heart-rate high . . . respiratory arrest'.

As soon as I was noticed I was ushered out of the room. I stood and watched as the whole emergency team continued to work on him as he was rolled towards the lift. Dad saw me and said, 'Take the boys away, Con. Take them away. They don't need to see this.' He reached his arm out to me as the lift door closed on him and he disappeared from view.

A nurse took hold of my hand and led me to a couch and Mike took the boys away.

'Your father is a very sick man,' the nurse said. She explained that Dad had been taken to ICU and that they were going to try to keep him alive, but my brain wasn't taking it all in. I just kept hearing that same phrase over and over again: 'Your father is a very sick man.'

The nurse left me to check on how Dad was going and I started making phone calls to let the family know what was going on. I called Sam, then I called my Aunty Marg and Uncle George. Dad was the youngest of nine children, and George is the next youngest. Their mum died shortly after giving birth to Dad, so George and Dad were brought up by other family members and the other seven children stayed with their dad. George was really close to Dad, and Marg was like a sister to him, and had been his biggest supporter for many years. When I was young I spent weeks at a time with Aunty Marg after Mum died, and she was like a mum to me. I knew she would know what to do.

I called my brother Dave and told him that he should get here as quickly as he could. I didn't know whether to call Richard in New York or not. He was so far away. I decided to wait until I knew more. When I'd finished and knew everyone was on their way, all I could do was wait and hope. I sat on the other side of a very big door, unable to go in to Dad, unable to do anything. The wait was interminable and the helplessness I felt was crushing.

—

I don't know how long I sat there. Every second felt like a minute, every minute like an hour. I sat and watched the clock tick, staring at the doors wanting them to open but terrified at what could happen when they did. Every time a nurse walked out of the doors I stood in expectation, only to have her walk past and address another anxious family, or wheel another patient in or out.

Hilde eventually arrived and it felt like days had passed but it had only been seven hours. We still weren't allowed to go in. Hilde was angry with me for calling the family. When Dad spoke to her he'd asked her not to call anyone. He didn't want to make a fuss. I understood that Hilde was following Dad's orders, but to my mind I had done the right thing. They had a right to say goodbye and I was only fearful that they wouldn't make it in time.

Finally a doctor and nurse approached us.

'Your father is very unwell,' the doctor explained. 'We've had to resuscitate him, and he's now on a mask to help him breathe. He is a very sick man.' That phrase again. 'He has a lot of tubes and wires attached to him and it might look very scary when you see him, but he is awake and he can talk to you briefly. It is important that you don't wear him out. We are going to put him into what is called a medically induced coma so that his body can have a rest while we fight the infection for him, and then we will wake him up in a few days once he has regained his strength and has had some time to recover. Eighty-five per cent of people who come into ICU go back to the ward. We're just keeping him here as a precaution and to give him the best chance of recovery. His lungs aren't strong, and he needs some pretty serious help to recover from this, but he should be okay.'

I almost collapsed with relief. I had heard what I needed: he'd be okay. I started to follow Hilde through the doors and I was shocked that she pulled the folder out of her bag. We didn't need that anymore, hadn't she heard the doctor? Dad was going to be fine.

Dad was on the bed looking pale and a little fragile but he was sitting up. His whole face was covered in a plastic mask, and a machine by his bed was breathing for him. He still seemed himself, and his fingernails were a normal pinky-white colour once again. He and Hilde started talking about final wishes, changes to his will, and funeral arrangements straight away. I was horrified.

'Dad, they said they're going to put you in an induced coma so that you can recover more easily. You're going to be fine. We don't need to talk about any of this.'

Dad smiled at me and patted my hand, which was gripping

the bedrail so tight my knuckles had turned white. 'Just in case, Con, just in case.'

There were two nurses by Dad's bedside at all times, constantly reading the machines, and writing down numbers on charts.

Dad and Hilde kept talking, and he signed some cheques and some other paperwork. His signature was wobbly and not even recognisable as his usual elegant, cursive handwriting. But he was still talking and smiling normally. He seemed calm, as always, and I knew he was going to be okay. I felt like I could breathe again. It was scary but he would get better.

'Sorry to interrupt, but we have to intubate your dad now, so you have to go. You'll see him again when we wake him up in a few days,' one of the nurses said.

We had only been with Dad for about 15 minutes so I was shocked we had to go so soon. Dad was still looking okay and if it wasn't for the beeping machines and the hovering nurses I could have fooled myself into thinking that he just had a cold. It was hard to say goodbye but I wasn't really worried. I knew he'd be okay. Dad gave us a wan smile as he waved goodbye. We walked back out through those doors and I turned to see him one more time but the doors had slammed shut.

—

Sam, Dave, Aunty Marg and Uncle George all started arriving at the hospital but they weren't allowed in to see Dad so we all went back to my house for a bit while the doctors and nurses did what they needed to do. Aunty Marg made sandwiches for everyone and we all sat around talking. It felt painfully real and acutely distressing but, at the same time, I felt like I was watching us all from up above. It was surreal.

We hugged. We cried. We talked. Willoughby toddled around and Hammy crawled around our legs. We took turns reading them stories: *Hairy Maclary* and Dr Seuss to keep them entertained but also to remind ourselves that life goes on. Willoughby patted me on the back while I cried and then walked off to get the tissues. He was looking after his mum. I wondered how much he understood. After a while he wandered off and resumed his work with his Thomas the Tank Engine tracks.

The next day we all went to the hospital and took turns sitting with Dad. It was confronting to see him lying there in a coma, with a tube down his throat and wires and drips connected to every part of him. I didn't know if he could hear me but I liked to think he could so I talked. Dad had recently told me that he loved listening to me read to the boys, introducing them to the wide world of fiction and fantasy, facts and stats that books open up to people, so I recited children's poetry to Dad, trying to remember all the lines.

Em was back in Melbourne looking after the shops so that Hilde could stay in Canberra. I knew she'd be hurting. I called her and asked if she wanted to talk to Dad. I held the phone to his ear and gave her the chance to speak to him. His oxygen saturation went up a peg and I saw his hand move. He was listening. He could hear us. I was sure of it. Dad would have been worrying about the shops and to know Em was there keeping things running would have been a comfort to him.

After I hung up, I sat and told Dad he was going to get better. 'You are going to come home with us. I will look after you, Willoughby will push your oxygen bottle around for you and it will all be okay.'

He was unresponsive and looked so still. The machines kept beeping.

I told Dad how much I loved him, that he was my hero and my mentor and my best friend. I asked him to hang in there.

Shhhhhh, Shhhhhh, Shhhhhhh, the machine kept breathing for him.

I think he squeezed my hand, but I wasn't sure if I was imagining it. Hoping. I really wanted to support him and tell him that I would be okay if he needed to let go. But I couldn't, I wouldn't be okay. Nothing would be okay. This wasn't okay.

'I love you, Dad. You have been the best dad in the world. There is nothing you didn't do for us. You have brought us up well. I love you, Dad.'

His oxygen kept dropping, the machines kept breathing for him and his heart rate kept rising.

—

The helplessness felt like it was eating me alive. The nurses explained that he was not recovering the way they had hoped. We were told to prepare ourselves for the worst. They explained that if he improved, he would still be compromised because he'd had such a long period of time with insufficient oxygen getting to his brain. I didn't care. As long as we could keep him. I would look after him. Just don't tell me this is goodbye. *Prepare yourself, Con. Prepare yourself.*

They moved Dad to a private room, and I knew what that meant. The nurses gave Dad a shave and put him in clean clothes, combed his hair and swabbed his mouth. He would've hated this. I wondered why the body insists on growing a beard, when clearly the energy could be used more efficiently elsewhere, concentrating all resources on recovery.

It was Dave and my turn to sit with Dad. We talked quietly to each other and to Dad and Dave played his guitar for him. He is a great guitarist. He'd only recently decided that he wanted music to be his life, so he bought every book on guitars he could find, and taught himself to play. Dad was so proud of his sheer determination, and persistence. Dave also wrote music, and he played Dad a beautiful song written just for him. The gentle melody filled the room with peace and beauty.

Beep Beep Beep! The machines went off and nurses ran in from everywhere. Dad's body jerked on the bed. The nurse heading up the team shouted across the room, 'Connie, do you want us to resuscitate him?'

My body froze but my mind was going at a million miles an hour. I didn't know what to say. I couldn't respond. I wanted to call Hilde and Sam but there wasn't time.

'Connie, we need to know. Now! Do you want us to resuscitate your dad?'

I knew Dad wouldn't want to live a life where he wasn't in control, where he needed help to do everything. We'd talked about this. He'd had to make the same decision years before about Mum. I knew what he wanted. But I couldn't let him go, could I? I knew that I had to, but every fibre in my body wanted to hang on to him.

'Let him go,' I heard myself say. 'Let him go.'

After a few minutes the machines were turned off. The room fell quiet except for my sobs. Dave held me tight and we both cried. Our darling Dad was gone.

CHAPTER 19

LIFE IS GRAND

That's the hardest thing about love. It gives you so much but the price you pay is too great when you lose someone. From a young age I'd known this but losing my dad was the hardest thing I'd ever had to face up to that point in my life. Sure, I'd lost my mum. I'd had cancer, faced the devastation of miscarriage and lost too many of my friends, but this was different. This was the person who loved me unconditionally for all my faults and made me feel good about myself. I struggled for a while but I knew I had to pull myself together for Willoughby and Hamilton. I had to be the woman Dad knew me to be. In honour of him I had to make a good life for them and for me and Mike. So I did.

Mike and I had been together for just over ten years at this point. We forgot to celebrate our 'got together' anniversary but that was okay. Anniversaries don't matter. Birthdays don't matter. It is every day that counts. And every day was a good day for us now.

A typical day in the 'Life of Connie and Mike' meant getting up early with the kids and getting them ready for preschool. They were going to the French Australian Preschool in Canberra, where they'd get a bilingual education. Despite our best efforts at learning French, the kids were already more fluent than us, and that made us proud, though playing catch-up to a couple of toddlers is a little more than just embarrassing.

I'd drop them off at preschool, then head off to my new job, just around the corner from their school. I was working as an administration officer at a disability organisation. It was the best job I'd ever had. I'd get to meet and talk to heaps of people with disabilities every day, but I worked regular nine to five hours, which was so much better for our family life.

After work I'd pick up the kids and we'd go home. Every night was pretty much the same routine and I loved it. We didn't have a bath, so the kids had a baby bath in the bottom of the shower each night. They'd both fit in, and they'd giggle, laugh and splash. It was a pure joy to watch them at bath time. Sam and I were the same at that age – the best of friends.

The boys slept in the same room. Willoughby would go to sleep the minute I finished reading to them. They loved *Where is the Green Sheep?* and *Hairy Maclary from Donaldson's Dairy.* They'd memorise the lines and once I'd read the start of each page they'd finish it for me. Little Hammy would sit up late, leafing through something, often a pictorial encyclopaedia. That book was so heavy he'd tip over if he tried to lift it, but he looked at all the pictures and pretended to read it, making up stories to match the pictures, talking out loud. He'd finally fall asleep, sprawled out wherever he was when tired proved too hard to fight. He might be playing trains, reading his encyclopaedia, or sitting chatting to his teddies. Mike or I would go in and move him into his bed. He'd stir, say a few garbled words and then curl himself into a comfy little ball in his bed.

After the boys were asleep, we'd cook up a meal for ourselves, and eat it together over a glass of wine or two. We didn't have a television, so we'd just talk all night and hang out, like teenagers. We spoke about how happy we were, and how lucky we were. We'd just managed to save a deposit to buy an apartment. The bookshop was finally supporting us, so Mike only had to work one job. All of our hard work had paid off. We weren't rich, but we weren't poor. The boys were happy and healthy. There was nothing we wanted for. I could hardly believe my good fortune. Life was grand.

Then . . . BOOM!

My iron count was low so I started taking iron supplements. But it remained low even after that, dangerously low. The doctor suspected it could be a symptom of bowel cancer. The low iron levels combined with the fact that I had been bleeding down there rang alarm bells. I needed to have a colonoscopy quick smart. If it was cancer we had to catch it quickly. I protested weakly, I don't want anyone sticking anything up, well, umm, there! The doctor convinced me to do it.

I had had cancer twice, once as a 12-year-old, once as a 22-year-old. I was 33, and I was worried. The thought of going through surgery and chemo frightened me. My life was settled and perfect. One thousand and one thoughts flitted through my brain. What would it mean? Would I lose my job? How do I explain a bald head to a two- and a three-year-old. How much would I tell them? I was terrified but I held it inside.

I took the day off work and Mike asked a staff member to cover him at the bookshop and we went on a little hospital day trip. I hate the colours of hospitals. Apricot, pastel green, grey and white. The hospital gowns aren't any better, urgh. All the patients wait in recliners in the waiting room, in their white gowns, white cotton dressing-gowns, paper slippers and hair nets. Our partners and friends are even more uncomfortable, because they have to sit and wait on plastic school-style chairs next to the recliners. And they have clothes on.

People around me were getting agitated, I was getting agitated. We'd been there since seven in the morning; it was now approaching two and still no one had called my name. The number of patients dwindled; it couldn't be that much longer, surely.

'Constance Johnson,' a doctor with a clipboard called out my name. She guided me down the apricot corridor to a double-doored room and explained that this was where the procedure would take place. I was nervous, but more than anything I just wanted it to be over, and I wanted to eat. *Countdown from ten. Ten, nine, eight, seev* . . .

Next thing I knew I was awake, feeling a little hungover, with a doctor and nurse in front of me. Mike was there as well. The procedure had gone well, they'd got a good view of everything, and they said there was nothing of concern there.

I breathed out, and felt like I'd been holding my breath for days.

After a while we were allowed to go. Out in the corridor Mike picked me up and swung me around and around. Mike, the ever quiet and calm one was ecstatic, and not afraid to show it. It was only then I realised how worried he'd been. 'You're going to be okay.' He kissed me on the cheek. 'We are going to be okay.'

———

I was feeling invincible. It was not bowel cancer. I just had to change my diet and I'd be fine. I'd been vegetarian for the most part of 15 years, and the iron supplements weren't being taken up by my body so I had to start getting my iron straight from the source. I had to start eating red meat.

I didn't want to but it was important, so I'd have to force myself. Mike took me out for dinner to celebrate, and I picked at his steak, slowly reintroducing red meat into my life. It could be worse. I could be dealing with a cancer diagnosis.

Within two weeks I had another blood test, and the introduction of red meat into my diet had fixed my iron-level problem almost immediately. But something still wasn't right. I had a bad feeling. My right breast was sore. It had been lumpy for some time, and I'd had it checked by a doctor about a year before. She'd said that it was nothing to worry about, so I put it to the back of my mind. There were more lumps now, and my breast was red, swollen and painful so I had to do something.

Back to the doctor. After an examination and several questions, the doctor concluded that I had mastitis and prescribed some antibiotics. I thought that was a bit strange. Mastitis is an infection of the milk ducts in the breast, and it is most common in breastfeeding mums. My children were two and a half and three and a half and I hadn't breastfed in about 18 months. I was surprised to hear that it was possible to get mastitis when not breastfeeding. The doctor assured me that any woman could get it, even an 85-year-old who had never breastfed.

Two weeks and two courses of antibiotics later, I went back to the doctor because nothing had changed. If anything, it had become worse. There was a sinister thought at the back of my mind. I tried to suppress it, but the voice kept coming back. 'You've had cancer twice, you have a lumpy, sore breast. It could be cancer.'

I tried to ignore the voice. No one, not even me, could be that unlucky!

When the doctor called my name I snapped out of the daze I was in, the inner discussion and ponderings. It's scary in there. In my head. I don't like it. I wanted the doctor to tell me it was nothing to worry about, but he examined me again and asked more questions.

'Do you have a history of breast cancer in the family?'

'No.'

'How long since you stopped breastfeeding?'

'Eighteen months.'

'Is it painful?'

'Yes.'

'Did you take the entire course of antibiotics?'

'Yes.'

'Did you take the repeat script?'

'Yes.'

'How long has your breast been red and swollen?'

'About four weeks.'

The doctor prescribed a different antibiotic, a stronger one. 'I want you to take the full course and see how that goes. It is mastitis, it just didn't respond to the general antibiotic I gave you last time. This should fix it up.'

Then it was my turn to ask questions. 'What if it isn't mastitis? What if it's breast cancer?'

'It doesn't present like breast cancer. It presents like mastitis. It's a common infection. This should fix it up.'

'I'm worried. What if it is cancer?'

'It's not cancer, but if you want we will do a scan if it doesn't respond to this course of antibiotics. You're too young for breast cancer anyway.'

'I was too young for cancer when I was 12 and 22 as well. I would like to rule it out.'

'You are too young, you have no family history and the clinical signs don't point to breast cancer. You don't need to worry.'

For a while this news kept me quiet, but my previous history of random unrelated cancers fed my fear. My inner voice started making itself heard again. I reluctantly took the doctor's advice, and began the course of antibiotics, but the malignant thought that it could be cancer didn't go away. I was about to find out what I had always known deep down to be true – my inner voice is rarely wrong.

CHAPTER 20

BOOM, CRASH . . . CANCER

Another two weeks and another course of antibiotics and still my breast was lumpy, sore and red. I wanted a scan. I explained that we didn't have a lot of money and it would be preferable to get a bulk-billed scan. The doctor told me that wasn't possible and gave me a referral for an ultrasound.

That nervous, sick, something-is-very-wrong feeling got stronger. Fear. It hurt like hell having the ultrasound wand pass over the sore bits. The look of concern on the radiographer's face wasn't good either. She explained that there was something, possibly an infection, blocking her view. She needed to get a doctor in to look at it; she wanted a second opinion. She disappeared. The wait was torture.

The radiographer and a doctor came back and they stood close together, looking at some of the images and talking in low voices as if I wasn't there. They looked at each other several times with very earnest expressions on their faces. I couldn't stand it and asked what the story was, even though I knew they weren't supposed to tell you anything.

'Well, there may be a mass, maybe even two back there, but because of the inflammation in the front, we can't get a proper look at it. And the inflammation itself is complicated. When we see inflammation like this we would normally think mastitis, but we know you aren't feeding so that's unlikely. We need you to take antibiotics and come back for another look when that inflammation has calmed down.'

The panic I felt ramped up another few notches, into the red zone. I'd googled breast cancer and inflammation of the breasts, and come up with some pretty scary results. Inflammatory breast cancer is the worst sort of breast cancer. It's a diagnosis that no one wants and, of course, I concluded that that was what I had. As people say, a little bit of knowledge is not a good thing. Access to 'Dr Google' must drive doctors mad because patients constantly self-diagnose. Most of the time they're probably wrong and I'd hoped I would be too.

My GP wasn't impressed when I asked if this could be breast cancer, that was for sure. He brushed me off, telling me I was too young, I didn't have a family history of breast cancer and it wasn't presenting like cancer. When I said, 'But what if it is, and it's going undiagnosed, for weeks, months even?' he told me that it would make no difference if I was diagnosed now or in two months' time.

That's when I decided to get a second opinion; though I guess, technically, it was a third opinion, because I had been to a doctor 12 months earlier who'd said that my lumpy breasts were nothing to worry about. This couldn't go on. It was painful, worrying and causing me to have to take time off work, something I didn't want to do because I liked my job so much.

The third doctor examined me, and came to the same conclusion. But I'd had enough – I wanted answers and I wanted a treatment that would work. I asked the GP for a referral for a scan. He recommended that I wait ten days until after I'd finished this new course of antibiotics. I ignored his advice and decided to go to emergency the next day.

I turned up at the Canberra Hospital emergency department at nine in the morning. After waiting four hours, a nurse came over to ask if I was the mum with mastitis. I explained that I didn't think it was mastitis, that's why I was there. She told me to keep doing the right things while I waited to see a doctor. I asked, 'What are the right things?'

'Feeding regularly, and expressing if you can't feed.' Exasperated I explained that I was NOT breastfeeding, that my children were turning three and four, that I hadn't breastfed for years!

It was useless, I was just a number and the staff at emergency didn't want to see me anymore than my local doctor wanted to hear my concerns. After waiting nine hours without seeing a doctor, I left. But when I got home, the pain was bad and it wasn't getting any better so the next day I tried again. Someone had to help me.

I turned up to the Calvary Hospital emergency department, hoping that I'd have a better experience there. I was surprised to hear my name called after waiting just 45 minutes. The doctor examined my breast and took my past history. She was very concerned, and ordered a scan immediately. She asked me to come back to emergency as soon as the scan was done so I did, relieved. The doctor called my name again. All up, I'd been at the hospital less than 75 minutes.

'I am so sorry, but there is definitely a growth there. It looks like cancer. We need to do a fine needle biopsy as soon as possible to find out what sort of cancer it is, then you will need to have a mastectomy,' she explained. 'The cancer looks like it has spread through the ducts as well as being in two distinct lumps, so you will need a full mastectomy, but I'll let the surgeon talk to you about that. You are going to need chemotherapy and radiation, which will be organised by your oncologist. I'll do referrals for you now.'

I sat there shell-shocked, nodding and listening carefully but all the time a voice in my head was screaming.

The doctor organised an appointment the same day for me to have the fine needle biopsy. She told me that I would have my surgery within 28 days.

So in less than two hours, I was tested, diagnosed, booked in for a biopsy, booked in for surgery, and booked to see an oncologist. There was a lot for me to process. My mind was a mess of thoughts. I was brimming with anger, full of doubt, parts of me were trying to grasp onto the hope that it wasn't cancer. Maybe the fine needle biopsy would show that it was benign? How can I have cancer? How can this be happening again? Fuck, what if I die? The kids will be left without a mother. It was at this point that I remembered that I had to get Willoughby a present. It was his birthday.

I made my way to radiology in a daze, wandering the corridors, not really knowing where to go or what to do. A kind man with grey hair and smiling eyes stopped me and asked if he could help. I told him that I needed a fine needle biopsy as I'd just been told I had breast cancer. He put a hand gently on my arm and said, 'I'm the doctor who does those and I have a vacancy right now. If you'd like to get it over and done with now, we can.'

I gratefully accepted his kind offer. I watched the whole procedure in a bit of a haze, as if it was happening to someone else, then thanked him for his kindness and went on my way.

I realised I was going to have to tell Mike what was happening. I HAVE CANCER! I couldn't believe it. Not again. For a moment I thought I would not go through chemo, that I'd refuse to go through that hell again, but of course I woke up to myself and realised it was different now. This time I was a mum. I had two beautiful little boys who depended on me every single day. I had to fight this. And I had to win.

I made my way to the mall to buy a present for Willoughby. It was his fourth birthday and we were celebrating that night with cake and presents. I had to buy him something good. He was really into Buzz Lightyear, despite never having seen the *Toy Story* movies, and I saw some Buzz stuff. I grabbed a toy and a T-shirt, some wrapping paper and headed for the door. Somehow it had hit six o'clock and there was a partition up in the corridor of the mall. I was locked in.

How can somebody get locked in a mall on the same day they get diagnosed with cancer? I needed to get out of there. Not only did I need to get back to Willoughby before it became too late, but my head was spinning and I was spiralling into a panic at the thought of being locked in a shopping mall overnight!

I finally found a security guard, and he explained that the door I had come in through had been closed so I had to walk to the other end of the mall, leave via the supermarket and walk back around the outside of the mall. It was about a kilometre. I stared at him in disbelief. 'But my car is just there!' I pleaded. 'Can't you just let me out? I can't walk out there in the dark, and it'll take ages. My son is waiting for me. It's his birthday.'

He wasn't willing to budge.

'Please, I just found out that I have breast cancer, and it is my son's birthday, please, just let me out of this door so I can get home.' I started crying. I was totally defeated.

At the sight of my tears, the security guard softened, 'I'll let you out this door now, but don't let this happen again. In future, you have to leave via the other exit after 6 pm.' As if this would ever happen again!

I wrapped the present in the car so I could walk in with it in my hand. Willoughby ran up to me as I walked in the front door, hugged me and grabbed the gift. He took the parcel into the lounge room and opened it slowly, savouring the suspense and drawing the thrill out as long as he could. He loved the toy, but was extremely impressed with the Buzz Lightyear t-shirt. The t-shirt was just so cool he couldn't wait to put it on. He wore it all night, and then refused to take it off to put his PJs on. I realised that we'd have to prise it off him every few days so we could wash it but I was so happy that he loved it so much.

Mike had baked a cake, and we sat down and lit the candles. We sang 'Happy Birthday' in English, then 'Joyeux Anniversaire' in French, then Willoughby blew out the candles. Both boys shoved banana cake into their mouths, completely forgetting their manners and just enjoying the moment. Willoughby fed his teddy as well, because it was his birthday too.

After the boys went to bed, Mike and I sat up at the table. I steeled myself. If I said it out loud it would be true. But it was, so I had to. I told him I had cancer again. We cried. We hugged. We talked about what lay in store for us over the next few months. Neither of us could believe that it was happening again. The sting of the 'why me?' question burned fierce, it's not that I wanted this to happen to someone else, it's just that I couldn't believe it was happening to me.

Again.

———

Initially I was treated 'to cure'. This news came as a massive relief to me; it wasn't terminal, I was going to survive. I might have to go through hell to get there, but at least I would be okay and the kids would get to keep their mum. The thought of going through chemo again frightened me; I wasn't sure how I would cope, but it had to be done. I had to survive. I had to live to tell this story to my boys when they were adults. I accepted that I had to lose my breasts, that I had to have six months of chemo and two months of radiation, but at the end I would at least walk away from it all with a life to live with my kids.

The biggest factor in surviving breast cancer is early detection. The key is getting to the cancer and treating it before it has a chance to spread to other parts of the body. When I first got diagnosed they did full body scans to check that it hadn't spread. It was in my lymph nodes, but it looked like it hadn't spread further than that.

But there was a big question mark hanging over my lungs. There were some nodules lurking around the edges and they couldn't quite determine whether they were of concern or not. The doctor hoped it was scar tissue from a previous bout of pneumonia or a remnant from the treatment I had as a child. The only way to tell if it was cancer was if those nodules grew or shrank, during the treatment. If they grew, it meant that the cancer had spread, and if they shrank it meant that it was cancer and it was responding to the chemo. If they stayed the same then it was nothing to worry about. It goes without saying that we all wanted them to stay the same! So although I was being treated to cure, the nodules on my lungs hung heavily on me. I just hoped and prayed that they didn't change.

The chemo was hard and the radiation was tiring, but I endured it all. I'd do anything to survive. My kids needed their mum. Sam and I were aged three and four respectively when our mum had died. I thought about losing her at that age, and remembered what it was like growing up without a mum, and without any memories of her to carry with me. I was so relieved that they had treatment available. I could endure this.

—

I drastically underestimated the impact losing my breasts would have on me.

Prior to my mastectomy I hadn't thought much about losing my breasts, but as every woman does, I *had* thought a lot about the size and shape of my breasts, and was never entirely satisfied with them. Mike loved them, but I always felt like they were too small. I think every woman wishes that her breasts were bigger, better, perkier, smaller, with bigger nipples, smaller nipples, et cetera. We always want what we can't have.

In the back of my mind were the taunts from school and my days as a checkout chick and waitress, when my colleagues felt it appropriate to say things like, 'You would have a perfect body if your tits were bigger', or, 'You should put a couple of oranges in your bra, you look like a 12-year-old boy.' I look back on those comments now, and know that I wouldn't tolerate them, and nor would I be concerned about them. Now, I would be more likely to say, 'You're not a supermodel yourself, so perhaps you can keep your appraisals of my body to yourself, you twat!' rather than going home and crying about it.

Like them or hate them, our breasts are part of our body and part of our identity as women.

First they help us attract a mate, then they nourish our young. They're part of us. I hadn't thought that much about it when I was told that I would have to have a mastectomy, I was just determined to do anything I could to make sure that I would be able to watch my kids grow up. If my breasts had to go, they had to go. I had never thought about what a mastectomy involved. For some reason, I thought that the nipple wouldn't be removed too. I thought I'd have a chest like a man's, with muscles and nipples. Not so. The nipple is nourished by the breast, and when I begged to keep my nipples the surgeon explained that if you kept them without the surrounding breast tissue they would die and shrivel up like sultanas. That convinced me that I could live without my nipples! Whatever I had to do to stay with my kids. Surely it couldn't be that bad? I mean, it wasn't like losing a leg or an arm, or a finger. We don't use breasts other than for feeding and we can live without them.

I just wasn't prepared for the immense feeling of grief and loss I experienced when I looked down after the surgery and saw where my breasts had been. Intellectually, it didn't matter if I had to lose them, but emotionally it mattered a lot. I didn't expect my chest to look so flat that it was almost inverted. I didn't expect the shape of my whole upper body to change as much as it did. I didn't expect the feeling that I had lost what had made me a woman, and differentiated me from men.

Neither was I prepared for the pain following the operation. I figured that I had had a whole bone removed from my leg when I was a child, and assumed that this couldn't be that bad, but it was. Because the surgery is on the chest and under the arms, it hurt every time I took a breath, coughed or sneezed. I found myself praying that I wouldn't get the hiccups as the pain was unbearable.

Once the physical pain settled down I tried to wear normal clothes again, but nearly all of my tops and dresses were unwearable now. Anything with darts or gathering in the chest area no longer worked, 'cos you just ended up with big sacks of empty fabric on your chest. Most conventional necklines didn't work either because you could see the prosthetic or the bra. I ended up having to buy clothes that I never would have considered wearing before, clothes that would normally appeal to an older age group.

I wore prosthetics as soon as my scars healed enough for me to be able to stand them. They stick on so every night when I pulled them off it felt like ripping off a bandaid. It was lucky some of the skin in that area was numb. But then my right arm started to swell up – fluid was gathering in it – and it was not going away. It looked a lot fatter than my other arm. My hand went numb by the end of each day. I could usually feel it again by the next morning but then I'd get shooting pains down my arm. It took me months to realise that all of these symptoms were caused by the bras I was wearing. I experimented, trying to find a bra that wouldn't cause these troubles, but my nerves and lymph nodes were so damaged from the surgery that there was no bra that I could wear comfortably.

My oncologist joked that she wished that curing breast cancer was as easy as telling your patient not to wear a bra. So my arm was cured by not wearing a bra, which meant I had to go flat and proud, whether I liked it or not.

My oncologist said in passing one day when I asked if I could have a reconstruction, 'Keira Knightley is flat chested and she is beautiful, and famous. You don't need big breasts to be beautiful.'

I didn't want 'big' breasts, I just wanted some shape so I could fit into women's clothes! I smiled politely, but inside I was furious. How dare she compare me to someone with breasts like that? I didn't have nipples, I didn't even have little lumps. My chest was actually inverted. I didn't even have chest muscles anymore. It was *not* the same, and it was *not* okay to make that comparison. I knew that it didn't matter to other people whether I had breasts or not, but it mattered to me, and more than anything I just wanted people to acknowledge that it sucked.

Maybe if she had said, 'It must be really hard to adjust to a new body shape' or, 'I don't know how it feels to lose your breasts, but it can't be easy', this would have at least validated the difficult emotional nature of the loss.

I sacrificed my breasts, and endured all of the treatment, and it came time for my last check-up. The oncologist was confident that the treatment had gone well and sent me on my way, saying that I needed to come back in six months for a follow-up check-up.

I couldn't believe what I was hearing. And I didn't trust her. 'Aren't you going to do a scan to confirm that it hasn't spread?' I asked, incredulous.

'No, we don't scan as a matter of course, but given your history, if you want a scan, you can have one.'

'But what about those nodules on my lungs?' I asked, anxiety building. I had spent the previous eight months of my life having all this treatment, hoping like mad that nothing had changed, it was all I could think about, and here she was, willing to wave me off without a scan?

'Oh, yes, I forgot about that, thanks for reminding me. Yes, I'll order a scan and see you for the results afterwards.'

I was beyond furious. I couldn't believe she simply 'forgot' something that had been hanging over me for months. I had a bad feeling and that inner voice that fed my anxiety started to get louder.

—

The phone rang and I picked it up quickly. 'Constance, I have your scan results here.'

'Oh, what's the story?'

'I really think you need to come in to discuss it. Can you bring Mike? You'll need to have support with you.'

That's when I knew.

The cancer had spread.

I went to the hospital with Mike and his mum, Chris. We were prepared for the worst, but it didn't help. When the doctor said that the cancer had spread to my lungs, spine and pelvis, and possibly my liver and that it couldn't be cured, I felt like I couldn't breathe. It was like iced water rushed through my veins and chilled me to my core.

This can't be happening. I did everything I was supposed to do. I had all the treatment. I had the surgery. I did everything right. How can this be? How do I tell my kids? How do I say goodbye?

There were extra people at this appointment. A breast care nurse, a senior nurse and another intern. I heard the words and I comprehended the answers, but I couldn't believe it. I could not bring myself to believe that I was going to die.

There. Is. No. Cure.

I fumbled, desperately trying to find a mistake in the diagnosis.

The doctor repeated. 'There is no cure.'

Mike cried. Chris cried. I was crying. How could this be real? My kids. What about my kids? How do I tell my kids that I am going to die? Will they even remember me? I don't remember Mum. Not at all. How can I love them so much, and yet they'll grow up not even remembering me?

'How long have I got?'

I was told that the average life expectancy for a young woman like myself from diagnosis to death was often about three years, but given the aggressive nature of my cancer, and its resistance to all of the treatments, I would be very lucky to live that long.

I was told to quit work and to spend as much time with my kids as I could. I was told that my outlook was grim; I was not what is medically referred to as 'riddled' with cancer yet, but my prognosis wasn't good.

Over the next few months we tried more treatments with the aim of delaying the spread of the cancer, and none of it worked. The cancer kept proliferating. I became very sick a number of times and made quite a few visits to ICU. I also spent some time in Clare Holland House – Clare's Place, as the kids call it – a hospice. A place where people go to die. I was told that I was not 'actively dying' yet, but my health wasn't good. My mental state was even worse.

Something had to change.

CHAPTER 21

THE DARE

So, it looks like I am dying, and quickly. I am weak. I am tired. I am just plain sick. I have breast cancer and it has spread. I have to come to terms with the fact I am not going to beat this cancer.

I am scared. I cry and scream and rant and shake my fist at God, but none of that will change things. Watching Mike struggle with the news breaks my heart. Watching my kids and knowing I won't see them grow up almost breaks me completely. I have to keep going until I can't, for them. I am what they call terminal. Such an ugly word. But somehow fitting because all I can do now is wait. This isn't a cancer you fight. There can be no battle, no positive outcome. It has already won.

Sam, Em, Hilde, Chris and Dave all come regularly to see me. Every time they visit we all wonder if it will be the last time we will see each other. We all wonder, but never do we dare to ask the question out loud. Dad is gone, there is no one to tell us what is right or wrong. We're all grasping for meaning, and trying to work out the right way to deal with all this.

In my desperate search for peace, I want to make some kind of difference for my family. I would like my death to mean that something gets better somehow. I don't know quite how so I make plans.

Hilde is on her own, trying to pay a mortgage and to provide for her kids. I would like to help relieve her financial pressure just a little bit, so that things can be that little bit easier for her and her boys. My super will allow me to be able to give them a bit of a safety net. Easy.

I want Dave to be able to follow his dream and keep writing music. He just needs a little financial kickstart. Some of my super will provide him with a little bit if that's what he wants to do. Easy.

I want Em to be out of debt and in a position where she can start to save for something she and her partner, Charlie, want. Super will take care of that. Easy.

But Sam wasn't so easy. Sam was tricky. Sam couldn't be fixed with a few bucks. All the money in the world wouldn't fix Sam. How could I fix Sam?

I desperately want Sam to be happy. Truly happy. I'd lost him over the last few years. Since before Mike and I got married and even before that, if I was honest. I wanted him back but I wasn't sure I knew how to find him again.

I had such emotional happiness and stability and I really wanted Sam to experience some of the happiness that I had found. I'd lost my way back in my late teens but I had consciously changed my life and made decisions that had made me happy and fulfilled. I wanted Sam to be able to feel some of the happiness, contentment, togetherness and pride that a good decision brings. How could I help him do that?

Before he was lost, Sam had a huge heart, a generous spirit and a love for life that was infectious. He'd wandered off down a road and ended up somewhere dark and all-consuming, at the bottom of a hole so deep and so steep that it was near impossible to claw his way back out. Losing Lainie was hard, but the slide had begun before she took her own life. Thinking about it now, maybe my first cancer had started things. The ground underneath both our feet began to crumble back then.

Losing Lainie was another devastating blow for a soft-hearted man who cared too much. Maybe he didn't want to say goodbye anymore. He'd distanced himself from his family, and made it very clear that nothing we could ever say or do would change his mind. He was not going to have a career, get married or have kids. He knew what he *wasn't* going to do, he knew how he *wasn't* going to live, but that didn't mean he had the answers for what he *would* do, for how he *would* live. I think that somewhere inside Sam felt that we didn't understand him, and that he was going to show us that if we couldn't understand him and accept him the way he was, then we couldn't have him at all. It was a self-imposed period of exile from his family, and none of us really understood it. I missed him.

I remembered the bubbly Sam, magnanimous and gentle, generous and loving, but I couldn't see that Sam anymore in the doubting, negative man my brother had become.

Just before Dad died we all spent the day together and that day, Sam caught a glimpse of something he had been blind to for many years. The irresistible tug of family. It could pull you back from the deepest of holes, the roughest of storms and somehow we all put on our game face and refused to give up on him. We were going to get him back. And together, slowly but surely, we did. But Sam still sat dangerously close to the edge, too close to temptations I didn't even pretend to understand. I was worried. I knew he could topple into the abyss at any moment.

Yes, he was back, but he didn't trust us, he didn't trust anyone. Everyone had motives, and no one was on his side. Now that I'd found out I was dying, I so wanted him to travel along a path to health and happiness. No need for wealth or riches, just good health and a smile would be enough, more than enough. How could I make him smile again? How could I help him find the Sammy Seal Johnson that he once was, and embrace that? Could I use my impending death to his advantage? Could I play the cancer card and help him?

It might not work, but I had to give it a crack. If I was to find any peace before I died, if my death was not going to be for nothing, I had to try. Try anything I could think of to find the old Sam and somehow help him to enjoy life again. I wanted to go to my grave knowing that he was on a better track.

I had a secret idea. I didn't tell Mike. I didn't tell Em. I didn't tell Hilde or Dave. And I didn't tell Sam. Especially Sam.

I had figured it out. The way to get Sam out of the quagmire and into life, was to put him on his unicycle and get him to ride around the whole country. In 2003 he rode from Sydney to Melbourne on a unicycle and raised $500,000 for CanTeen. He was at the height of his fame with *The Secret Life of Us* and voice-overs and had a lot more traction then, but I knew it was still possible.

I knew this one had to be epic. It had to be something big enough to get him fit and healthy for a year. It had to keep him busy long enough for him to remember that there is beauty in life and that people are nice. It had to restore his faith in humanity and himself and, maybe, at the end of it, he might be able to focus on getting his production company really happening.

I had fantasies about it. How far he would ride, how much money he would raise and how good it would be for him to talk to people in every town he visited. But how on earth would I bring it up with him? How do you ask someone to ride around the country on a unicycle as a favour? I knew that I held a powerful card, the ace of all aces, the cancer card. If I used it like a weapon, I could get what I wanted, but did I want to leave behind me people who resented me for forcing them to do things they didn't want to do?

I had to be very careful what I asked for. I know that a dying wish is a powerful thing, and I had to use it wisely. This was not something I could waste on myself – I'm dying anyway, I don't need it.

I'd sorted out my super and who would inherit what, and how it would help everyone to make their lives that little bit easier. I know that Hilde will be okay. I know my nephews will be okay. I know that I will have done what I can for my brothers and sisters, by leaving them some of the money that I won't be around to spend. I know that Mike and Willoughby and Hamilton will be okay. I know Mike will make sure my boys never forget me and they'll know how much I loved them. They'll know that I would never leave them if I could change things.

But that still left a big question mark over Sam. What could I do to ensure that he would be alright, to ensure that he would be on the right track?

Hilde has just gone home. Dave was down the week before that, and Sam has just arrived. We order pizza. I don't want to waste time cooking, I just want to spend the time I have left with my family.

Pizza and a few drinks. Perhaps more than a few. Sam is blunt. He tells me that he won't be there when I die, that he hates hospitals and that he knows I understand. He wants to know how I am. He isn't after an answer about my blood counts, or tumour marker counts, he just wants to know how I feel. He isn't interested in the cancer, and that's refreshing.

We sit in the kitchen, talking about the past. Talking about the future. It's hard for Sam to say anything without putting his foot in it. He tells me how keen he is to spend time with me by saying, 'I've been wanting to come and see you so badly, I've just been *dying* to come up.' We both burst into laughter. He tells me how he understands the whole cancer thing, but doesn't want to focus on it. 'Look, Con, I know you're sick, that's all I need to know, I don't need to be *abreast* of every medical development.'

I look down at my newly flat chest. 'Nothing to be abreast of, Sam!'

The laughter doesn't stop. Mike comes home from the bottle shop; he's bought a slab of bourbon and coke, a slab of premixed vodka, and a slab of beer. Let's not beat around the bush, we all know that tonight we are going hard.

'Good on you, brother. Gee, you've laid on the supplies, you've got enough to last a lifetime,' Sam says.

I start laughing again. 'Well, Connie's lifetime anyway!'

The hours pass and Mike checks on the kids and leaves us alone. We laugh a whole lot more than we cry.

Sam asks me a question I thought he'd never ask. 'So in the face of all this nonsense, Con, what do you want your legacy to be?'

His question hangs heavily in the air. It reverberates around my head several times and we both go quiet. Sam isn't into all this stuff, legacies and the like. He lives life in the present, unconcerned about what other people might think of him now or in the future.

Sam: The idea of leaving a legacy can kiss my arse. If I had kids I might feel very differently, sure, but if you had a semi-automatic directed at my temple and forced me to articulate what I wanted my 'legacy' to be, I'd hope for nothing more than the tiny pocketful of people close to me to agree among themselves at my remembrance, 'Well, Sammy tried. He sure did try, that kid.'

That. Would. Be. It.

Then they'd move on with their lives and promptly forget about me. The idea of legacy is too dependent on the notion of permanence, which I have little faith in because as far as I can tell, very little lasts in this world. Permanence can make itself over and instantly gratify my balls. The very nature of time doesn't allow for permanence – isn't it obvious? Sure, Shakespeare or Mozart fly in the face of such an assertion, and somehow the Bible slipped through too, but there's always exceptions, and there's nothing about Connie or me or anyone else

I've ever met that says anything greater than 'blip', as far as I'm concerned. Fuck 'legacy' and all its shitty little implications. The very word only serves to reinforce my sense of smallness . . .

See what I mean?!

It was the weirdest question Sam could ask me. But I wasn't going to let this chance pass me by.

'I don't want my death to be meaningless.'

Sam looks at me across the kitchen expectantly, his head tilts to the side slightly.

'None of us want that, but life, and ultimately death *is* meaningless. What do you mean, you don't want your death to be meaningless?' he asks.

'Well, I would love to save just one other family from going through this hell. I would like to prevent just one other mum from having to say goodbye to her children because of this bastard of a disease.'

'Gee, Con,' he pauses. 'How the hell do you think you can do something like that?'

This is my chance to ask Sam to change his life. For him to do something huge in my name, and change his life in the process. Should I do it? Can I really ask him to do this? Can I really expect that he would give up his entire life, his career, his friendships, his family, to do this for me?

The doubt in my mind is huge. But I'm determined. I want him to have an opportunity to do something beautiful, and to see the beauty inside people in the process. To see the beauty in life and to find some peace.

'Sam, I think you should get on your unicycle again. Not

just Sydney to Melbourne, but the whole country, to raise money and awareness for breast cancer.'

His face says it all. Disgust is written in his eyes, across his brow and in his hard-lined mouth. I steel myself for what is to come.

A few vodkas later he's standing up, arms gesticulating, face alight with the possibilities. I've lit a spark and he seems wildly excited at the prospect of unicycling around Australia.

'Just imagine, Con, we could raise a lot of money, we could make a difference. I could remind women to check their boobs. We need a motto, a boob motto! I could even break the record for longest distance travelled on a unicycle.'

After a few more vodkas the doubt settles in. 'But I don't have the profile, we would need some real celebrities to help us out.'

And, 'I shouldn't be away from the family at this time. I should be here with you, not gallivanting around the country on a unicycle.'

And, 'It's a hell of a commitment. What if I don't make it? Then the whole country would be laughing at me, and rightly so.'

I sit there and listen. Nodding, letting him think out loud. Occasionally Sam asks a question and we get the computer out and search 'The Google' for answers. But we both know what is happening. The idea has taken hold.

PART II
LOVE YOUR SISTER

CHAPTER 22

A DYING WISH

It felt like I was slumped forlornly in the shadows of my sister's terminal diagnosis. I was, in fact, sitting in Connie's kitchen, trying to present well.

'If you're ever going to sit up straight, Samuel, do it now,' said my brain for the millionth time.

My mind was drifting but I had to focus on Connie. This wasn't about me. We were having one of our silences again. We are full of gaps, me and Con. I can be on the phone to her and there'll be lengthy silences. Very lengthy silences. I've never experienced it with anyone else over the phone. Sometimes I wonder whether they're little Mexican standoffs or whether they're what's termed 'comfortable silences' – I've never been too sure. I usually opt not to fill the silence, and Connie waits too, eventually conceding via some weighty utterance. The silence on this day was different though, it held the weight that accompanies a death sentence. This time it was my turn to drag us out – head on.

'So what do you want your legacy to be?'

I knew the question would appeal to her ego. Connie has always maintained a stronger sense of self than I have; that's why I asked. I knew the idea of a legacy would be pleasing for her to think about; it would help provide meaning or a purpose to what was essentially a senseless situation. I was consciously steering the conversation towards what mattered to her, and to what we could still change or affect, because so much was out of our hands by that point. It was unhelpful to talk of the helplessness of it all. There were at least parts of this saga that we could still determine. I didn't want to just be a shoulder to cry on. I've never shown that kind of support to Connie. Over the years I've slowly learnt to listen better, but if she wants full-blooded empathy she can find someone else and she knows it. I offer Connie a more brutal, less complicit love. I'll listen and make the right sounds, sure, but I do it poorly enough for her to tire of it. She's sentimental enough without me needing to drip it on top, and besides, Dad was dead and there was no one else who had the balls to ask her the hard stuff. I stand before Connie in a way that many others can't. It's small stuff, but it takes balls because Connie is a one-way woman. Leading questions. Expectations. All that stuffy properness.

'So what do you want your legacy to be?'

I watched her absorb the question. She breathed in. Connie breathes in with more gravitas than the Queen of England, I'll tell you that much right now, but this was one unique inhalation. I could see that she wasn't beaten yet. Her eyes became clearer as she focused hard on the footprint she wanted to leave. I started to worry. She had that Connie look. The one you don't fuck with. She looked at me, her eyes full of strength and daring . . . 'We've gotta do something.'

And that's when I knew. She needed my profile, fading though it was. She wanted her death to mean something and I was her man. 'We've gotta do something' meant 'We've got to do everything we can, and by "we" I mean you, kiddo.' It wasn't enough for her to fight silently for her kids. No, Connie wanted to be bigger than that. Connie's kids needed to know that when the fit hit the shan, their mum fought for more than one family. She fought for every family. Connie never knew her mum and she would make God Damn Sure that her kids would be left with more than she had been.

I was to hop on my unicycle and go to every town. Every city. No matter what it took. We would fulfil our goal of reminding every young mum in the land to be breast aware. We would raise a whole million dollars for breast cancer research. And we would break the World Record for the longest distance travelled on a unicycle. I couldn't say no now. She was dying and this was what she wanted her legacy to be. Who says no to a dying wish? She had me by the balls.

I instantly regretted asking the question. Now I was implicated. I had, by uttering that question, unleashed a dream that depended almost entirely on me. I had already repaid the debt we owed to the cancer charities that had helped us out so much as kids, by riding my unicycle from Sydney to Melbourne in 2003, raising $500,000 for CanTeen – I had closed the book on the whole cancer thing. It was finished. Now there was to be a sequel? I just didn't like it. The idea wasn't new and I've never been one for rehashing. I didn't want to be away from my family when it mattered most and my profile was middling, at best. I'd plateaued and was now well and truly on the other side of the crest. I simply hadn't 'kicked on' and I didn't have the leverage of a decade earlier. I'd burned a few bridges along the way and it wasn't like I had a lot of people to call on. And Connie was talking about something truly epic. Something on an enormous scale. I knew, right from that moment, that we were in for a complete shit fight. And it scared me. Why did I have to fight her battles for her? Resentment crept in. Fuck her and her sense of entitlement. Fucken stupid me for opening up a can of worms. Fuck that question being so precisely weighted. Fuck everything. Give Me Her Cancer So I Can Die And She Can Look After Her Kids. How do you like that for a legacy?

—

On the way home from Canberra I've got plenty of time to think about Connie's idea. I try to separate myself and be objective. Mind Over Heart.

It's a good solid concept. It's got the elements needed for it to work. There's a comic hook in the unicycle; it's unique, and hasn't been done before on this scale. It's got tragedy, in that Connie is a young mum who won't get to see her kids grow up, with the brother who will bury his sister no matter how far he pedals. It's got a goose at the front with a profile — sure, not an A-lister, but not quite yet a no one. As a narrative and also from a marketing perspective, it stacks up and I know it. There's also the detox journey I know I'll need to go on to get road-ready; I've been around long enough to know that there's an angle there too. I'll need to bring in some bigger profiles to help me sell it to sponsors and to a network. Without A-list support we're unlikely to score a TV deal. Without a TV deal we don't stand a chance of attracting enough sponsors to pay for the thing — Connie was very clear about one hundred per cent of all donations (hereafter known as 'doughies') going towards research. The operationals would be astronomical and it would fall on the corporates. A whole year on the road? The cost of producing a TV show by its side? How does one even start to budget something like this?

My heart kept interrupting, of course. What of the familial implications? What impact would this have on the family unit as a whole? Was this really the right way to handle Connie's illness? What about my other sister? There was a lot about Connie's dream that made me uncomfortable. Firstly, I didn't want to be away during such a critical time for the family. I felt this very strongly. My instincts said that we should be fighting this among ourselves. It felt personal, not public. I didn't want to be off playing the hero while the family suffered. What if she died while I was in the middle of nowhere and I couldn't get back to her in time? Couldn't we just do what normal families do and fight it together without tabs on it? My belly wasn't stirring. My heart didn't beat for the cause. I didn't want to help other young mums living with breast cancer – I wanted to help Connie, Mike and the boys. And did Connie fully understand the implications of 'going public'? I had gone public about my partner's suicide on *Australian Story* a few years earlier and I've never felt that that was worth going through, for me or her family. How far was Connie prepared to go? Would she willingly be photographed topless after her double mastectomy, for example, if it meant a donation from a glossy? There's no middle ground – you either maintain privacy or go all the way. You're either open and advocating or shutting the fuck up. What about her husband, my dear brother Mike? I expected that he, along with my other sister, would have preferred to fight it privately. But Connie had everything to lose and everything to gain and no matter how I spun it, I always came back to those eyes of hers, so full of strength and daring. Something changed when she said, 'We've gotta do something.' Just because this was her dream didn't mean it couldn't become mine. But I couldn't avoid the gaggle of lawyers in my head purporting to represent my conscience, or my sense of self, or my sense of duty, or my self-esteem, screaming, 'OBJECTION, YOUR HONOUR, OUR CLIENT IS NOT IN A FIT STATE TO ATTEMPT THIS CHALLENGE!' And that there was the problem.

Without quite realising it at the time, I was looking for any excuse *not* to do it because deep down I knew damn well what it would take to get myself road-ready. A lot would have to change. I'd have to get real. And don't think Connie didn't know it. Fucker.

———

I also had to consider a friend. He's not a secret, but he kind of is. I call him Henry and he's a bi-polar bear. That doesn't mean I've *got* bi-polar, I just know a bear who has and his name is Henry, that's all. He's not like my best friend or anything. I quite like him, but if I'm really honest, I don't always want to see him – he's like one of those friends who always turns up when you've got other stuff on. He's pretty good though, as far as bi-polar bears go. He lives outside my house, but that's okay because he keeps to himself mostly. Except for this one time when he had a big fight with a scary black dog, but he won easily and the dog never came back. So Henry protects me too by roaring very loudly sometimes. At least he doesn't live inside, I figure. He's nice enough, just a little sensitive, and sometimes he gets so upset with the way the world works that he gets a little angry, but all bears get sad and angry, right? Just like humans really . . .

Sometimes I'm not sure whether Henry is even there. I know it sounds weird but I just can't help but think he may not actually exist at all. When I forget about him though he reminds me that he's still alive because sometimes I get home and he's sitting right there on the couch. I don't like it when he comes inside without asking. It's very rude. But I can be rude too, like him, so I try to say nothing. Sometimes he can be a bit alpha-bear and become very demanding but as I've got older I've been able to tell him off better and I'm not so scared of him anymore.

CHAPTER 23

I DON'T CARE IF YOU LIE TO ME, JUST DON'T LIE TO YOURSELF

It was post GFC and the corporate world had reacted by strangling itself with its belt. The boom had passed and the bottom had fallen out of the sponsorship market. During the 18 months I was out selling Love Your Sister, the Victorian Government sold the *international* naming rights to the Australian Grand Prix to Qantas for a meagre $100,000 and here was little old me trying to net up to $250,000 for a poky little local event. It would take a killer proposal and a very sympathetic corporate but I remained convinced that we could provide value at that price. I just had to be strategic. A lot needed to go right and I needed to stack my proposal with Zing! Pow! How to do that? I needed celebrities. Like it or not, you need them. We needed an elite A-lister to give us real oomph. Any old Logie winner or Moomba Monarch wouldn't cut it – no, we needed a woman who stood at the core of Australia's cultural identity. There was a shortlist – Kylie Minogue, Olivia Newton-John, Cathy Freeman. My heart screamed

Cathy. And I needed a sponsor to target. A perfect fit for Love Your Sister. A brand that existed for young mums like Connie . . .

I had fronted an unconventional advertising campaign a few years earlier for the bra company Lovable. They put a guy at the head of what has nearly always been a woman's domain – a fairly bold marketing move at the time. I was deemed non-threatening and metrosexual enough to score the gig and it kinda worked. It was irreverent and fun – it turned heads and did what it was supposed to. Breast cancer. Women. Bras. To me it was perfect, who better to 'support' breast cancer research than a brand that prided itself on the 'support' it already provided to women?

So I needed Cathy and I needed Lovable. I would work everything around that. I knew two people who knew Cathy, and I had a small in because of my past with Lovable – it seemed the smartest play.

I cold-called Lovable and was lucky enough to connect with Dianne Taylor, the Group Brand Marketing Manager. She remembered the campaign I'd done for them and she had lost her mum to cancer two years earlier after a fifteen-year struggle. She thought it a fabulous idea and pledged to take it on high with all the gusto she could gather.

There is one adage Dad espoused that will stay with me forever. It may well be the best advice I've ever received. You're Only As Good As The People Around You. I knew that for Love Your Sister to work I'd need a killer team. When Henry went on his next day-trip I got on the blower to an old mate of mine, Tony Jackson. I begged him to come on board and take over the production side of Love Your Sister. Tony Jackson is a gun as a guy, and as a craftsman. He shoots, cuts, writes, directs, designs and has a producing history that I can only dream of; he knows an awful lot more than I do. I'm a reluctant actor who's never really put his mind to anything before and he's a fucking wizard. I was seriously buoyed by his willingness to take Love Your Sister to market, *and* he could get on to Cathy for me to boot! I'd need a bunch of Tony Jacksons and a swag of luck for it all to come together, but I felt like I was giving it the best chance – as long as I remembered that You're Only As Good As The People Around You.

Cathy's agent's number trickled down to me. Tony Jackson had briefed Cathy; she was keen to help and the agent was ready to talk. The trick was not to ask for much. That's always the trick. These type of people get bombarded on the daily – it's no wonder they have people to say 'no' for them. All I was asking for was a 30-second video testimonial for private use only to be shown in one boardroom, one time. I could meet her wherever she liked, the agent(s) were welcome and I would need no more than ten minutes of her time. Well blow me down if she didn't arrange to meet me at the very park where I played most of my tennis as a junior! And dang and blast if she didn't bring her newborn and her mum with her! I had the opportunity to meet the whole clan – three generations!

I've met a few famous people before but this one took the cake. I, like the rest of the nation, was right there with Cathy through that famed 400 metre sprint. She captured me like she captured everyone else. She stirred a pride in me that I've never felt before or since. Sure enough, on the day I was to meet Cathy, Henry popped up in his fancy duds thinking he had access all areas. I barely kept him at bay. I was all over the shop. I only had a brief window, and I was so anxious that I got pretty manic and pretty much slapped her across both ears with our Love Your Sister dream; I was all enthusiasm. Somehow she locked in from the start. I suppose it was Cathy calling me an inspiration that sent me right off the edge. I'm lucky I didn't faint. She told me three times, so it can't have been an accident. She was genuinely enthusiastic about what we were trying to do and wanted to see it succeed. I told her this was my 400, and then back-pedalled furiously, saying that I wasn't comparing what she did to what I was going to do, I would never *dare* do that, but it's just that I felt that Love Your Sister was as important to me as the 400 was to her, you know – faaark! I tried to re-balance by simplifying – I've learnt to do that when my brain goes fuzzy – I told her a lot could go wrong, and that my primary hope was that we would all complete the challenge safely within Connie's lifetime.

She looked at me with peace and warmth and said, 'You'll make it. The spirits are smiling on you.'

Well, coat me in honey and feed me to the lesbians. You think that didn't shut Henry up. My insides went outside for a smoke. I reassembled what was left of my compass. This was the first of many spin-me-out moments that I can attribute directly to Love Your Sister. Cathy did a killer piece to camera, effectively telling Lovable that it was incumbent on them to fight for women's health on behalf of all of their customers – it was superb. Driving away down the highway I had a big cry. It was all very overwhelming. Keeping Henry away had been exhausting and the cry tired me out. Now I knew the spirits were smiling on me, there were less and less places to hide.

The Lovable meeting was fast approaching and I needed more than a 25-second testimonial from Cathy to smash this one over the line. I needed a video package that detailed the whats, whens, wheres, whys and hows and my mate Tony Jackson, the killer craftsman, came through with the goods like a champ. I added Tottie Goldsmith, Asher Keddie, Claudia Karvan, Catherine

McClements, Chrissie Swan and Noni Hazlehurst to the mix, and I went to Lovable knowing I'd done my best. It'd been a mad scramble to get there, but we were as ready as we could be.

I walk into the boardroom feeling more nervous than when I walk on stage. More nervous than when I present a Logie. More nervous than doing live TV. More nervous than being on 774 with Jon Faine. More nervous than fronting a media pack outside a Magistrates' Court! This isn't just a primary presenting partnership to me. This is personal. I care way too much, but then again, it's my passion that will sell this. It's the fact that it *is* so personal that'll make it work. Henry is at his most vociferous during heightened times like these. He knows I've put all of my eggs in one basket. If this doesn't work out, I can't exactly go back to all the women who helped with the video each time I target a new sponsor. They are very busy people and hard to lock down. They tailored their pieces to camera for Lovable, and I hadn't had the foresight to get generic testimonials, so single-mindedly focused on Lovable was I.

My eyes dart from person to person, looking for clues, as the video is played. Then comes the punch, the personalised testimonials from my bevy of notable Australian women, each of them down the barrel, directly urging Lovable to join Love Your Sister in the fight against breast cancer.

As they were playing, the CEO, Michael Gazal, looked at me and said, 'You can't do this!'

I smiled, and said, 'I'm doing it.'

Cathy slammed it home. The lights came up. A butter knife would have cut the air just fine. Michael gave a furtive glance to his 2IC. 'I think it's safe to say that we, as a group, are very interested in taking this further.'

'Great.'

'What are we looking at in terms of budget?'

There was, of course, no budget.

'Well, it's not going to be cheap. It's a whole year on the road. A sustained campaign like this can't come cheap, and we're aware of that so we're in the middle of lining up a mountain of contra and in-kind to help offset the cost of operations. Gatorade, Fitness First, Asics and others are already on board. Then there's the TV special on top of that. We're working through the broadcast agreement now with Ten. We should have a budget within the week, we're just putting the finishing touches on it.'

'Keep us looped in.'

'Thanks for your time.'

'Thanks for thinking of us.'

'It's a perfect fit. That's why I came to you first.'

'Send our love to your sister, from all of us here.'

Boom. We were away! On the flight home I ordered two bourbons and one Coke. I had a serious amount of work to do now, and I knew I wouldn't be able to live with myself if I didn't give it my absolute best. We were a real chance now and I needed to be on my game. If I was to tackle the challenge of unicycling around the country I would first need to tackle a challenge of my own. It was time to choose Connie and Love Your Sister. It was time for the miscreant in me to take an extended leave of absence.

—

I've self-medicated since I was 15, initially as a way to moderate my energy levels and behaviour. Pot and booze, mostly. That's not all of me though. I've tried to balance out my base hedonism with volunteering and sizeable helpings of drug and alcohol counselling; I have always tried to be honest with myself about my problems, or my need to seek help. By and large it's a battle that I consider myself to have mostly lost, though I have the consolation of at least being a functioning addict. I still get shit done. I've got an in-house Critical Incident Response Team that tends to keep me from straying too far over the line, but I've given the boundaries a decent push in my time. I don't advocate it, never have, and while I like to believe that mental health and addiction issues need not ultimately be a barrier to success, they certainly don't *help* – they will *always* exact their toll and have the last laugh.

Stay the fuck away from drugs and alcohol would be my advice. The happiest people I know aren't dependent. Which is why I was entering a seven-day detox program at the hospital I was born in. I went to my doubles partner and local doctor for a referral – I hadn't had an Alcohol Free Day in I don't know how long, never mind the other stuff and I needed a permission slip to function. I wrote myself off the night before the program began, not giving a single hoot about the breathalyser I knew awaited me at 8 am the next day.

The hangover was bearable, I was that used to them. It was my favourite kind of morning. My hometown sits atop a hill in the mountains and is found guilty of being too stunning to believe with startling regularity. As was their wont, the mountains were refusing to wake up and fog coated everything. I shuffled my foghead through a mystical morn to face myself and couldn't help but smile at nature's gift; an obvious reward, I was sure, for getting myself to that very point. The spirits were smiling on me, reminding me to be calm and peaceful. I walked in, ignoring Ken Kesey in my head and thinking that my life was starting to feel a bit like a poem.

I took my laptop to write down any thoughts that might come to me during my 'journey to wellness'; some books, a few clothes and a small camera that Tony Jackson, the master craftsman, had given me. I almost felt relieved at the thought of giving things a rest for a while. I'd been giving it a right old nudge in the weeks leading up to this day. I was about as ready as you can be, I suppose. I'd done this once before, so I knew what I was in for.

I Don't Care If You Lie To Me, Just Don't Lie To Yourself.

Another pearl from the Oracle that still nestles near me. Well, I knew my limits. I knew I didn't have enough discipline, or 'self-care', to get clean on my own. And I knew once I walked away from the program that I would take an out if I saw one. So the trick was to put myself in positions where there was no way out. Detox was the first. I could walk out any time, but that would mean I had failed. Failed my sister. I might not do it for myself but I could most certainly do it for my dying sister. I'd thrown away many of my initial misgivings and was running with my promise to Connie and using my verbal will to create a whole web of promises around it that I had to keep. I turned a promise to my sister into an open declaration that I couldn't escape from if I tried. If you're going to make a promise, you might as well make it an almighty one and finally, after years of fighting to be clean, I had found the best excuse in the world not to fail.

For someone who hates promises and legacies in equal measure, I had found myself squarely in the middle of both. If there weren't so many empty promises floating about the place maybe I wouldn't have such an issue. Promises rely on the premise that the future can be controlled by an individual (the promiser). Sure, you might be able to influence the future, but you are a fool in my book if you think you can determine it. And promises are determinisms, aren't they? I can't promise to take you to Disneyland because I might die before I get the chance, or lose the airfares in a Ponzi scheme. I can't promise to love you till death do us part because you might end up interfering with our children and I might be left with no choice but to hate you. You don't ever know what's going to happen, is my point. I Fucking Hate Promises. But that doesn't mean that they're not good for you sometimes. As long as they're kept. Be careful though, they're dangerous. A broken promise is something nobody enjoys.

———

As soon as I get out of detox I lean on the two near to me who can wrestle the best out of me without offending me. And I add my secret weapon. I know if I don't substitute my usage with exercise then I might as well have not done the program. There's Nothing More Dangerous Than An Idle Man and I know I have to keep my body busy to keep my head right. I have a haven built just right. No outs.

Luckily, I feel a stronger sense of community at my local gym, The Fighter's Factory, than I'll ever feel at a Town Hall, or even a local footy field. Murray Thompson, who runs the joint, is the Statesman; a former champ who lives and breathes the sport just as he did when he was a kid. Steve, who works pads with me, is my sensei. He's got massive guns and an even bigger heart. He *knows* boxing. He trained me for free, he just wouldn't let me pay. It was his way of helping out Love Your Sister. Everyone else at the gym is a compadre; we are all siblings in this tribe and the ring is our church. Now I can't box for shit, but that's really not the point – it's what you get out of it and, like everything in life, the more you put in, the more you get out. Boxing will expose you. It's another place I can't hide. Steve won't let me. He takes me through thresholds I didn't know existed. He believes I'm stronger than I think I am, and he's right. He sees a champion in me where I do not yet. I figure he's my man when it comes to thresholds. You're Only As Good As The People Around You, right?

When I'm not doing pads in the ring, I'm doing regular circuit work. I keep to myself there, my headphones keep me safe. I don't want to talk to anyone, but I'm really glad they're there. It's one of my most private spaces, but it's full of people. At The Fighter's Factory I feel like I can be a warrior because here, it's about *trying*, and that's about the only thing I happen to be really good at. It's a place that makes me want to try my heart out, skills aside. It's so much more than a workout. It's proof that you're tough. It's proof that you can survive. It's a community that celebrates *sheer willpower*. It brings out and then satiates the animal in you. It helps you believe in yourself. Through raw human power you actually somehow find empowerment. And nobody is measuring dicks, like you get at normal gyms.

It's got everything a gym should have. Photos, posters, clippings and quotes cover the walls, separated only by cracked mirrors and shitty brick. The building has worked as hard as the people in it. The walls, floor and ceiling have endured intense human force for years on end. Paint stands no chance and peels under the pressure; cobwebs provide further structural integrity. It's dirty and dusty in just the way it should be. No windows. It's a safe house for the junkies that hate the middle. Women and men evenly mixed, from all walks, all colours, all there for the same reason. Lawyers and high-end professionals, tradies, artists, young mums, the unemployed, the single, the desperate, the broke. Everybody's equal at The Fighter's Factory, because it's not about the individual – it's about hard work, discipline, hanging in there, pushing through and never saying die. You can purge yourself of all of your anger, resentment, hatred and self-loathing. It provides structure to the aimless, or at least it does in my case.

—

So she's all basically going to plan. Slowly, deliberately, bit by bit, I was constructing a place where success was the only endpoint. I slid more smoothly than anticipated into sobriety and was backing it up in the gym. The miscreant's remnants had been sweated out and I was getting cleaner and stronger, physically. All that was left to attend to was the mind. My 'temperament', as Dad so delicately used to put it.

For me there's only one person to consult when it comes to matters of the mind, and her name is Banu. She's elite in her field and incredibly good at her job, along with her husband, who specialises in paediatrics.

You're Only As Good As The People Around You.

She's seen me through some of my worst and is the best person to assess the madness of Love Your Sister objectively. It's been a while since my last confession and she's expensive, but you can't put a price on peace of mind. I was a little worried, to be honest, about one of my self-imposed conditions. Two of my three prerequisites for fully committing to Love Your Sister made sense. I wanted my 'other' sister's blessing – that made sense. I wanted a qualified psych, who knew my history, to give me a professional opinion on my likelihood of success, given my 'temperament' and somewhat patchy mental record, which is where Banu came in. But my third prerequisite was what worried me. I just had it in my head from the very start that I couldn't do it without Cathy Freeman's blessing. Sure, I asked for a testimonial, but it was her blessing I truly sought, almost from the first moment. This very fact worried me no end. Why would I need to get Cathy Freeman to approve of Love Your Sister? I'd never even *met* her before I asked her to provide the testimonial. It smelled like a grandiose delusion and made me think I might be, well . . . a little *crazy*.

I had an hour booked. I condensed everything from when I'd last seen her, through to my dear sister's terminal diagnosis and the Love Your Sister dream. It took 19 minutes, which I thought was pretty good because I'm such a chatterbox.

It took Banu less than a single minute to give me her assessment. 'Sam, I think this is perfect for you. You've got the energy for it, it gives you an outlet; something to focus on. I have no doubt that you'll succeed, and make your sister very proud.'

One big, suspicious pause. 'Is that it?'

She was meant to tell me I was bonkers.

'That's it. Go for it.'

'But what about the Cathy Freeman thing? Doesn't that worry you?'

'It's important to have role models. It's great that you met her.'

She didn't let me pay for the session. She told me it was her way of supporting Love Your Sister. And so closed another escape hatch.

CHAPTER 24

ONE STEP FORWARD, THIRTY-NINE STEPS BACK

It was all coming together, but the two most essential components hadn't been locked in – our primary presenting partnership and our broadcast agreement with Ten. Tony Jackson pulled together a package that detailed Connie's story, my 'journey to wellness' and a training sequence – we added snippets from our Lovable testimonials and had ourselves a decent pitch-reel. There was one guy on high at Ten who had put up with me for years. He would at least give us an audience. We flew to Sydney to meet with him and he reacted positively to the pitch-reel and promised to take it to the next level, which was encouraging, given that he was a heavy hitter himself. At the very least we were after a one-hour special, but we were pitching an episodic series to run for the year. My old mate took it to a commissioning meeting and it got shot down. It wasn't a flat-out rejection though; we were told that they would provide us with a broadcast agreement for a one-hour special, within the network (which meant no guarantees of being on Ten – they could put us on at midnight on One, for example), but with no production funding. Unless there was a rabbit somewhere, that left Tony Jackson with no choice but to pull out. With a full brood and a new company to nurture, he couldn't put everything on hold for nothing, which was disappointing but understandable. At least I did have an agreement for some air-time though; it kept me in the sponsorship mix. Obviously that wouldn't solve the problem of finding the production funding. I had relied on favours and funded the remaining production costs myself to that point. Apart from income from the odd voice over, I had no money to my name. Raising the operationals for the event was proving problematic enough, let alone the associated production costs. And there was a serious cash flow issue. The $20,000 I had saved in the bank when Con got sick was well and truly gone. I didn't have enough cash to keep covering airfares, and most of Love Your Sister's business was happening in Sydney, and I'm a Melbourne boy. I couldn't afford to keep the ball rolling. For the first time, I started to feel that I was well out of my depth.

It was time to bounce back with Lovable and lock away a deal to cover event costs. I called Dianne Taylor and could immediately tell that the game had shifted. Lovable was in the middle of a takeover, and she told me if it happened it would throw our deal into somewhere near limbo. She would do her best to take it over the line with the new mob should it get to that, but she was always just one woman in the middle of an amalgamation that had nothing to do with siblings, unicycles or Dianne's lost mother, and everything to do with cash in slacks. My stomach sank. Surely any new company coming in would be looking to trim costs, if anything? All of my voices told me that we were highly unlikely to survive the transition. There was no back-up either – we had pitched the life out of it, without any nibbles. We accrued some contra along the way, but that was it. Too much was resting on this and it was starting to quack like a duck.

It had taken months to get to this point and I was only just beginning to get a taste of the pace of corporate Australia. If I wanted to get a few stakeholders together it would take weeks to coordinate. It would take weeks if not months to hear back from corporates, if I heard back at all. I found myself reacting badly, due largely to my pre-existing allergy to bureaucracy and inaction. Plus my sister was dying. Time was not something we had a lot of. This wasn't a promise I was willing to fulfil in memoriam. It would be morbid and awful. Love Your Sister needed to be a jaunt, a jolly old show, not some ghostly parade for a lost sister. No, it had to happen while Connie was alive so she could enjoy the spoils. But companies don't run on sentiment, do they? Unless it comes at the right price, of course. And we were way too expensive.

While I was wrestling with red-tape Connie got really sick and this whole unicycling business suddenly seemed very fanciful indeed. Not wanting to traumatise her children, Connie had somehow made the impossible decision to die away from her home, husband and children, at a 'hospice' in Canberra – Clare Holland House. While we didn't think we'd be needing the place for a while, Connie experienced a sudden deterioration and before you could say 'ride around the country on a unicycle', she was admitted. I was summoned. Clare's Place, as Connie's little boys call it, is a place for those 'actively dying', but my adaptive subconscious told me that this wasn't the time – not yet. I trusted my gut. I figured if this was her time then, as her brother, I would somehow sense it. Like when we were kids. I knew she wasn't going to die then, and I knew she wasn't going to die now. This was all nonsense, of course. I just didn't want to say goodbye yet. Still, I had to go.

The term 'palliative care' holds no sway when even Connie's little ones can sense that it's a place where you go to die. They haven't been told as much, but death smells the same no matter who's near and we all know kids aren't stupid. Everything was right about Clare's Place. The staff were genuine, caring and keen for a laugh. The building itself was as lovely a place as any to conclude your business; it sits abreast Lake Burley Griffin and the grounds are swollen with flora and fauna. There's peace to the place. I just can't avoid the fact that this is where I'll have to say goodbye to my sis. The place forces me to face the truth of it. I start to think that I'd rather be on a unicycle in the middle of nowhere. Slowly, piece by piece, the promise is growing in me. Her dream is becoming mine, because the truth is worse.

To be honest, I'm a bit of a denier when it comes to Connie's illnesses (typical male, I suppose). I've never been the brother to lock arms and say, 'Well, we're in this together', and off we trot to the hospital. Connie would laugh at that thought. Sure I've been to hospital to see her – more times than I'd care to remember, but less times than you'd think. Thankfully, Connie understands what it does to me. I'm pretty open about avoiding her cancer wherever possible. In fact, I've pretty much embargoed the old cancer chats. I don't want to talk about it. I don't want to chart her test results or follow her platelet counts. I don't want to hear about how she feels about losing her nipples. Never have, never will. It's too upsetting, because I can't change it. I can help by being there, but I can't help her get better. I can't give her her breasts back. Or time with her children. To take me through the details is torture because it only serves to amplify my sense of futility and I end up distressed because I'm a sensitive sod, so I digress to stuff we can change or affect. Just because there's an elephant sitting in the room doesn't mean you have to offer it a cup of tea and scones.

Cancer will not compromise our relationship. It will not cost me my sister. Well, it *will* cost me my sister, but you know what I mean. When I see Connie, I have zero interest in talking to a cancer patient. This might sound a little odd, given I'm now somewhat of a poster boy for brothers out there, and it probably seems on the surface of it that I'm an incredibly supportive brother, but I don't care for her cancer journey one bit. I was starting to like the idea of pedalling away from it. It was a natural extension of my avoidance syndrome – implausible deniability! There was no avoiding it at Clare's Place though. Watching Connie confront her mortality made me wish for a death of my own, and much more instant.

Coming away from Clare's Place I remained convinced that Connie still had a bit in the tank, but I was starting to doubt whether I could pull Love Your Sister together in time. Even if I did, the likelihood of Connie seeing the event through looked grim. I had to move quickly.

———

Even before Connie got sick, I was an aspiring minimalist. If I was to be volunteering for a year on the road with no income, I would have to make sure I wasn't carrying any debts. Luckily my credit rating was shot, so I didn't have any credit card debt to worry about. I don't own a car or a house – so no repayments there. I did have a bit of stuff that I'd been lugging about the place since my twenties though, and Love Your Sister provided me with the perfect excuse to get rid of it. After all, I wouldn't be able to afford storage while I was away. I gave my paintings to my friends and sold the rest of my stuff at a garage sale for $1500. What wasn't sold went to the tip, where it would be on-sold at their onsite store. I kept my futon, my CDs, my bicycle and my laptop, plus some paperwork. I moved into my 'other' sister's book shed in Melbourne to keep my living costs down and to be closer to Love Your Sister meetings and training facilities. We rearranged the bookcases in Hilde's shed to create a beaut little hide-out which I could access separate to the house. The only bill I had to worry about was my phone, which was doable.

—

Love Your Sister is essentially about a promise I made to my dying sister, but to achieve our stated goals, I needed to go and sell that promise. It was wearing me down. I was riding each phone call or email as if my life depended on it, because Connie was on limited time and I was desperate for the dream to be realised within her lifetime. I was putting myself under much more pressure than I was actually under partly because that's my habit, but also partly because I'd never worked on something that meant so much to me. You see, there's the hitch. I'm emotionally driven. The process of publicising something I hadn't yet dealt with privately was proving to be tough going. I was spending all of my time talking about Connie and her situation, and it's my least preferred thing to think or talk about. Having your verbal will on full throttle leads to run-down, leads to go-down, leads to stay-down. I had to remove myself and my sister from the equation to give it a better run. There was no way it was all going to come together on emotion. I needed to be smart. Mind over heart.

In keeping with my newfound minimalism, I stripped Love Your Sister back to its core. To sell it, it needed to be well branded, and to brand it for market we needed sound bites and catchphrases. Simplification. Minimalism. Less is more. I had to break it down. It all boiled down to our three stated goals, listed here in order of importance:

1) Remind every young mum in the land to be breast aware.
This is a great primary aim, I think, because it is an aspirational goal with no ceiling. To get as close as we could to achieving this primary aim, we would need to go face to face through as many communities as possible. One generally skim-reads the paper, if it is read at all. One often does other things while the television and radio are on. TV, print and radio are extremely effective, but they don't necessarily guarantee that next-level engagement that we were looking for. Connie and I were convinced that sharing our story person to person remained the most effective way to remind young mums to be breast aware. We would go old school, from town to town, with our pink soapbox and scream our story out to anyone who would listen. Any media would be the icing on top, and help take us to the places we wouldn't be travelling through. And what of our catchphrase? We needed a simple message that encompassed all that we represented. What was our message, in just a few words? It didn't take too long (I'm a sucker for wordplays).

Don't fall into the booby trap – be breast aware!

We had our catchphrase and our bumper stickers. (Connie would later trump me with 'Save a life, grope your wife'. It's much funnier, but is skewed towards males, doesn't cater to our core demographic and doesn't encompass our primary aim!)

2) Raise $1 million for the Garvan Institute of Medical Research.
I thought Connie was bonkers when she proposed a $1 million target. I have a fairly good understanding of how hard it is to raise money for charity and when I looked at comparable events I saw totals that were nowhere near that. One advantage would be that we would have an entire year to reach it, giving us time to build momentum. We would need to nail our community engagements, get loads of media, earn word of mouth and maintain a strong presence on social media to be a chance. I liked it because it was lofty. Never would I have agreed with Connie to a target that I thought was realistically achievable.

3) Break the world record for longest distance travelled on a unicycle.
In a way, this was the easiest part because all it entailed was pedalling and not giving up. I'm a stubborn fucker and when I was a kid I thought my bike could fly, so in a way I was the perfect candidate. We would sell it as impossible, but it would, of course, be built to be achieved. The record holder at the time had taken only 8–9 months to go across every state in America *and back*. I decided we should take a whole year for a couple of reasons. Taking a year allowed for mishap, injury or illness; I didn't need the pressure of having no wriggle room. Also, I wasn't attempting this as an athlete. I was, first and foremost, an advocate; our ethos rests on community engagement, face to face. We would not just visit a town, take their money and shoot through. We would stay long enough to engage at multiple community events, with time to say thanks at the end. If we were going to be about breast awareness then we might as well stay long enough to beat the drum.

That was it at its simplest. The other essential tenet was *tone*. No one wants another hard-luck story so we based the entire tone for the event on this premise. Sometimes the media would take us there, but we never started it. We had to be fun and irreverent. We would be grass-roots, accessible and keen to take the piss. I was determined that the event simply would not work without this flavouring. Every time I drilled Connie on it I was reminding myself too. We were in Australia where there is zero tolerance for victims. Connie was to be the stoic cancer patient, smiling in the shadow of death, and I was to be the goose on the unicycle tackling an extremely absurd challenge in the name of his sister. We could feel sorry for ourselves until the cows came home, *in private*, but publicly we had to keep it light. Ask anyone close to Love Your Sister and they'll laugh when you mention 'tone', for they are *very* well drilled in my opinion on the matter! Poor Connie had to hear it over and over again – sorry, Sis!

—

There was a niggle that wouldn't go away. When I had held my garage sale after detox, I found myself watching a bearded man walk rather dismissively past my things. As I was thinking that he must be looking for tools or spare parts, of which I had none, I wondered if I'd actually met him before. And then it twigged. He looked like Jon Faine, from 774 ABC – indisputably the greatest radio broadcaster I've ever listened to. Seriously, I worship this guy. I've never heard anyone hold our public officers to greater account; he provides perfect balance by pitting himself evenly against all sides – he's terrific. Could it possibly be him?

'Has anyone ever told you you look like Jon Faine?'

He sized me up and to my astonishment, replied, 'It's me, Sam, you idiot.'

I couldn't believe he would even remember a flea like me. He's had so many people through his studio.

'Got any tools?'

No, but I had one heck of a story. I showered him with my verbal will and scored his email address. Taking another step towards minimalism was proving to be of immediate reward, it seemed.

I emailed him promptly, asking for a written expression of interest:

'Given that the event lasts an entire year, and therefore costs a fair whack, our sponsors understandably need some hard evidence that this event will attract some media interest. I understand that you can't necessarily guarantee coverage, but I'm wondering whether I might be so bold as to ask for a letter from you or one of your producers that may vaguely refer to being interested in chatting with me beforehand and/or along the way? I'm fully aware that we can't mention brands on the ABC, I'm more trying to prove that there is interest in the event. I'm sure you'll let me know if I'm out of line, which I hope I'm not . . .'

And he got back to me. 'Yes, we would talk to you about your journey. Would envisage one studio interview before you leave, along the lines of "How crazy is this guy?", then an occasional chat along the way, and after you have SMASHED the record. Am not able to do a weekly chat or anything – I reckon the audience would not want that much of you. And yes, it would be a breach of ABC rules if you banged on about brand names all the time and we would have to cut your tongue out for that.'

Vintage Jon Faine. I was bloody thrilled.

Weeks later, Jon Faine's email was still niggling away at me. Given that he's as media savvy as they come, I thought it safe to apply his opinion more broadly across the media landscape and ultimately I gleaned that there would be a degree of media interest at the start of the event and at the end, but the in-between was arguable. So the question was raised – how would this maintain relevance while I was in the middle of the desert for weeks on end? I would spend literally months in between some capital cities. Why cut to the goose on the unicycle if all he's doing is pedalling every time you speak to him? Now that I thought about it, it would get old pretty quickly. The unicycle gave us an initial hook but we would need more. A point of difference was good, but it wasn't enough. We had Connie's bucket list. I was to do all the things that she never got time for, but I couldn't sell it. It was a nice personal thing to do, but hardly newsworthy. A bit morbid if anything. I wouldn't want to cut to a guy in the middle of nowhere doing something his sister can't be there for – it just didn't sit right. No, we needed something fun and irreverent, in keeping with our tone. Something media-friendly to keep any potential audience engaged. I could try to get some celebrity presence out on the road, but it's hard to lock celebs down, especially outside the major centres. It's hard enough to get an hour out of them, let alone a couple of days. I ruled that out. We needed some set pieces. Out of necessity, and from Connie's bucket list, came the Love Your Sister challenge system.

It felt wrong to just rock into a town, preach for a bit then beg for doughies. Arriving in a town on a unicycle isn't enough to inspire next-level engagement, which was at the centre of our community engagement ethos. We were in their hood. Was it respectful to just roll up and roll out some fundraising template? We had to respect that each community is unique, right? So what better way to get the locals involved than to invite them to challenge me to do something *particular* to their area? If we are in sheep-shearing country, I'll shear a sheep. If we are in croc country, I'll swim with the fuckers! I would do *anything* for a donation and we were offering the chance for communities to get together and have a laugh at the city-slicker slash fish-out-of-water. Although the challenge system was born from the need to maintain relevance and feed our 'content' for the duration, it quickly became the centre-point of our 'next-level' community engagement plan. After all, everything came back to goal number one. Remind every young mum in the land to be breast aware. We would stop at nothing and never forget that as *the reason* we were bothering to ride around the country on a unicycle in the first place. If we wanted their attention, then we would have to earn it.

So, after plenty of time, thought and consultation, we found out who we were and what we stood for. We had three clear goals, a hook, a point of difference, a challenge system, an ethos, a kick-arse community engagement plan and a fucking slogan. It had taken months to get there, but it was a start.

———

I'm sitting at a restaurant that's way above my pay-grade, with the CEO of the company that just swallowed Lovable. His name is Justin. He seems a slick sort of character. Expensive phone cover, shiny watch, clothes that aren't worth what they cost. But he doesn't come from that. He's self-made, which makes him much more magnetic. He tells me that Lovable were very passionate about Love Your Sister and that he'd promised them he'd take a look at it, which is why we were there. I thanked Dianne Taylor in my head for pushing it to the new mob as promised.

I started my 'pitch' but every time I got some rhythm going he'd check his phone. Now I do understand that we live in an increasingly connected world and I concede that it is quite easy for a lot of people to do more than one thing at a time, especially these high-functioning CEO types. Nor was he being rude. He looked at me intently as I spoke. But he kept checking his damned phone. It reminded me of my first Logies experience, when every single person I spoke with spent the entire time looking over my shoulder. I felt like asking, 'Are you seriously much busier than the rest of us, and do you really have a constant stream of people desperately needing you to sign off on something mega, or is it a corporate dick thing? Tell me, please, for I am a mere mortal.'

Again, I was taking things too personally. Not only has that tendency helped ruin each of my relationships, it was now threatening to unsettle Love Your Sister. I tell myself, *This is just the way the world works, Samuel.*

We stood at the end of the dinner, Justin shook my hand, looked me in the eye and said, 'Sam, we will underwrite this event for you'.

I walked off my fine cuisine and my misgivings along the Yarra River in Melbourne, from Crown's boulevard of broken dreams up to the majestic Flinders Street Station. The city lights bounced off the river, helping me realise that now, with a broadcast agreement and a primary sponsor in place, we looked like we were a goer. A lot would still need to go right, but the odds had definitely shifted. I kind of wanted to scream. I may actually have snuck a fist through the air. Imagine. Just imagine if you pull this off, Samuel. Maybe I could provide Connie with something to really smile about. Just maybe.

ONE STEP FORWARD, THIRTY-NINE STEPS BACK

—

I was quietly panicking about the production costs. Having a camera guy on the road for a year, let alone the gear we'd need . . . it was a real amount of money and I had to find it from somewhere. I'd promised a schmicko TV spesh to all of my sponsors, in stone. All my friends were practitioners fighting for their own morsels of funding, so my industry contacts couldn't necessarily help out. I didn't have a bunch of skilled guys on hand that could afford to devote their time and resources to this for an entire year. I needed help. It's one thing to know when you're out of your depth, it's another to know that you're never out of options. I minimalise. I start from scratch. I make lists. I sift through my past in search of an exchange, a moment, a person, a point of contact. Someone to help me with my production dilemma. I think back to my first unicycle ride in '03, from Sydney to Melbourne, to one of my many spin-me-out moments on my day of departure, which I remember as 22 October. When I was leaving Andrew Denton turned up, completely unannounced, to wish me well and call me a mad bastard. Then, a couple of weeks later, at my halfway point, he emailed me: 'Chafing along with you, love Andrew'. It was the equivalent of my Cathy Freeman moment with Love Your Sister. If I could find Andrew Denton, who had built Zapruder's Other Films into pretty much the most shit-hot production enterprise going around, then surely he would be able to give me some *advice* about where to go from here? He would remember what it was like to get productions up from nothing. He was perfect.

I cold-called Andrew Denton's production company and verbal willed my way to his email address. He was away at the time, but they put me onto one of his guys who heard me out then promptly convinced me that I could do the lot for 20k. He reminded me of the basics. Forget 'broadcast quality', just buy a couple of decent cameras, point and shoot the fucker. The story told itself. Well, 20k should be do-able. Although I didn't know anyone with 20k. Or did I? I sifted again. There was one guy. He was an extra I'd met on *Home and Away* in '95. He'd gone on to the London School of Economics and married the daughter of a Russian billionaire. He'd then gone on to make many more kabillions of his own. I emailed him and he promptly pledged 20k for production costs and made a 100k donation to the cause. Boom. Just like that.

Advice is free to those who seek it truly. Then I add my verbal will. Then I add my theory of going to the best, because You're Only As Good As The People Around You. Then I add my philosophy of asking for less and mostly just seeking advice. I knew not much of nothing about many of the facets of Love Your Sister but I could reach out to those who did, actively seeking their collective wisdom. It's got me out of all sorts of pickles. The kind of pickles created by reckless use of verbal will. Because once I started really believing in verbal will I started using it, well, at will – I tried it on strangers and, sure enough, I began to forge alliances from nothing. Sure, there were a lot of dead ends, but the results were irrefutable. I was constantly taking numbers. I would rarely ask directly for help. I would ask if they knew someone who might be able to help. This took the pressure off them; I was asking nothing from them but a contact to talk to. I was applying my theory about coming in small, using my verbal will, actively seeking the best in their fields and it was yielding results.

But it only works when you go in small. It's a different story when you're asking for the world. As our meetings with Lovable, now Bendon, progressed, it became clear that they were looking for an extra partner to help shoulder the cost. The original commitment from Lovable before the takeover was substantial. But after Justin and Bendon gobbled Lovable they reduced that commitment and requested another partner. Bendon was understandably cautious. If we could find a supporting partner, they would step up and take front and centre. That was the upshot. We needed another taker.

—

Stewy at Vodafone would cover handsets and all phone and internet charges for the entire team, courtesy of the fact that I was appearing in their ads and doing their voice overs at the time. Stewy put us on to Brian at Pivotel, who was straight up and very easy to deal with, happily providing a satellite phone and coverage. Brad Moller from Asics would provide shoes for the team. Glenn at Schweppes guaranteed all of our drinks. I did a corporate, in-house voice over for Swisse and at the recording studio I met the clearly very capable Lauren Armstrong, International Business Manager for Swisse, no less. From that, Swisse would provide protein bars, powders and vitamins. Ralph at Unicycle.com would give us two unicycles. Tony, a beaut bloke from Clever Bits, reached out to us and offered to help with web build and design. I teamed him up with Jacob Zhivov who had done all the tech stuff with me on Ten's *Rush* for three years, then Tony brought in Marc Brewster, who designed our logo (we settled on Marc's after rejecting four other designers – I was so obsessive about the design because I was in the middle of the Steve Jobs bio at the time!). Fitness First and The Fighter's Factory were both providing trainers for free to get me road-ready. Dion was an absolute delight; I met him randomly at a function and we forged an alliance from nothing, and as one of the heads at Print Design Australia he would print all of our fliers, posters, stickers, business cards, banners, etc. Mel, bright, brash and beautiful, looking very much at home in her souped-up Commodore, would pump every outlet in Adelaide through Deventer PR and Communications and provide fundraising support and accommodation in Adelaide as well. Justine Bloome, a right gun at the helm of The Village Agency, was mentoring me (I made her, after seeing her TedX speech) and providing about 100k of real value – everything from social media to design, messaging, marketing and communications and volunteer networks. She brought in Nicole from EndToEnd who was full of great ideas to bolster us further. Chris and Shannon, about the loveliest couple you could ever meet, would use their MooMedia empire to smash it for us in Geelong. Andrea from the Australian College of Massage would provide massages for me and the team Australia-wide. The humble Cousin John organised us the biggest van you can get, a Mercedes Sprinter, later to become known as 'The Boobmobile', to tow the Jayco caravan and hold all our gear and support crew. He threw in a motorbike too. There's a man with a stunning black mane named Andy. He had a way of asking that was very different from mine, and more effective, I think – he just told them! Kaos Custom Bikes took it to the next level for us and got Park Tools, Oakley, Schwalbe Tyres and Garmin on board to create the best batch of bike gear we could have dreamed of. Andy the mane man then organised Big John from Antique Motorcycles to fit out our motorbike to be a support vehicle. (He's such a unit, our Love Your Sister wristband doesn't even fit around his wrist!) Andrew Ryan at Jayco continued the company's tradition of giving back by throwing 20k at the cause and providing a caravan for the year, with a freezer and a generator thrown in. We had 20k committed for doco production, which was enough to start with. We had written expressions of interest from ABC Radio, Nova 100, *The Project*, *The Circle* and an agreement to feature Love Your Sister riding through Erinsborough on *Neighbours*. We had written or filmed endorsements from Asher Keddie, Claudia Karvan, Noni Hazlehurst, Cathy Freeman, Catherine McClements, Ashleigh Brewer, Tottie Goldsmith, Molly Meldrum, Susan Boyle, Kate Langbroek, Dave Hughes and Chrissie Swan.

But there was an awful lot we didn't have. We had no provision for support crew, and covering their costs would prove expensive over a year, not to mention their expenses back home while they were on the road. There was little likelihood of finding an administrator who could work the logistics fulltime for the year, so there was another slab of cash to cover an annual wage. If we wanted a PR agency to cover the east coast we were looking at a heavily discounted rate of 15k. We had hit up all of the major fuel companies to no avail and one of the fuel estimates floating around was scarily high at 65k. We had no luck with any of the supermarkets either and food was estimated at 35k. The production budget of 20k was begging for a boost. But most pertinently, we didn't have another sponsor to match Bendon's 100k. We had hit up every company we could think of. I was aware of how long a large supporting partnership like this could take to build, given my experiences to that point, and I wasn't running any leads. Nothing even lukewarm. Everybody was coming back with contra but no one was holding any cash. That was the reality. It was post GFC. There was goodwill, but never a real way.

And so it stalled. It looked good on the face of it but you didn't have to scratch too deep to see the holes. I couldn't go back to Bendon for their 100k until I'd found someone to match it. I'd scraped the barrel dry. I'd exhausted all of my contacts and all of my verbal will. This was as far as I could take it. There was only one option. It had been mentioned to me months before, and I had dismissed it out of hand. It was my least preferred path. It was against what I stood for. But desperate times, right? I had to compromise and bite the bullet. I had to go to family.

CHAPTER 25

A FAMILY AFFAIR

According to Oscar Wilde, the world only belongs to you for a season. Connie's terminal diagnosis certainly helped highlight that for me, and indeed for the wider family, who we'd seen too little of over the years. We'd stayed in touch on occasion, but the occasions had proven rare. When Connie got sick we all just flocked back together. It was beautiful. Another one of the positives to come from Connie's illness; a timely reminder to us all of how brief our season can be.

I've got cousins coming out of my earholes. Cousin John and Cousin Jamie front the pack. They're a formidable brother combo, with way more runs on the board than me and Con. They show great leadership in their professional lives, which has led to great successes for them both, and it spills right down the line into family and everything else they do. I look up to Cousin John and Cousin Jamie primarily because they've done such a good job at keeping their family unit together and providing for their kids, but also because they're just such darn decent people. Their kids lead amazing lives and have experienced stuff most kids could only dream about, but they remain incredibly grounded and grateful (this also has everything to do with Sue and Alison, who do a phenomenal job of holding the lot of them together somehow). To my mind, Cousin John and Cousin Jamie hold an elevated status because they've worked their cracks off to earn it, and because they take the responsibility of it extremely seriously. They're also quietly very charitable, and have been supporting MS in a big way for years. They're generous to many other groups too, and have an unassuming bank of extraordinary kindnesses to their name. Which is why I'd rather have them appreciate Love Your Sister in its own right, without having to chip in. They've done enough and I respect them too much to go asking for a bloody handout. I want them to pass me the baton and to run with it over the line. I don't want them to pay for the bloody race. It feels rigged, but I'm out of options and I figure that sometimes you have to sacrifice one principle to feed another. For the millionth time I remind myself of our primary aim – remind every young mum in the land to be breast aware. *It's not about you and your hang-ups, Samuel.*

Cousin Jamie had indicated that his door was open from the start, and Cousin John had already been mentoring me in small ways. Cousin John is a very humble and fairly quiet guy; he doesn't talk much, which gives his words extra weight. And when he does speak, he says what he thinks. It's a frightening combo for a waffler like me and I get all twisted up when we talk Love Your Sister because I know he'll see straight through my verbosity. He meets me at a cafe in the city. I'm late and we have a narrow window. He breaks it down into such direct sentences and he talks for Cousin Jamie too. As long as Lovable match and formally agree to a primary presenting partnership, he'll provide the necessary support and bring in up to 100k through Web Lease and Cousin Jamie's Money Now. 'Good luck', he says, and he's off. It was never a familial plea for him, which is what I was worried it would look like. He treated it as a business proposition, straight up, on merit. Sure, he wanted to help family, but he was very clear about me proving that we could hit the target. Provided I could find adequate corporate support, he'd throw his weight behind it. It was time to go back to Lovable.

So I went back to Lovable, now Bendon. I told them I'd found two major partners that wanted nothing in return, who would provide 100k and effectively halve Lovable's commitment, as per their request. I outlined the other contra and in-kind sponsorships we'd lined up to help offset the operationals and reminded them of our media agreements. As far as I was concerned, we were ready to pull the trigger.

To and fro we did go, for many more months from that point. To sum it up in a subdued fashion, the process was disheartening. There's not much I can say really, other than that ultimately, our package wasn't enough to convince the board. Bendon is a large company, ASX listed, with shareholders to consider, and Justin, who had the decency to ring me himself, finally told me that the board wouldn't commit and there was no cash. After well over a year of wrangling. As he mentioned wanting to become a donating partner, and talked about a cause-related marketing campaign that could raise potentially 500k, I wondered whether he even took it to the board. I thanked him for the call and hung up. Time slowed. My heart wilted. We've all felt the sting of 'no' many times before, but this one cut deep. Stupid me had told people it was in the bag. Why had I believed him? Just because he shook my hand?

I should've listened to my gut when he kept checking his phone. Could I have asked for a clearer sign? What kind of dumb sucker ignores his adaptive unconscious? Did Malcolm Gladwell teach me nothing? Didn't I see the flags? Maybe I wasn't the budding entrepreneur after all.

The guts had been ripped out of the event. I felt like I'd gone to a high-stakes table and been exposed as a fucking chump. Despite how I felt, the fact remained, primary presenting partnerships don't grow on trees. In over a year of sifting through a depressed market, I'd found only one. Would it take another year to find a replacement, or longer? Would one be found at all? Cousin John's and Cousin Jamie's 100k was contingent on the Bendon deal. We were back at zero and I couldn't see a way out of it. Was it time to feed the red rover?

I knew that this was the part where my back was against the wall. I'd anticipated it before taking Love Your Sister on and properly committing. I knew that these things don't come together easily, otherwise everyone would be doing it. This was always going to happen. I knew I was meant to fight through it, re-gather, bounce back and go on to win the prize. I knew this was my moment of truth. I sensed that this moment was more challenging than any I would face on the road. But it's one thing to know something, and another to do something about it. (Yes, that's the Oracle talking.) So what did I do? I got the whip out because old habits die hard and leopards don't change their fucking spots, no matter how much their sister might be dying.

I went to the pub. After a few beers, I spotted a gateway. Henry was there, waving me over. In counselling circles, they don't call it a relapse anymore, they call it a 'slip'. So I didn't relapse (that holds too many negative connotations and sounds too much like failure), I just 'slipped'. As if it were a fucking accident. That's about the best euphemism ever. I'd say it's more like I snuck furtively into my local shadowlands, determined to camp sullenly beside oblivion. I nestled into my private cavern where I could float numbly through safe tears and rainbows. With the world on mute, music would play narcotic too, nursing me through painlessness . . .

If addiction provided no succour, then we would not bother, I suppose. I did more than let it take hold. I committed to it like I commit to everything: with full blood and rigorous abandon. I would try to swallow myself to spite my life. But this time was different. However hard I pushed, I couldn't get away. Sure, I got trolleyed, but the events of the last year stayed near. The masking agents were on an RDO, it seemed. It wasn't much fun, because Love Your Sister kept gatecrashing.

—

I went pretty far down but I limited the damage by not staying there too long. It just gets boring after a while, especially when there are other interesting things in your life, like places you *haven't* been before. After a while I shaved my face, combed my hair and stumbled down the stairs to meet the day, Kristofferson style. I felt pretty sheepish, but had been around long enough to know that beating myself up wasn't going to help. I did my best to put the whip away and walked through that point I hate the most. The point where you know you're starting from behind, you know you've un-done a lot of your hard work and you know that it's not going to get any easier any time soon. A couple of sessions at The Fighter's Factory and a heart-to-heart with Cousin John would take good care of that. It's good getting older – you learn to help yourself better. Caring for Connie in the ways I'd done over the last year was bleeding into some sort of self-care too.

Cousin John was pretty clear, which I always value him for and forms part of why he's such a good mentor. He was totally unconvinced that we could raise the one million as we stood. He believed we had to achieve some kind of partnership, cash or not, with a group or company that could provide *real* help on ground level.

'You're not gonna get there by shaking tins.'

If he wanted to throw 100k at breast cancer, he'd just donate. What could I do that would convince him that his 100k towards our ride would result in a million? He argued that there was no use wasting anyone's time, especially with Connie so sick, unless we had a real way forward. I went over our community engagement plan, our challenge system, our media deals.

'But who's going to do all that, Sam? You'll be on the unicycle. You're telling me the what, not the how.'

Who was going to do it? We had been fully corporatised to that point. All of the key people, except for me of course, were going to get paid – event management, support crew, logistics, PR. They'd all gone, as soon as the money disappeared. We were back to me and my Gmail and my mobile phone. How could we raise a million dollars with no money and no team? The contra we'd lined up would never be enough on its own. Cousin John knew the answer, but like any good mentor, he needed me to work it out for myself. It seems obvious to me now, but at that time I couldn't tell the forest from my knees.

CHAPTER 26

COUNTDOWN TO LAUNCH

After the meeting with John I was due up in Canberra. I hadn't told Connie about Bendon falling over because I was too busy sucking my thumb in a corner like a pathetic little wimp, but there would be no way around it once we caught up. She would invariably ask for an update.

Connie wasn't well at the time. She was on some drug that puffed up her face pretty severely and I called her Moon-Face, for we were both Enid Blyton junkies as kids. I remember thinking that it might hurt her feelings, but you have to be kept honest in our family, it's the rules, like with most true Aussie families. I do what I do best and put the blinkers on at the sight of Connie's ill health. No matter how sick she gets, I just tell myself she's having a bad day and will feel better tomorrow. Mike was busy with the kids so I was on bath duty. The bath is one of the few places Connie has that really helps alleviate her pain, so she was in there, bubbles and all, and we were talking things through. I told her it fell over. I told her I was out of aces. I noticed the scars from her double mastectomy and looked away. I told her I couldn't see a way out, I'd used everything I had and it just wasn't enough. I brought up again that I didn't want to be away from the family for a year.

'Sam, this is bigger than us.'

She was right. While I was riding the emotion of it, she was thinking outward.

'As a family, we've said all we've got to say.'

She was right there too. We had found enough time over the last few years to establish a love devoid of any past grievances. But it didn't change my thinking that we couldn't make the trip work. I was, of course, looking for her to say, 'It's alright, Sammy, I know you tried your best', and I'd be off the hook. She had no such plans, of course.

'I know I'm not allowed to say this . . . but I'd be really upset if this didn't happen.'

Damn straight she wasn't allowed to say that. I hurtled straight towards indignation and made it extremely clear that she wasn't allowed to lay it on after the effort I'd put in. If I said we were done, I didn't say it lightly. I can be quite bullish at times, and it's a brave person to challenge me while I'm in the middle of 'making my point', but Connie faces up to me in the same way I do to her, and she wouldn't be deterred. She also knew not to fight fire with fire and lightened the tone. Ever hopeful and quite brightly, Connie said, 'What about we go back to the Bendigo?'

What the actual fuck? We had approached Bendigo Bank a year earlier and they had passed. Why go back? What, were we now going to re-approach all the companies that had said no? It seemed madness to me. I was just through 12 months of pitching the thing dry, and now she wanted to go again? I was no such glutton for rejection and had no intention of matching her optimism.

'You can if you like but I really don't see the point.'

Out of hand was where I left it.

—

She did, of course, raise a salient point. The Bendigo Bank was high on our list from the start for a reason; we share a similar community engagement ethos and they had established contacts within the communities we'd be going through. It was exactly the thing that John had told me we needed. It was a perfect fit. Of course I had no chance of seeing that at the time.

A couple of days later, well after I'd harrumphed my way back to Melbourne, I came to respect Connie's handling of me. She was right. It was too important to lose. Of course it would be upsetting if it didn't happen. We had done too much to throw it all away. It's a good sister who can talk me off the ledge, because when I convince myself of something I usually cling to it as gospel, for good or for bad. I'm lucky to have a sister who doesn't really tolerate defeatism, for sadly, it's long been too prominent a feature of my 'temperament'.

I was dodging most of my training commitments, sending the odd email, avoiding my phone and teetering far too close to the objectionable. I knew I had to reload, but I lacked my typical vigour. Henry had been over for ages, and he never gets the hint. Then I got the call.

Connie called to tell me that the Bendigo Bank wanted to meet. Turns out that her local branch manager, Ralph Hawkins, took it to his contact at Head Office, Callum Wright, who had loved the idea from the start, but they were flat out with bushfires, floods and drought all across the east coast and just didn't have the capacity to help at the time. Mother Nature had since abated and they had a bit more room to move now. He was glad 'we' had come back to them. There was nothing else to do but look for the nearest hat. Connie hadn't given up, and she was facing a death sentence. I felt like a proper sook.

We met up and Bendigo Bank offered us an official partnership. They would manage our banking needs and provide their community branches with an opt-in to hold fundraisers for Love Your Sister in the lead-up to and upon my arrival in towns all along the way for the entire year. Some branches would inevitably pass, due to their existing community commitments, but they were confident that the take-up would be quite high. Bendigo Bank have managed hundreds of appeals and boast an impressive record of connecting with communities. If you coupled the Bendigo Bank deal with our plans to independently engage with councils, cancer support groups, information centres, schools and community groups, we were starting to look the goods.

Connie had scored us a major community partner that would help shoulder the considerable load of trying to raise a million bucks, right when it counted most. She gave me a proper lesson in persistence, which I would need to learn from if there was a chance of completing the challenge she'd set me. It provided the necessary fillip and I got straight back on the horse.

Cousin John drove me to Bendigo for the meeting in his white Calais. I looked into the passenger side window and there I was, quite literally beside myself. It had been more than two months since the Bendon deal had collapsed. We had breached our start date twice. We had been at it for nearly 15 months. The future of the event depended on Cousin John's reaction to the Bendigo

Bank deal. On the drive up I couldn't help but feel that this was our last play. Cousin John wouldn't entertain it forever, and Connie wouldn't be around forever either.

All that really mattered was that the Bendigo Bank team outlined to Cousin John, very clearly, all the ways they could help. It was all he needed. On the way home, after we had dissected the meeting together, I threw it out there. 'So is that a green light?'

I looked across at Cousin John. He nodded almost imperceptibly and gave me the smallest of smiles. 'Go for it.'

—

When I set about building Love Your Sister I made the mistake of only considering the event in two forms. To me, it was always an event that was either 'supported', or 'unsupported'. I would either do it with the help of sponsors and a full support crew or I would do it solo and unassisted. I thought I was a long shot at achieving the distance un-supported and was realistic about how severely it would reduce my chances. Even if I did somehow complete the distance solo, the fundraising and awareness would suffer greatly. It would become almost solely about survival. Our primary aim never had anything to do with unicycling, in fact, unicycling doesn't even rate a mention until you reach our *third* stated goal. If the unicycling was all I could manage, then would it be worth it? There seemed to be no point in doing it for its own sake. I wasn't trying to prove anything to myself, it was about Connie's dream of trying to prevent one other family from experiencing the pain of saying goodbye to their kids. So I committed to doing the event 'supported', to give it the best chance. It was the percentage play. I applied my theory of only being as good as the people around you and sought out the best event management group

I could find. I went through dozens of candidates, all very well credentialled, before deciding on a mob that had worked with Jessica Watson and Oprah Winfrey on her tour Down Under. I can't budget for shit and I don't exactly have a lot of experience with corporate sponsorship or event management, so it was the right play to pull in people who knew more about the process than me, but the problem with going to the best, for anything other than advice, is that they cost the most. They budgeted the administration, operationals, PR and production costs at 288k, which required sizeable corporate commitments. Despite feeling strongly throughout the process that we were going in too high, I deferred to the 'experts' and ignored my adaptive unconscious. We didn't need 300k – what the fuck was I thinking? The 300k had been invented by event management companies that wanted to get paid! It wasn't all or nothing. There was a place in the middle of the two that, for 18 months, I'd been completely unable to see. Why blow a fortune on a Rolls when you can cover the same distance in the same time in a Datsun 180B?

Now that we didn't have to map the ride according to Bendon store locations as we weren't going to every Bendon store and didn't have to spend time trying to put big pink bras on all the 'big things' around Australia, we could concentrate on what *we* wanted to do. We were beholden to no one. Cousin John and Cousin Jamie had decided to place their trust in me and Con, and it was up to us. We could be *independent*! Grass-roots! Family-run!

And that's where Emma Rooke came in. Embo has been Connie's bestie for, like, forever. She's a Johnson really. Has been for years. I can hardly remember Em not being around. When Dad was alive she ran his business for him, and she's the first person Hilde and Connie call too. While I had built a solid enough foundation, I'm

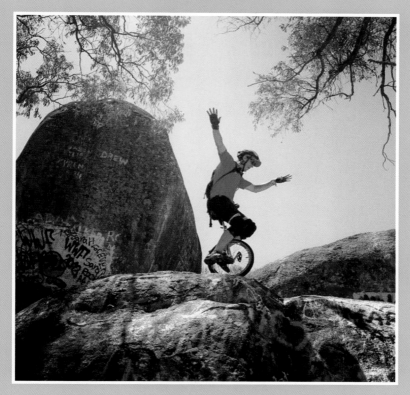

ABOVE: Sam proving his unicycle skills balancing on rocks at Stawell, Victoria. Still early days.

BELOW LEFT: Our trusty Boobmobile – merch storage on wheels.

BELOW RIGHT: Sticking to the far left of the road and fighting the wind.

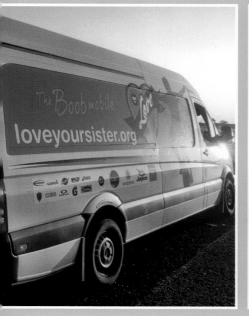

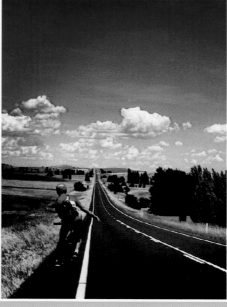

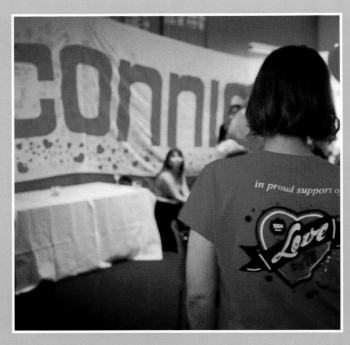

Getting ready for the Mornington Sisterhood event. This was the very first Sisterhood event to raise funds for Love Your Sister. It was the start of something good. And yes, that's my back!

BELOW: Every day on the road was different.

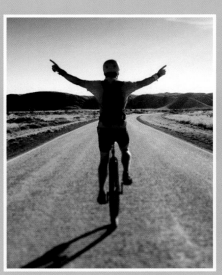

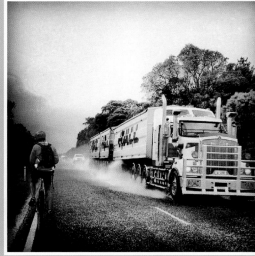

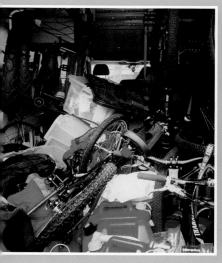

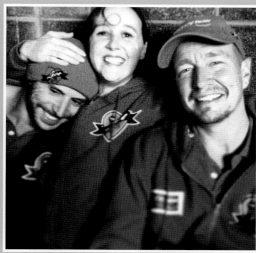

TOP LEFT: The inside of the Boobmobile looked like a bachelor pad threw up in a bike shop.

TOP RIGHT: Me with Al (left) and Leighton (right).

BELOW: Sam talking to students at a school visit in Albany, WA.

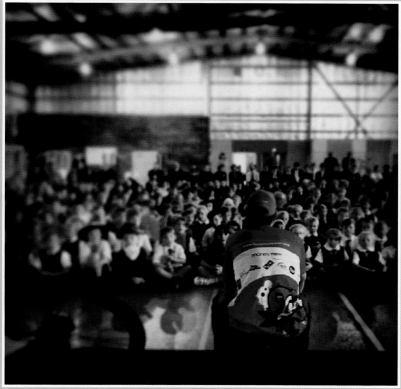

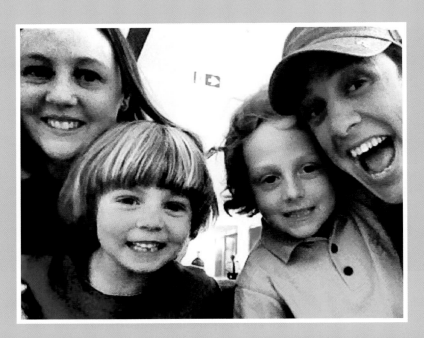

ABOVE: Me, Hamilton, Willoughby and Uncle Long Legs at a *Who Weekly* photoshoot in Canbe

BELOW: Hilde and Sam. I love my brother and sister!

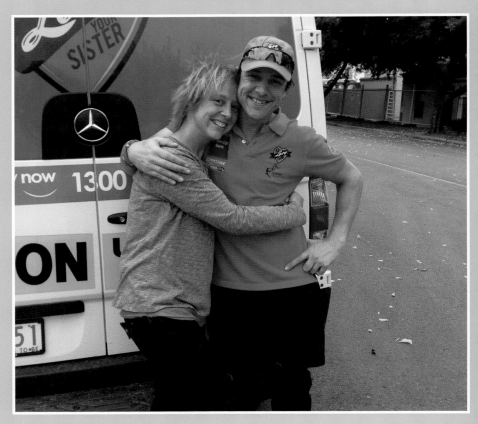

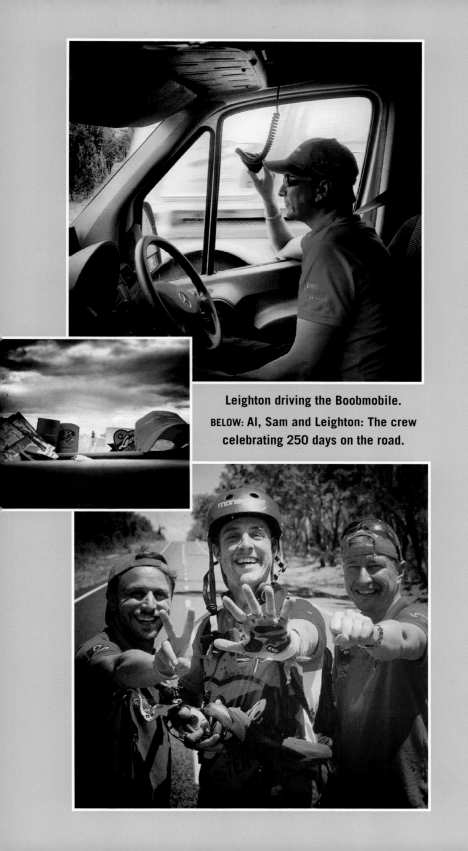

Leighton driving the Boobmobile.

BELOW: Al, Sam and Leighton: The crew celebrating 250 days on the road.

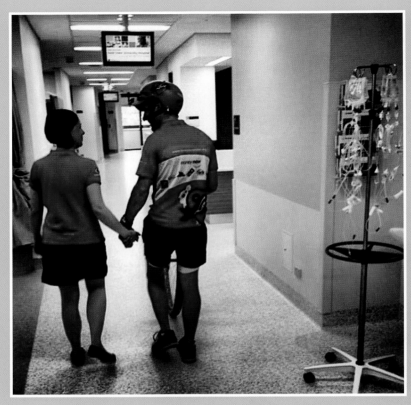

Me and Sam at the Gold Coast University Hospital.
Who says you can't ride a unicycle in a hospital corridor?

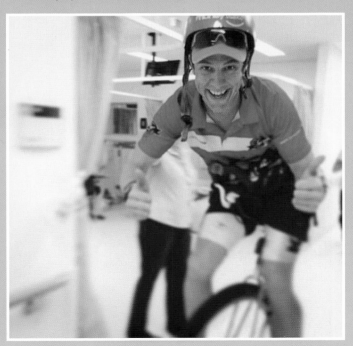

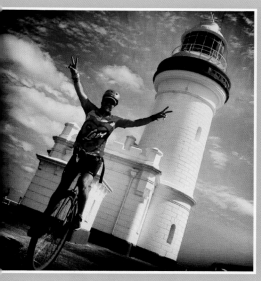
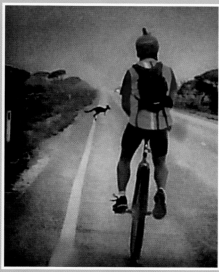

ABOVE LEFT: Sam at the easternmost tip of Australia: Cape Byron.

ABOVE RIGHT: You had to keep an eye out for the locals on the Nullarbor.

BELOW LEFT: Skydive the Beach – me and Sam getting ready to skydive in Wollongong.

BELOW RIGHT: Sam hanging off the side of the Gordon Dam in Tasmania: the world's highest legal commercial abseil.

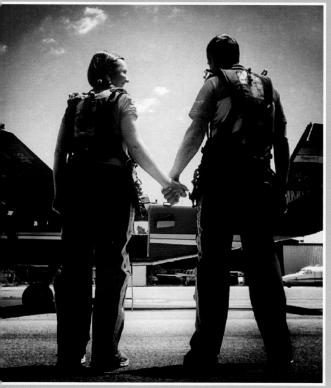
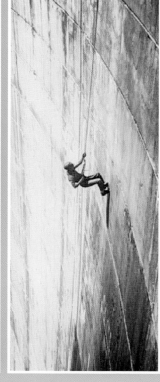

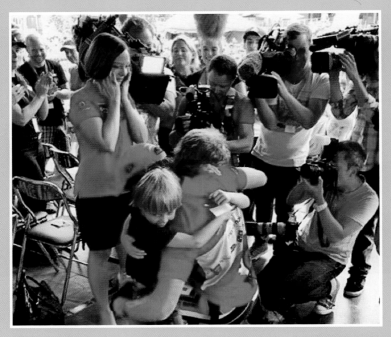

The return: the day brought a mixed bag of emotions for me and Sam. But I had my brother back.

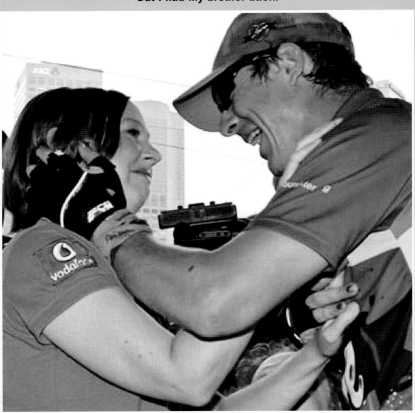

not the most organised person around and we needed someone to take it to that next level and that fell to Embo, again, to help save the day. I'll eat a small portion of my hat if she doesn't care about our family more than we do! She had a fulltime job, but that wasn't going to stop her. She'd finish at her paid job and then work into the early hours on Love Your Sister. All of our partners got used to their emails being replied to overnight. It didn't take long for Cousin John to see that we couldn't survive without her and he sponsored her to become Love Your Sister's administrator. After months of no sleep, she was able to leave her job and throw everything our way. Schedules. Mapping. Logistics. Fundraisers. Community events. School visits. Accommodation. Food. Fuel. Vehicles. Safety equipment. Tools. Camping equipment. Satellite phone. Merchandise. Uniforms. Signage. Two-way radios. Water. Printing. Web design. Social media. Collection tins. First aid. Motorbike licences. Sponsorships. Public relations. Embo took control of all of it. In Embo we trust!

The few weeks leading up to departure were a heady mix of nervous anxiety and sheer terror. I was out of outs. We were all doing a lot of different things for the first time, and plenty went wrong. I didn't have enough time to train properly during this period, so a lot of my physical preparation was undone in the immediate lead-up. We were totally exhausted by the time the event started, but eventually the day came . . .

PART III

DISPATCHES FROM A UNICYCLE & NOTES FROM HOME BASE

15 FEBRUARY 2013 — 13 FEBRUARY 2014

THE ROAD CREW

Samuel Johnson aka Uncle Long Legs – determined unicyclist

Jonathon Hinton aka JonBonJonno (Hilde's eldest son) – Jonno of all trades

Leighton Thomas aka Ley-Ley/Uncle Tippy/The Guru – bike mechanic/ driver/warhorse

Alistair Marks – director/producer/cameraman/sound recordist/ filmmaker/support/all-rounder

Stuart Liddell – cameraman/sound recordist/filmmaker/editor

Amanda Nelson – community liaison/organiser/Jill of all trades

Dion Szer, Nathan Wentworth, Gemma Green, Sarah Hallam – you gave us what you could when you could and we're really grateful for your amazing help.

All the crew volunteered their time, put their lives on hold and made massive sacrifices to make the Love Your Sister road trip happen. Sam and Leighton were on the road the whole time. Jonno, Alistair and Stuart alternated support and filming duties.

HOME BASE

Constance Johnson aka CJ – sister, mother, organiser, merchandise, media and bossy boots

Emma Rooke aka Little Miss Get-It-Done – everything but the bike stuff

CONNIE

Sam had done it! This was really happening. Several departure dates had come and gone, but this one was the real thing. He was actually leaving on a crazy year-long odyssey that we'd cooked up in my kitchen. The words had become a reality and I knew it was going to be everything we hoped it would be and so much more.

I went down to Melbourne to help out a week before the scheduled departure date. The boys kept asking me why I had to go away and wanted me to explain what Love Your Sister was and why I was doing it. It wasn't that easy to explain without telling them the brutal truth. They knew that Uncle Long Legs (Sam) and I were working together on a project to raise money for breast cancer. When I was explaining it to the boys, Willoughby said, 'Just like you, Mummy, 'cos you have breast cancer, don't you?' Oh, they are so innocent! They looked forward to the launch because they wanted to say goodbye and good luck to Uncle Long Legs before he left on his unicycle.

When I arrived in Melbourne, Hilde's house was taken over with the madness that is Love Your Sister and I realised that we had already achieved so much. To me it felt like Sam had already succeeded because it had been such hard work just getting him to the starting line!

Channel Ten did a big feature on us on *The Project*, and all of a sudden it seemed real. This wasn't just a brother and a sister working together on a little project anymore. Love Your Sister *was* real. It was a thing now. We had gone public, and there was no backing out. Sam had made a promise to me, and we had promised the country that we would do this. We had to follow through.

Just going on a camping holiday takes a lot of planning and preparation, so this, a year-long unicycling odyssey, was epic. It was like a camping holiday on steroids times infinity! This was four guys, four unicycles, a motorbike support vehicle, a Mercedes Sprinter van and a Jayco caravan going away for a year – with a message to spread, a record to break and a million dollars to raise.

I knew if we wanted people to listen to us, to open their communities, their hearts and their wallets to us, then we had to be professional. And we had to look professional if we wanted to gain the trust of a nation. I didn't think the iron-on logos on the cheap t-shirts that I had stayed up all night to make for the photo shoots were going to cut it, much less last through more than one wash, but they'd have to do.

SAM

Leighton's mind is like a computer. Mine is like a hornet's nest. I need Leighton. He's pragmatic, good with his hands, geographically savvy, mechanically gifted, has great recall, good people skills, a very solid work ethic and a positive disposition. No task is too small and he gets a buzz out of solving problems and saying 'yes'. About the only thing he can't do is cook. He's basically everything I'm not, and that's why I need him. I'm not looking at his weaknesses because I need his strengths. You're Only As Good As The People Around You and if I'm a chance to achieve this thing in a practical sense then I need people with a solid sense of self who can think their way out of any given drama. While I try not to let emotion sweep me away and concentrate on basics like behaving well without losing my shit, I need someone to actually help. He's the man. JonBonJonno is young, and he has Johnson blood, so he's never going to be the anchor we need. Leighton had shone during Lifecycle (my Sydney to Melbourne trip in '03) and there was never anyone else. I had approached him when the Bendon deal was looking like a goer and he had said no. He couldn't manage it. When I rang him a year later, with no money, no resources and nothing but a promise to have the time of our lives, he thought about it for 24 hours and came back to me with a yes. He had reached the top of his game in the bike world. The world's leading bike brand had hosted him and only a few other reps in Switzerland the year before and he'd been involved heavily in cycling, on all levels. He had a bunch of retail experience which would prove invaluable when it came to our community work, or even shifting merch. He was a retail master, and we needed someone up front to take the hits, because, while I was the flag bearer, I never had the set of skills he did, and they were skills that me and JonBonJonno needed help with.

CONNIE

Jonno, Leighton, Al and Sam had organised everything they thought they needed for the road. They covered things I hadn't thought of, like water storage, a back-up generator and a freezer. I did a quick inventory of the van. I inspected all of their hard work and I was impressed. They had custom built storage to house all of the merchandise they were taking with them, their living supplies and the motorbike and unicycles. There were shelves, hooks and plastic tubs. Everything was strapped down for safety. No one was going to get hurt if the boys had anything to do with it. Safety was their number-one priority. They had a juicer to make Sam healthy, unicycling-inspiring drinks, they had a sharp hunting knife in case they needed it (I never did understand that – or find out if it ever got used), first-aid kits and tools to repair the unicycles with. They had little trick bikes to take along for the kids to play with at school and community visits. But they didn't have any food! Or sheets! Or towels! Or toiletries! There was nothing in the freezer, and they hadn't packed anything to wear.

The bossy older sister/mother in me kicked in. I was horrified at the thought of the smell that four bachelors stuck in a caravan would generate. I started to worry more about communities smelling us coming than about generating interest in our event. At this point I was relieved I had the excuse of chemo, hospital visits and kids to look after, so I wouldn't have to go on the road with them!

Without wanting to make them feel bad, I pointed out there were a few other necessities to consider, like food. We had a gaggle of friends and family volunteering to help, and we called on every last one of them in the week leading up to departure. We sent friends off to the grocery store to buy heaps of healthy food, as well as long-life food that could be eaten with little preparation in the middle of the desert. Another friend went off to every op shop in the area to buy pots and pans, can openers and plates. Another went on a mission to buy the cheapest towels and toiletries available. Sunscreen and bug spray were stocked up on.

With the help of Nat Clemmets and Nat Fielding, two inspiring young women who went through my first cancer journey with me, we managed to get the caravan stocked with everything we could think of that the boys might need to get them through the first couple of weeks. Nat and Nat are both cancer survivors who have gone on to have families of their own and lead amazing lives. Both have struggled with numerous health problems resulting from the side effects of the treatment we had as kids, but have faced these with strength and fortitude. Both had also been helping in a huge way with preparations for the Love Your Sister launch.

It was 10 pm on the night before it was all supposed to start and we were all cutting up vegies. Every pot in Hilde's house was being used to cook some big batch of food or another. Then we realised we needed containers to put it all in, so someone rushed off to the supermarket. They were given a list of last-minute things to grab at the same time, like batteries. Amid all the chaos a photographer turned up to take 'last night' celebration photos. We still had to pack the van!

Then Em pointed out we needed signs to advertise the merchandise the boys would sell on tour and price lists had to be made. Paper, scissors, paint, textas, and every spare shoebox we could find were employed to make the price signs and display boxes.

The van was packed, repacked and packed again. How was all this stuff going to fit? How were they going to be able to access any of it? It was an exhausting, logistical nightmare and we were all running on pure adrenaline. We were ironing logo patches on clothes (printed at the last minute by Ian at Copperhead Screen Printing) at midnight. At one point someone asked, 'What about wet weather gear?' That set more people off on searches for raincoats and the like.

There were about 30 of us rushing around when our cousins rocked up to celebrate with some champagne. It was the only time during the whole preparation period where we all stopped and gathered as a group. Jamie toasted the year ahead and we all took stock of what we were working on. It was pretty humbling that so many people had stepped up to help me and Sam make this happen.

We finally accepted that if there was anything else to be done, we hadn't thought about it and even if we did then there was nothing we could do at this late stage, so we all crawled into bed, onto couches or the floor for a nap at about four in the morning.

We got 90 minutes sleep before the alarm sounded and we were on. Sam and I had back-to-back media to do. We showered and got into our uniforms as quietly as we could, then tiptoed around all the sleeping bodies and snuck out to get to the radio interviews.

I fell asleep in the car, and was woken when Sam whispered to his girlfriend, Sarah, 'I can't believe this is actually happening.' I was dozing, but listened to their conversation. Sam told Sarah he was feeling worried and wasn't sure he'd done the right thing. 'What if something happens to Con while I'm away?' His words flowed in a gentle whisper. 'I'm going to miss everyone so much.'

It hit me then that this was one of the last times we'd be together for a year, and that was if I survived the year. I started to feel a bit sick and anxious at the thought. I took a deep breath and tried to focus on the moment I was in and to not think too far ahead. Our first radio interview was in about ten minutes so I had to pull my thoughts together.

I was hopelessly nervous about being interviewed on live radio, such a contrast to Sam, who, as a voice-over artist, heard himself on radio stations all over the country every day. I was surprised that morning because Sam seemed nervous too. I told him how weird it was to see him, an actor and stage performer with 20 years' experience, looking anxious. He let me into a little secret, telling me that the nerves never go away but that was a good thing, because if you're nervous it means you care. He reminded me to be light and irreverent. 'Don't depress them, inspire them, make them laugh.'

I wondered how I was going to be light, engaging and funny when talking about cancer and death and he read my mind. He said, 'This is about life, it's about finding meaning in the madness, it's about making something positive out of something negative, it's a happy story.' He was right!

As we were shown through a rabbit warren of corridors and offices to the studio, I was getting more and more nervous. I got to meet Dave Hughes, who I find hilarious, gregarious and charming, and Kate Langbroek, an entertainer whom I have followed and adored for years. I clasped my hands together in front of me to stop them shaking.

The interview came and went in a blur of excitement and anxiety. Kate and Dave were so nice and accommodating, and they were genuinely excited and inspired by Love Your Sister. They asked questions that were easy to answer and are expert interviewers who know how to get good breakfast radio out of their guests, even if they are as inexperienced as me, so it all went without a hitch. Sam grabbed me and hugged me as we left. 'You did so well, you are born for this!' I was grateful for the praise and enjoyed it while we searched out a café. The

Old Paper Shop Deli is a long-time favourite of mine, and it had a TV, so we went in and found that they were playing *The Today Show*. Perfect.

A few weeks earlier, Karl Stefanovic had come to my house in Canberra to interview Sam and me about Love Your Sister, and it was going to air that morning. We ordered and sat down in a good pozzy to watch the interview. Silence fell as the other customers and staff realised that the people on the TV were in the café with them. Everyone stopped and watched the telly and people kept glancing over at us watching ourselves. It was a surreal experience, something I'd never experienced before. I thought this was normal for Sam but Love Your Sister means so much to him that it really mattered to him how people saw us. He cares so much about this project. The piece finished and a customer clapped, looking at us with tears in his eyes, then everyone started clapping. People came over to us and hugged us, handing over five- and fifty-dollar notes, whatever they could afford. Before we'd even launched we had raised a few hundred dollars, and the café gave us our brekky on the house, thanking us for what we were doing. The fuss subsided and we were finishing up our breakfast when two girls in aprons came into the café. They were carrying huge bouquets of flowers and they headed straight for us. The owner of the florist down the street had been in the café when the piece had aired and was so moved that he wanted to contribute something. For the tenth time already that day, my eyes welled up. I was completely overwhelmed by the generosity of these people who had walked into the café at the same time we did that morning.

There were more interviews to do, so there wasn't much time to contemplate what had happened. We did an interview with Matt Tilley and Jo Stanley on Fox FM and again I was surprised by the level of interest in our 'little engine that could', and in my side of the story. I didn't really expect that anyone would want to interview me; I thought it would all be about Sam. He's the famous one. He's the interesting one. It felt nice that we were interviewed as a pair, and that I got to talk about my part in this. I was grateful to have new experiences that I'd never anticipated having.

Once the interviews were over we headed to Federation Square. I had my make-up done while Sam went off to talk to Chrissie Swan and Jane Hall on Gold FM. Preparations were well underway and the excitement was building. The Mornington Secondary College drum corps was there, practising for the big moment. Busloads of students arrived and hung about, waiting for the launch. People wearing pink started to arrive. I breathed a big sigh of relief. I hadn't realised that I was stressing about not having a crowd attend our big event until the sight of people arriving made me relax . . . a little. Although I felt sick with anticipation. It wasn't the chemo making me sick, it was the buzz!

Every moment of the day was planned down to the second. Brigitte Duclos and Molly Meldrum were hosting. I'd first met Molly when I was a kid with cancer so it was lovely to see him again and tell him that. The drum corps was providing the pomp and ceremony. Justine from The Village Agency was looking after all the social media and Tanya Singleton Event Services was coordinating the whole event. Kate Radford, make-up artist extraordinaire, made me feel like a movie star, so I felt less nervous about going out and talking in front of a huge crowd, not to mention the interviews for the news and documentary.

There was a heart-shaped path sectioned off, with the press in the middle and the public around the outside for Sam to ride through when he left the stage on his unicycle. A helicopter circled above with aerial photographers to capture the heart and the crowd.

The Boobmobile and the caravan were parked in the square, ready to follow Sam when he rode off. The merchandise stand was set up and staffed. Dion from Print Design Australia was there with all of our brochures and signage. Some of Sam's best friends from TV and radio had come and volunteered their time for interviews and endorsements. Claudia Karvan, Deb Mailman, Catherine McClements, Tottie Goldsmith, Jennifer Hansen, Jo Stanley and, of course, the brother of the year, Samuel Johnson, were all there for a photo shoot with the media. There was little old me in the middle. How out of place was I? Willoughby and Hamilton were in the mix, and while Willoughby seemed to take it all in his stride, little Hammy was a bit stunned, and who can blame him – so was I!

It had all happened because hundreds of people and businesses had helped us get here, for free. I had been involved in the planning, but I was still genuinely shocked by the magnitude of it all.

In the back of my mind a thought nagged at me. 'This is goodbye. I hope it isn't goodbye forever.' I was ushered to the stage for the ceremony and I could see Sam dressed in his riding uniform, ready to depart and I was overwhelmed with sadness. What had I done? Why did I say it was okay for him to go away for a year? What if I died while he was away and I never saw him again? We must be crazy. There was no time to wallow, it was all happening and before I knew it Sam was about to ride off. I buckled his helmet straps together and then sent him on his way.

Sam made it down the steep ramp and rode through the heart-shaped path in the crowd, high-fiving everyone on the way. Everybody was yelling and cheering, some people were crying. There were cameras everywhere. Before I knew what had happened, Sam had gone.

SAM

I thought finally setting out would be the best day of my life. All of the hard work over the last two years was finally coming to bear. All of my friends and family were together. But I had absolutely no idea how hard it was going to be to say goodbye. I've always done the 'ghostie' to avoid goodbyes. I'm that guy at the dinner or gathering who disappears without a word. I've always hated goodbyes. I don't know why I thought this would be any different.

The day itself was an amalgam of frenetic snapshots. Anxiety at no one turning up, fear that I'd fall at the first hurdle (a motorbike ramp coming down off the Fed Square stage), photos for everyone, smiles, thank yous, not enough time to see my family and friends, so many news cameras (you mean this whole thing might actually work!), more people than I could poke a stick at, Mornington Secondary standing stoically through the heat (onya Mitch!), Molly anointing my sis with a pink akubra, my nephew Willoughby on stage, grabbing my hand and saying, 'Will you ride extra quickly so you can come back soon for me?', my sister and her amazing speech (I can't believe how much she makes me cry sometimes) and then that beautiful moment at the end where everything crystallised into one moment of colour and clarity.

The human tunnel! Riding through that love heart of people, all saying yay for Love Your Sister, gave me an incalculable amount of joy. Hats off to every single person who came to Fed Square. What a send-off! Connie and I felt most special.

The first stop after 42 kilometres was Bacchus Marsh. I competed in an 'Apple Pie Triathlon' upon arrival. First leg – bobbing for apples; second leg, peeling and cutting; third leg, pastry, flour and sugar. Well, whaddya know if the whole thing didn't turn into a massive food fight!

I loved the challenges that communities set me along the way. We raised $500 that day and I had such a renewed faith in humankind. All types of people in all types of places and situations were stepping forward to donate. There's nothing more encouraging than having a carload of people pull over on the highway, rush out and shove notes in your tin. All of a sudden you don't feel your legs burning anymore. All of a sudden you're not wondering whether you've bitten off more than you can chew. All of a sudden you're drowning in joy and generosity. It made my legs lighter and it lifted the whole team too.

We were having all of the teething issues you'd expect us to have at this point. One of our caravan cupboards was a little loose, which resulted in tomato paste EVERYWHERE! We hadn't quite managed to get the water going. Our storage system was barely coping (invariably what you need is at the back and bottom of a pile), we were still trying to get our freezer to freeze properly, my body wasn't coping as well as I'd have liked and we didn't meet our kilometre quota on day three, but all of that kinda stuff would iron itself out in due course.

I competed in a Tim Tam challenge and found out that I could balance 15 or so packs of Tim Tams in my hand while on the unicycle! Afterwards I met a guy called Dimitrios. He lost his sister to breast cancer at the same age as I was then and he brought along something for me to sign. It was the tie he wore at her funeral. I didn't want to wreck his beautiful tie, but he wanted me to, so I signed the back of it. That way he could still wear it. He still missed her pretty badly and my heart bled for him. It was meeting other people, also directly affected by breast cancer, that was wrecking me.

In a good way, of course.

—

On the fourth day of the ride, riding from Beaufort to Ararat, I realised what I'd got myself into. The heat alone was crippling enough, without the northerly headwind! The cramps went to another level, despite my best efforts. I was unsteady on the bike and the mind games started. If I was tired now, what chance did I have? Had I really thought this through? What made me think I could do this? There was only one thing to do. Shut that crap out and soldier on. So I did. And I got there. Eventually! I knew I'd have to get a lot tougher if I was a chance going through the desert in a couple of weeks' time.

—

My, oh my, did Dimboola turn on a cracker show! This was a town with a very healthy sense of humour, my friends. Police escort into town – dingaling!

The main drag was closed off and lined with locals. We pulled out the trick bikes and the usual kid-frenzy ensued. I met the locals and shimmied with the Bendigo Bank team. Then, the moment

I'd been waiting for: The Emu Challenge! A horse float backed in. The emu was clearly ill-tempered, judging by how loudly it was thrashing about inside the float. I was pumped. But then I got worried. If this emu was feeling a bit testy, then what about all of the kids milling about?

'What about the kids?' I asked.

'This emu doesn't mind kids,' someone shouted back.

I didn't have time to give it a second thought as the ramp on the float was being lowered. I scooted off quick smart and after a few nervous moments, turned back to see . . . a guy dressed in an emu costume running after me.

COMPLETELY HOODWINKED!

Like the whole Santa Claus thing, I wanted to believe, I suppose. Then it was straight off to the lawn bowls club for a roll. The locals were in such bloody good spirits and it was infectious. Massive lid tip to the Brittons for making us feel so at home after an incredible day of family, laughs and community.

—

I never realised how much the community engagement would affect me. It just went straight through my heart. Sweating it out on a unicycle was such a tiny price to pay for the chance to engage with communities on a truly meaningful level. Channel Ten's *The Project* crossed to us in Nhill's Jaypex Park and that was absolutely nerve-wracking. Then we had a sheep-shearing challenge. Chippa the sheepologist kept everyone entertained while poor Josh (gun shearer) had to take me, the city-slicker, through it step by step. I did terribly, but it didn't matter.

The trip was already full of things I'd never have experienced otherwise. All these firsts tickled me pink, I tells ya.

When the Kennedy family dropped over a pav after it all was over I thought, if I die tomorrow, I die a contented man.

—

Arriving in Radelaide was a big milestone for the boys and me. It marked our first inter-city leg and went a long way towards proving we had what it took to get the job done. We needed this milestone. Melbourne felt like a world away. The leg to Darwin would be another issue entirely, but getting to Radelaide unscathed and having missed only one engagement (which was re-scheduled) proved a confidence builder going into what would be perhaps the toughest section. Cousin John, Cousin Jamie, Hilde and Connie were all scheduled to converge, along with Al, my filmmaking buddy, who had been on board since the very early days.

Our timing couldn't have been better. We arrived at precisely the same time as two of Adelaide's most iconic events – The Garden of Unearthly Delights Festival and the Clipsal 500, so we were across two of the city's most popular sporting and cultural events. Because Mel van Deventer is a PR guru, we had a broad bank of media commitments across the entire visit. In fact, it felt as if we were scheduled to speak to just about every media outlet in the city. I was pumped about getting some serious fundraising done and excited by the challenge of raising money in a big city.

I really didn't anticipate it not going well, but from the moment I arrived I was anxious. Henry started babbling. Nobody warned me about the possible culture shock and I felt dumb for not expecting it. Though I'd only been gone from a big city for 17 days, I'd effectively gone to another world and I didn't realise the sensory overload that re-engaging with a thriving city would induce. The schedule was hectic, but that wasn't the problem. I hid my anxiety during media calls and functions, but I was an absolute mess in between. My brain didn't keep up. And when I get stressed I internalise until I boil over.

Al was an easy target. He'd not been on the road with me and he'd pissed me off by taking too long to turn shit around, so I virtually massacred my relationship with him over the course of the visit. When I wasn't giving him shit I was giving him nothing. Although I had a point, I made it shamefully. I went into the red zone where everything I did and said came from a place of intense emotionality. I couldn't see reason and I got incredibly overwrought. Connie became invisible to me, I was so inward. The only time we spent together was doing press or functions and I somehow thought that was enough. I didn't even consider catching up with her to see how she was.

I felt for Mel and her family having to deal with me so blustery and tempestuous, but they handled us so kindly and seemed to somehow understand the stress. I was glad to get out and face the desert in the end, hopeful of being able to redeem myself come Darwin.

CONNIE

Sam had been on the road for two weeks. Reports were filtering back to me about how he was, but it didn't give me a complete picture. He was so focused on getting from place to place and making sure everyone felt involved and part of Love Your Sister that he didn't have time for much else. I was busy back home but planned to catch up with Sam in Adelaide. I'd been told that Sam had cramps so bad at night that he couldn't sleep. I was concerned that despite all of his training this was going to be too much for his body to handle.

The dares and community engagement had been amazing, but there'd been scheduling errors and miscommunications about where to be and when. It was so hard for me to understand life on the road, and I know Sam and the boys had no idea what was going on back home.

We were getting emails and offers of help but we couldn't get through to the boys to coordinate new opportunities so they would fall by the wayside. The trip to Adelaide was going to give me a chance to meet up with the road crew and we could hash out any problems. I really wanted to get a real picture of where Sam was at and how he was coping with this brand new, crazy life. We were only at the beginning and it was already so hard to coordinate everything, I wasn't sure how we were going to get through the year.

One of the amazing offers we'd received was from a woman called Mel van Deventer. She headed up a public relations business and when she saw us on *The Project*, she Facebook messaged, offering to manage the Adelaide visit. Wow! Their generosity was amazing and Mel was only one of many people who would contact us out of the blue over the next 12 months to give us assistance, money, their expertise and their support.

Mel and her sister had connected with our story and they wanted to help us make a difference. And they did! Mel picked me up at the airport and she and Em worked out the whole program, including interviews on every radio station, a trip to the Clipsal 500 V8 Supercars Race (Love Your Sister logos were on some of the cars at the race), she coordinated a community barbecue, a visit to The Garden of Unearthly Delights, which is an incredible outdoor arts festival, and much more. Cities are so much harder to make things happen in than regional centres and Mel helped us tap into the communities within Adelaide to make our visit a successful fundraising and awareness-raising event for Love Your Sister.

I was there for six days and Adelaide turned it on for us! Bella, aka Lil Miss Macaron, baked hundreds of macarons and organised a stall to sell them at the Bendigo Bank, which was advertised with posters, on social media and on radio. Lil Miss Macaron and Jess at Buggy Boo Designs coordinated the fundraiser and donated their time and their merchandise to Love Your Sister. They raised an amazing $5000. It was an unbelievable effort from these two young mums who wanted to help out.

Despite all that was going on, the thing I most wanted was to connect with Sam. It didn't take long for me to realise this wasn't going to happen. The schedule was so jam-packed that he hardly had time to shower and eat, let alone sit and talk to me. I had to accept that I wasn't going to get to see him one on one. My first glimpse of real life on the road astounded me. I didn't know how Sam did it.

He travelled from one fundraiser to another, taking every media opportunity he could find and unicycled in between all that. Everywhere he went he'd get stopped by people wanting photos, wanting to donate or to have a conversation about their cancer experiences. And he always had a smile and time for a chat. He went hours and hours without even having time to go to the toilet or eat, he was literally that busy. Now I knew why he didn't have time to take a phone call when I wanted to organise something with him. He was so exhausted, but he never complained about being sore, busy or tired, not having any down time or only getting four hours sleep a night. He seemed to relish every experience and said yes to everything.

When I wasn't doing media or fundraisers, I took over Mel's kitchen and cooked up huge batches of food, dishing it up into portion sizes for the freezer. All the food we had cooked in Melbourne was already gone, and it wouldn't be too long before Sam and the boys hit the desert, so I was determined that they would leave with a freezer full of yummy nutritious food. Fifty-six containers of bolognese, chilli con carne, beef strog and tuna bake later, I was satisfied that I had done all I could on that front.

The boys were loving all the home cooking they were receiving on their travels. So many people cooked up meals or cakes and biscuits for the crew. Again I was blown away by people's generosity, and I started to realise that they wouldn't do these things for us if they didn't feel something for Love Your Sister, some kind of connection. So many people emotionally connected with our story because they had been affected by cancer in some way. It really is the cruellest disease and it doesn't discriminate. Young, old, mums, kids, dads, granddads, brothers, sisters – it impacts on so many lives and takes so many people away from their families. Sadly, there are very few people who haven't been touched by cancer in some way.

The plan was for me to only visit capital cities while Sam was unicycling, because that way I didn't have to travel long distances to regional centres and I could stay close to a big hospital, just in case. Being on chemo lowers a person's immunity and any infection can be life-threatening. During the planning of Love Your Sister, before the launch, I'd been struck by an infection and it had hit hard and fast.

It was 10.30 at night and I was just having a cup of tea and a chat with Mike. I was fine, but within 15 minutes I started to get a headache. By 11 pm I was unconscious. Mike called an ambulance and they took me to the emergency ward. I came to, briefly, and asked if I was dying. I don't remember the answer.

Next thing I knew I was in ICU and a team of doctors and nurses were working on me. One was holding my hand, stroking my head, telling me that they were doing everything they could to keep me alive, but they weren't sure I would make it through the night. He explained that my brain and kidneys were failing, that my system was shutting down, and nothing they were doing could get my blood pressure or oxygen up. I let myself rest, just hoping the pain would end.

After many days in intensive care, and weeks back on the ward, I slowly recovered, but I was weak and tired. The pain was severe and my face was all puffed up and swollen from the steroids that helped save me. The medical term for this particular side effect is Moonface, which caused Sam many a laugh from our childhood days of reading *The Magic Faraway Tree*.

This sort of emergency trip to ICU happened twice within six months, so I was afraid of being away from medical care, and Sam felt happier if I was close to a big hospital. So I had to live the regional sections of the trip vicariously through my brother. When faced with a terminal diagnosis it is hard not to think about the things you would have liked to have done before you die, and it gave me peace that Sam was going to see our country, and meet so many wonderful people along the way.

At least one of us was doing it! I was happy to see the photos and hear what was happening during the occasional phone call.

Before the trip to Adelaide felt like it had even begun, it was over and I was saying goodbye to my brother once again. He'd seemed distant but he didn't even have time for more than a quick hug before he was off again. I wouldn't see him again until Darwin and that was a lot of days and a lot of kilometres away. I knew I was going to worry about Sam and the boys in the desert. The thought of him riding through the exhausting heat and dealing with the flies and the isolation and God knows what else was at the front of my mind.

But despite all my worrying I knew he was going to make it, somehow. It would take more than a little heat and a few blowies to quash his determination.

Mel was driving me to the Adelaide airport when my phone rang. It was Sam.

'Hi, what did I forget?'

'When you left I realised that I didn't spend any time with you while you were here. I feel like I ignored you and we didn't get to talk. Now you're gone and I feel really bad.'

'It's fine, bro, really. Don't worry about it. I had no idea what it's like on the road for you. It's crazy.'

'I am such an idiot. What if you don't make it to Darwin? I'm a fool, why didn't I make the most of you being here?' he said.

'It's fine, really it is, and I WILL be in Darwin, I will see you there. And, Sam, I love you, and thanks for doing all this for me.'

'Love you too, Sis, see you in Darwin.'

My quest to get Sam on a path to a happier, more fulfilling life was underway, but after seeing how he was in Adelaide I knew we still had a long way to go.

SAM

The good folk of Wilmington did a ripper job of things. I met with the kiddlies at their primary school and they walked me to their rodeo, where I was promptly put in a pink tutu, with pink lippy and nail polish to boot. And that was just the entrée! Thankfully, they had selected a steer for me to attempt to ride, as opposed to a bull. Even so, it was quite frightening at first, but adrenaline soon kicked in and after my first ride, I was begging for more. Luckily they had brought three steers with them!

I was then encouraged to go along to their bowling club to relax. It sounded like fun after a long day. Little did I know that they had concocted a secret 'bush-tucker challenge' for me . . . to eat a live huntsman. I thought they were joking until Geoff pulled out a jar full of them. Now I'm seriously arachnophobic. Not just a little scared of spiders; a lot scared of them. It stems back to a childhood trauma, as many phobias do. I tried to get into the spirit of it, but I could barely hold the damn thing, let alone crunch away at it. But it was for a donation to the cause, and I'm the silly one who asked towns to dare me, so there was nothing to do but push on, chew it and swallow. It was one of the most traumatic things I've ever been involved in, but afterwards I felt strangely liberated. As if I could do anything!

No wonder . . . I had just conquered one of my biggest fears in one of the biggest ways possible. Thank you, Wilmington, for helping me rid myself of the 'city-boy' tag!

Disclaimer: This was the last time I'd eat anything alive. No similar challenges would be entered into henceforth!

—

My wheel cracked its way through the dust, powered somehow by me. One unicycle frame had already fractured, leading to a three-day wait and an exhaustive game of catch-up. Dust was in everything. Our cameras were cactus. We didn't shower because there was often no point or no way. I pushed on slowly and steadily, averaging 11 or 12 kilometres an hour, through baking terrain where everything was disused, dishevelled or disheartened. The further north I pedalled, the more stark it became. Bush dogs lay listless, helpless against the flies. The tumbleweed wasn't tumbling. I felt like a winning applicant on Mars One. Out there nothing wins against the Big Mother Nature. She rules the joint with a molten fist. The faint-hearted don't stand a chance.

And there was I, pedalling by on arguably the most absurd contraption in the world, in my pink lycra, sporting bright pink nail polish courtesy of a dare from the local ladies in Clare, a surprisingly snazzy town further south that treated us to a cracking fundraiser and the most beautiful B&B I imagine I'll ever stay in.

My fetching pink nails proved quite the conversation starter the further north I travelled. Most of the outback towns we rolled through offered powered sites through their service station or pub. Our generator was being a little temperamental in the dust, so we stayed at pubs and roadhouses wherever possible, to keep the caravan, freezer and all of our comms charged. Sometimes we'd rather have stayed overnight in the middle of the desert, away from the townships, and sometimes we did, but power was vital and we needed to never forget our primary aim of raising awareness, *especially* in remote areas, even if sometimes it was a bit hard to blow the trumpet after a full day in the heat.

Where there was power, there was beer. It wasn't hard to trigger our community engagement plan in a town of 12 – they were all at the pub, or at the bar in the roadhouse. It was not like we were going to walk up to everyone with a brochure; the only effective way to get the word out was to sit at the bar, have a beer and wait for a yarn to unfold with the locals. The pink nail polish did the trick. Over and over I got told to take my nail polish off before I rode to the next town, because the folk there weren't quite so . . . understanding. The badness never seemed to exist where we went. It was always at the town down the road.

Not a lot of people know this, but the outback is full of young French women. It sounds outrageous, but I swear it's true. See for yourself. Drive from Adelaide to Darwin and you'll find a French woman running almost each and every roadhouse, bar or bistro along the way. Hang around at dusk and you'll meet a bunch more from cattle-station postings, clutching their beers in undisguised celebration at surviving another day in the desert. It's all courtesy of some visa stipulation that requires four months of labour in regional or remote areas. There was something special about unicycling through the outback desert for a day and then sitting down and ordering a beer in French . . .

As I rode up the guts of the country, I met all sorts. Weird desert-loving maniacs; travellers trying to get as far away from home as they could; folk who had finally found a place where no one asked too many questions; workers away from their loved ones; desert kids who had never known anything else; truckies who had seen it all to the umpteenth; mums that never once thought they'd end up out there; drifters who didn't care where they went; woofers chasing bread; grey nomads either showing grace in age or bickering the house down; maintenance guys and servicemen and women out with the Big Mother making sure shit still worked; other enduro-freaks like us and, of course, internationals doing their rural time to score their visas. So many transients, all sharing stories in bars in dusty-as-fuck outposts on the tail of a brutal summer.

JonBonJonno was 24 and in his absolute prime, so it was only right that he shared our message with the travellers. Leighton and I had been where JonBonJonno was, during Lifecycle in 2003, and we played our cards differently this time around. While JonBonJonno flirted with the exotic, Leighton and I found the local who had been there the longest. The true local. That local is invariably more unassuming than the travellers and tends not to impose. There's more at stake for the true local; they've got to live with the consequences of their actions whereas the travellers are out by morning with nothing to lose. The true local knows the politics of the place, the way the place *feels* about any given issue. Spot the true local who's been there longest and more often than not, as long as you're respectful, they're up for a chinwag. You can be down with it in under an hour; the neighborhood disputes turned violent, workplace mishaps, who's fucking who that they shouldn't, legal battles, land battles, stock battles, weather battles, guys with guns and lost minds, the broken and bankrupt, manhunts, those who vow earnestly never to come back . . .

Everything was amplified by our surroundings. The environment demanded it. Nothing was easy out here. Even the seemingly simple act of going somewhere for supplies could dramatically unfold into a 48-hour saga where lives became genuinely threatened. I come from the suburbs where I get bummed if they don't have my favourite flavour of ice-cream in stock, and I'd never been away from home for more than a couple of months before, so I was finding it all quite the eye-opener. At least when I travelled I knew how to get to know a place, thanks to Leighton. I'd strike up a robust conversation with someone who'd been there for ages and, above all else, be curious.

Riding into Parachilna with the biggest full moon I've ever had for company, I could smell a memorable one coming along. Connie was with me every day, but on full moons she was much closer. As I was riding in I clocked a sign that marked Parachilna as having an official population of two, so I wasn't expecting much, just hoping for some kind of access to power, really.

It turned out that this little beauty of a town boasted a proud and rather stately pub, the only thing I'd seen in weeks that hadn't been incinerated by the Big Mother's molten fist. The Prairie Hotel stands strong and proud, the sandstone matches the desert perfectly – verandah, water troughs and wine barrels out front. There was an art gallery inside, and wi-fi. It was the genuine article with all the trimmings. On Friday night, they did great grub and before we knew it, there were at least twenty people in the place – a small handful of locals and a swag of transients like us.

Leighton and I went straight for the local who had been around the longest and found Trevor the truckie, who was from 'down the road a bit'. He could tell me the make and model of every truck that drove past on hearing alone, and who was driving the rig, to boot. His surname was Driver, for crying out loud. He rolled out some ripping yarns about some of the more colourful people in the area and in the squint of an eye, the moon had drifted and it was last drinks. Me, JonBonJonno and Leighton were left with Trevor Driver and the two beautiful women who ran the town. The fattest full moon and its millions of bright cousins meant it didn't even feel like night. I could see each pebble beneath my feet.

Leighton the master fact-finder had caught wind of a whisper about a haunted house, and after a few enquiries, we were off on a mission to talk with the dead. We clambered to a classic ruin, suitably dilapidated and full of clues to its past; it still had all of its contents, buried under piles of bush dust. Sure enough, I found an old newspaper article about a local 'accident' laid out on a rusty bed. I fished around a bit more and before I knew it the gang had scampered and I was alone. I stood in the ruin, indulged in a rollie and took it all in.

On the stroll back to town, Alex, a bright and witty young woman with strong local ties, dropped a bombshell. There was a staff-only pool and she was willing to open it up to us! We had been days in the dust, and nothing could be finer. A swim in the desert is exactly as refreshing as it sounds. Just when I thought it couldn't get any better, the ever-inquisitive Leighton, who had discovered Alex had a passion for the violin, started needling her to bring out her violin and play. She was shy at first, but our urgings had the desired effect and before long we were bookending the stillest of nights with some dancing classical violin being played by a beautiful true local, as we bathed in cool water under a full moon in the middle of the desert.

You can't buy that shit for quids.

I floated on my back, wondering what on earth I'd ever done to deserve such riches.

—

I simply loved riding my unicycle at night. Our community engagements required a daytime schedule, so it was only really when we had a long vacant stretch that I could switch the clocks and indulge in the night. Daytime may hold majesty, but night-time holds mystique. In the night I am as a child, curious and un-knowing, brimming with wonderment. Daytime brings details devilish and truths too clear, offering false protection. Night slowly camouflages the scars of the day at the behest of the sunset, which, to me, is less a magnificent splash to end the day and more a mere suggestion of the magic the coming night will bring. Sure, there's fear and uncertainty in darkness, but what of its peace and mystery? Its quiet? What of its ability to heighten your senses? I don't just sense better at night, I *feel* more. I'm more connected with my environment, more in tune with myself . . . more like that scruffy little boy I used to know who loved whizzing down hills on his bike that could fly. The boy Dad called Mister Happy.

A road train wrenched itself past me into the night ahead. The two-way radio clipped to my shoulder crackled into life, 'Shouldn't be on the fucken road at night, ya fucken bozo.'

Leighton was first, 'We're more visible at night. You woulda seen us from a fair way back.'

Then it was Jonno's turn. 'That's why we're on channel two, mate, to make sure everyone knows we're here.'

My turn. 'Less traffic at this hour too. You heard the call-out, didn't you?'

We all wait for the reply . . .

'Alright, have a good one, boys.'

I throw a rare look back at the boys, to see them all grinning as widely as me.

Contrary to occasional opinion, we were not a bunch of cowboys with a taste for carnage. What we were doing was absurd, and very unsafe, which is why we understood motorists' reservations, because we shared them ourselves. It was not exactly the wisest call to unicycle at 15 clicks an hour on a highway with 65-metre-long road trains, no emergency lane and a 110 km per hour speed limit, but it was not illegal and we took every precaution. We were absolutely convinced that night riding was safer. There was less traffic, which meant less double-ups, and paradoxically, there was better visibility at night – we had two yellow whirlybirds going, special flashing L.E.D.s on the rear of the Boobmobile, hazards on all vehicles, plus I was lit up on the unicycle with a front light, helmet light and flashing rear light. So we were pretty much a rolling disco, giving plenty of notice to all around, including animals, that there was a hazard nearby.

Oh yeah, and on the back of our caravan, it said 'CAUTION, UNICYCLIST AHEAD!' in large reflective lettering. Safety was at the forefront of everything we did and our biggest fear every day was somebody getting hurt.

I didn't prefer night rides just because they were safer and less busy. My body preferred nights too, not only because I didn't get hot at night, but because of the slope, or camber of the road. Obviously, roads are built convex so that rain runs off them. During the day I was usually as far left on the road as I could get, where the camber of the road is greatest. This means that I rode with an awkward lean to compensate for the angle of the road, so my legs rode straight, but my torso was twisted in counterbalance. At night I rode evenly along the middle of the road where it was flat and my back could stay straight. Instead of feeling hostage to the traffic and hugging the left, as I did most days, at night I could feel almost complete ownership over the road. I could drift across its entire width if I cared to and sometimes I did, just for the freedom that going all squiggly brought.

So I loved nights because they were safer and less busy. I loved nights because they straightened my twisted back. I loved them because there were no interruptions – I was in a selfie-free zone with freedom to determine my own cadences. And I loved the night for sating my nocturnal yearnings and making me curious again.

But the real beauty of the night lies in its relationship between time and distance. While the night heightened my primary senses, it distorted my sense of time and space. The daylight provided an excess of clues and markers, so it was really hard not to gauge the distance in your mind, which created a longer ride. I ended up with a perpetual numbers game in my head.

At night, there were fewer markers, which made for less numbers, and when there were less numbers, time became looser. I was not measuring time, distance or pain, because the night disguised all of the yardsticks. So I kind of floated more because everything was more fluid and less exact. I was just riding, and before you knew it I'd travelled further and longer than I imagined possible. I'm no astronomer, and I can't read the stars or the moon, but even if I could have, I wore a peaked hat at night because it cut off the stars, which could distract me with their beauty and cause me to fall, which happened in Week One.

So I was at least 20 or 30 kilometres away from the two-way cackle with the truck driver. It was after 2.30 am and the boys were at the place where coffee no longer helped. The radio was silent. I was feeling fabulous, of course, with all that crisp night air and freedom to move, cutting my way through one of the best nights of my life. I pedalled over the crest of a hill and immediately noticed what looked like a car stopped a few hundred metres ahead to the right. I thought I saw it clearly enough, for my eyes were well adjusted to the night at this hour and I was aided by the Boobmobile's high-beams behind me, but the night robbed me of any great detail. As I rode closer I confirmed it was a car and noticed that the headlights were off, but the cabin light was still on. This wasn't just another abandoned car.

I pedalled closer still. I thought I could see a figure standing on the road. The boys started nattering, the radio suddenly awash with conjecture. I started to wish that we weren't so well lit, so I could glide up silently on my unicycle and get the jump on what was happening.

I mean, something had to have gone wrong for a man to be standing in the middle of the road at 2.30 in the morning, right? A split second of apprehension was cast aside – this was why I was out here, wasn't it? To see what really goes on in this mad, grand land of ours? And that was when I noticed it.

The man was holding what looked like a stick in his right hand. I hesitated. We had the numbers. It was like snakes, I told myself – they were always more scared than you were. But then I realised that it wasn't a stick, it was definitely not a stick. It was a baseball bat.

There was a man, standing in the middle of the road, in the middle of nowhere, in the middle of the night, *holding a baseball bat*. I was so close to him by that stage that there was no pulling out. This was just an everyday welfare check, I told myself.

'Howz it going?'

'Been better.'

As I pulled up I noticed a kangaroo on the ground beneath the man. I walked closer to see the kangaroo, completely disabled but still very much alert.

'Did you hit it?' I ventured.

'Nah. Just put it out of its misery.'

'Right thing to do.'

He was hesitating though. He seemed a little agitated. I was thinking he might be having trouble building up the courage.

I offered him an out. 'I'll do it if you want.'

'Nah, I got it.'

And that's when I noticed. He was wearing cotton gloves. White cotton gloves. Seemingly brand new white cotton gloves. I looked straight up at his eyes, which were focused hard on the beast. He raised his arms and brought the bat down in an almighty swipe. It was the cleanest, most cracking shot you could imagine, landing flush on the side of the skull. The sound sits with me now as clearly as it did then. It was another of those sounds I'll never forget, like when my dad wept on the couch after Connie first got sick.

The man moved almost professionally back to his car with the baseball bat under his arm, removing his new white cotton gloves carefully as he walked. He didn't acknowledge us at all. We muttered a couple of awkward pleasantries and we were out of there.

A few hundred metres down the road and I threw a look back. The car was still sitting there, cabin light on. All of us agreed that the sound had really shocked us. No one was expecting him to use as much force as he did and the resultant sound had effectively split the night. We were up and about after that one! I couldn't stop thinking about it as I pedalled away. I began to think that he wasn't agitated for the reason I thought he was. It wasn't that he had been struggling to go through with it. He was agitated because we had interrupted his *process*. His enjoyment of it. By offering to take care of it myself, I'd forced him into action before he was ready. I screwed with his timing and, in a way, killed his thrill.

Either that or he was just a bloke on the side of the road, doing what was right . . .

CONNIE

It's hard not to worry about your brother when he's in the middle of the desert, riding a unicycle, sharing the road with trucks so long you can't see the back of them. Vodafone had kindly offered to cover all of our phone expenses for the event, and put us on to Pivotel, who also climbed aboard 'our little engine that could', supplying a satellite phone for those areas where a smart phone just wasn't enough. This gave me great peace of mind, but I didn't realise that using a satellite phone was any different from using a mobile. Neither did Sam! Apparently, you have to be outside, you have to extend the aerial and point it to the heavens, or more accurately, the satellites.

Sam wouldn't have been worried about anything more than getting through the heat, the flies and the kilometres, so I was not sure if it was even switched on and charged a lot of the time. After days of trying all of the crew phones and the satellite phone regularly, I started to get worried about him and the crew, and really wanted to just check in and see that they were all okay.

So, it was back to a bygone era for us; to the old bush telegraph we did resort. Em and I jumped on 'The Google' and looked up every roadhouse, pub and petrol station within 400 kilometres of where they might be at that point in time, divvied up the phone numbers and started to ring around to see if anyone had seen Sam.

'Hi, this is Connie ringing from Canberra. I'm just wondering if you've seen a unicyclist at all in the last couple of days?'

'No. Sorry, love, can't help ya.'

Many of the calls went that way until we rang a roadhouse in the middle of nowhere. I repeated my crazy-sounding query, reassuring myself that they'd get calls like this from time to time out there.

The woman who answered said, 'Hang on a sec.' Then she called out to everyone there, 'Has anyone seen a unicyclist around these parts recently?'

I heard the crowd burst into laughter, then a lone voice answered, 'Yeah, Samuel Johnson. He's down the road a couple of days.'

We'd found him! And from reports on the bush tele, he was fighting fit. When we next spoke to him, we told him how to use the satellite phone, and thereafter we were able to rely on twenty-first-century technology.

SAM

The alarm harpooned my dreams at 3.30 am and I sat bolt upright. I woke up ready. That was one of the cool things about the trip . . . waking up ready. That never used to happen. The day was daring me, more than any other thus far, and I was not coming from a good base. The previous night's fundraiser in Leigh Creek had been a corker, but after finishing up there and prepping for the next day, it was well after one in the morning by the time I'd got to bed. I couldn't sleep because I was so nervous about the challenge ahead and so tired from the day before and the day before and the day before. The hugeness of our task had started to set in. I was beginning to realise that this thing we'd invented held absolutely no respite, and that I was always going to be tired and I was never going to have enough energy. But that excited me too. It wasn't meant to be easy. I needed to *relish* the tough bits. That was the whole point, right?

That day's ride was going to be epic. One hundred and eighteen kilometres down the road was a little town called Marree and I had to be at their local basketball court for a barbecue fundraiser by 6 pm. Sister June was bribing the locals with a free feed because she knew they wouldn't turn up otherwise. This one was not about the fundraising; it was a small Indigenous township where the issue of women's health was quite taboo, so I was looking forward to poking around in their business.

The weather bureau was again forecasting conditions of fucking hot, so there were no real surprises there. We planned to follow the Old Ghan Railway right up into the desert and to top it off, the bitumen would run out. I'd never ridden on gravel before so there was real doubt in my mind. I had no idea how much the gravel would slow me, or what toll it would take on my concentration or confidence, or even if I'd be able to ride through it properly. Well over half of the day's ride would be on gravel and I'd not ridden close to 118 kilometres in a day yet. I'd not even ridden a hundred. What I did know was that my body started to shut down after I'd ridden about 80–90 kilometres, so the day's last 30 was going to kill me and I'd have to bring it home in the hottest part of the day. I was not overly confident, to be honest; I had been absolutely hammered when I got into Leigh Creek the night before, but today was a new day and yesterday was no excuse.

JonBonJonno had hit his limit the night before and was wigged out a bit so I told him to rest up and meet us down the road late-morning with fresh supplies. The old warhorses, me and Leighton, would do the heavy lifting early. The town was dormant as we prepped our way through the dark; Leighton and I were both buzzing at the thought of conquering the day's milestones. We stacked the motorbike full of our pre-packed supplies, chucked in our big hunting knife for good measure (we were still at the stage where we went nowhere without it!) and we were off into the darkness with nothing but unanswered questions ahead.

As I pedalled out of town I realised why I was so jacked. It was fear. I was actually scared I wasn't going to make it to Marree. Fear's good, I told myself. It meant that I still cared.

We were not far down the road when traffic started to stream past us. Leigh Creek is a mining town and we were riding in the direction of the mine. It was all one-way traffic. A trail of mine workers passed us in their utes. A pre-dawn peak hour, one way, in the middle of nowhere and there I was, waving almost constantly back to every hand and honk. Once I rode past the turn-off for the mine we were well and truly on our own. I'd only ridden about 10 kilometres, and the sun was not even up yet, but fatigue started to hit, really bad. I panicked. There was 110 kilometres left to go, in the heat, with the gravel to come. The adrenaline of the late night and early rise had faded. I waved Leighton forward and he pulled up alongside me on the motorbike.

'I'm stuffed already!'

'Me too,' he screamed through his helmet.

I kept pedalling but my vision went all wobbly. I couldn't focus. I was crashing. My mind started unravelling. How could I possibly make it? It wasn't even dawn, the heat hadn't yet come and I was taxed to the max. I started to feel very uncertain on the unicycle. Two hours' sleep was never going to be enough. If I didn't stop, I'd stack it. Accidents happen around fatigue. I needed to sleep. Safety first. Willpower was getting me nowhere for once. My body literally shut down about 11 kilometres into the ride, with the first hint of the sun rising behind my right shoulder.

We curled up on the side of the road and slept where we'd stopped.

With the dawn came flies; Leighton put his motorbike helmet back on it was that bad, and I wrapped a garment around my entire head. Every now and then a car or truck stormed past and I thought to myself, through my delirious haze, how strange it must be to drive past a big unicycle, a motorbike, and two blokes curled up on the side of the road. Within minutes the sun was too harsh and the flies too dogged, but we'd managed to sneak in an invaluable 25 minutes of interrupted sleep and it was enough to push on.

Leighton was forever studying up on the areas we were passing through. Populations, elevations, the town's primary industries, important dates on the local calendar, landmarks, notable people from the area – nothing escaped his attention. For the past week he'd been regaling me with tales of Sir Sidney Kidman, the famous 'Cattle King', and his dream of running the Ghan railway all the way up to Darwin. It really was good having him around. He brought such groundedness. He has a real eye for detail and history and it balances my emotions out really well. Facts are what matters in Leighton's world; he finds security in them, he knows that information is power. I'm too busy reacting to everything emotionally to find such comfort in structure, but his inquisitive nature inspired mine and I was grateful.

Then we hit the gravel. Theories mattered for nought and all of our hypotheses were reduced to a mere roll of the dice. Thankfully, it was fairly manageable. Increased concentration levels were required and there was obviously more risk of mishap and injury, but I found I could get along alright. Once I'd travelled far enough along to convince myself that Marree was achievable, I pulled Leighton off the road for another break.

We were well into the day now and the heat for Leighton on the motorbike was probably unbearable, but he said nothing because we had a 'no whingeing' rule; besides which, he was too excited about the railway track running parallel to the long straight we'd stopped on. I was keen for one of Leighton's historical distractions and I followed him willingly across the road, over a fence and a hundred metres along through spinifex and crunchy ground to the track itself. We sat on the Old Ghan together, absolutely baking in the heat, no chance of shade, just revelling in the history of it, imagining what it would have all been like in its heyday.

A road train emerged from the horizon to our left. 'First truck on the gravel!'

Leighton loved trucks and I was beginning to see why. This trip was all about firsts; things we'd never seen or done before. I was lucky that Leighton had created a culture within the group that fostered a thirst for all things fresh and new.

It began with no sound, just a big lump on the horizon, warped by the heat, slowly edging towards us. The difference this time though was the dust cloud in its wake. Leighton and I just stared silently at it for the minutes it took to reach us. The sight and sound and speed slowly built into an intensified rush of raw horsepower, speed, and violent plumages of dust, volcanic in proportion. The earth shuddered under the force of so much tonnage.

Leighton and I decided instantly that watching a road train plough through a dirt road at a hundred k's an hour was one of the most beautiful and magnificent things we'll ever see. Not from the roadside, mind. From a good hundred metres back, where you can take in the whole scene. We eagerly waited for another truck, weighing the chances of seeing one before we had to get back in the saddle. I felt like I was somewhere in between a Dali landscape, a George Miller film and a Slim Dusty track. I didn't want to be anywhere else.

To our delight another road train appeared before I'd even half-finished my rollie. It slowed and lurched to a halt ahead of us, air brakes hissing, right where we parked our unicycle and motorbike. The driver hopped out, scanned, spotted us on the tracks and pulled a textbook beeline. It might as well have been Lee Kernaghan striding towards me. He was young and upright, strong and manly. Jeans, buckle and flanno – I felt like I was in a music video. He walked to us with purpose. What did this guy want? He was going to quite some trouble to reach us.

I started to worry about JonBonJonno – had there been some kind of accident? It was nearing midday and we'd been expecting him to turn up.

Me and Leighton stood to greet the guy, who introduced himself as Andrew. He produced three ice-cold cans of Coke – there was literally ice dripping right off them. He had a freezer in his truck cabin, of course.

'Figure you boys could do with a nice cold one!'

I didn't even drink Coke, but I was in an ad now and it looked really tasty quenchy. There was no way I was going to knock back a Coke. I wanted to knock back a Coke!

So there we stood, three blokes in a triangle on the fringe of the Simpson Desert, smashing back a cold one and steadying for a yarn. The bush telegraph worked pretty well around these parts. It turned out that JonBonJonno was safe and sound, last seen by Andrew at a roadhouse back-a-ways.

'I was hopin' to have a word with ya actually . . .'

'By all means,' I replied, keen as the proverbial to hear this guy's story. He started talking and in that laidback Aussie style, revealed that he buried his sister to breast cancer a few years back. He got through it mostly with the help of his brother, and he just wanted to say all strength to me. He knew what it was like to lose a sister.

I told him the truth. 'It upsets me to hear that, brother.'

He went on to tell me that the weird thing was that I'd always reminded him of his brother. We were virtually the same guy, according to Andrew. Same attitude, same approach to life, same black sense of humour. I was intrigued that Andrew felt he knew me so well. He explained that it wasn't just from the telly and the voice overs, it was from two weeks previously, when he'd heard me on the radio talking about Connie while he was driving through Adelaide. I freaked him right out, because he felt like he was listening to his own brother talking about his sister when she got sick.

Andrew then told me that a year ago, to the day, he lost his brother in a tragic accident. Andrew was in his thirties and it was the first time he'd not been with his brother on his birthday. He'd been hoping to see us out on the road and today, of all days, on the first anniversary of his brother's passing, he'd found me. Like any good Australian truckie, he kept a good lid on things, but he was speaking right from the heart and the emotion of it all was only just below the surface.

He didn't want to keep us, or take up anymore of our time. We urged him to hang around but he had a job to do and he'd said what he came to say. He insisted on taking the empty cans back with him.

'Got a bin in the rig, no dramas.'

I said thanks and it wasn't enough, but he was off back through the crunchy paddock to his rig in the distance.

I pedalled towards Marree with renewed vigour. I was going to smash this sector and get there with time to clean up before Sister June's barbie. Andrew had called me a champion and today I would prove him right – it was the only thing I could think to do in return for the inspiration he'd proffered.

JonBonJonno re-joined us and we all honoured our new Aussie Legend, Andrew the Desert Truckie. It didn't take long for reality to set back in though. I still had a half-day of dust ahead. I didn't think further than Marree, because I knew I'd got ten days of gravelly nothing along the Oodnadatta Track from there.

It was one thing for your body to overheat, but when your head got hot, it became pretty hard to take care of the basics. My breath sounded very loud in my head and everything was fractured by a light brighter than it should be. I constantly drank fluid, but I never needed to piss. My sweat did little to cool me. My body responded much more slowly to my brain, which, on a unicycle, was not a good thing. The heat was ringing in my ears; the scrunch of my tyre through gravel was the only sound from outside that got in. I focused as hard as I could on the road's surface, trying to avoid any stone or rock big enough to unseat me. It felt like an Atari game. I was riding on the edge of nowhere, and it felt like it. The Flinders Ranges were gone and there was just open desert ahead. I pushed and pushed. After what seemed like a foreverness, I finally hit the sign that indicated Marree was within reach – only five kilometres to go. The pain felt as intense as the heat, but I knew I'd get there now. Most of the work was done . . . the road work, at least.

As I pedalled into Marree I noticed a few things out of place. There was a bunch of guys surrounding a massive roll-cage to my left and there were two guys up on a roof to my right, but the building had no rear, it was just a facade. It reminded me of the old Hollywood Westerns, then I realised that they were shooting a film here.

There had been two talking points in this neck of the woods for the last couple of weeks – Love Your Sister and *The Rover*. For days, everywhere we went, locals were proudly talking of having Guy Pearce and Robert Pattinson in the area, shooting a film called *The Rover*, David Michôd's follow-up to the internationally acclaimed *Animal Kingdom*. I was excited. I used to live with David in a share house in Collingwood nearly 20 years ago and one of my best mates had a role and might be in town, with a bit of luck. I was hoping I'd get to meet Guy Pearce too . . . turned out that the middle of nowhere was quite busy!

Sister June was at work but found time to give directions to her house, which would provide us with power to recharge everything before our Oodnadatta run. As we pulled in and started setting up, I noticed a shed in the corner of the backyard. A weary, sun-baked sign struggled to announce 'Mortuary'. After a quick sniff around I determined that there was no possible chance that this ramshackle shed, barely standing under the desert sun, contained any kind of refrigeration whatsoever. Death out here would be pretty messy, it seemed.

Thanks entirely to Andrew the Desert Truckie, I somehow busted through all of my thresholds in time to allow for half an hour of spare time. We spent it swimming with two teachers and three young Aboriginal kids. Their smiles infected me instantly and brushed away all my fatigue. They looked like they were having more fun tumbling into the pool than I ever had as a kid on my bike. We splashed and played and laughed. I showed them a move they hadn't seen before. I dunked my head and got half a moment of silence before a big splash pierced my senses. I opened my eyes underwater and saw my new friend, a young Aboriginal girl no more than eight, smiling and waving to me. I waved back and rushed back to air. I breathed in as clearly and deeply and cleanly as I ever would. I thanked Andrew in my head. Without him I never would have seen that beautiful young human wave and smile at me underwater . . .

The basketball court in Marree was in tatters; it had no chance against the blistering sun. It stood, soundly beaten, in the middle of the town, kerbed by a few trees offering precious shade and a brick barbie. A small mob turned out for our little fundraiser; they gathered in the shade on the court's fringe, leaving me on court and a little uncertain. Me, JonBonJonno and Leighton jumped on our trick bikes knowing that they'd bring the kids. If I get the kids involved I'd be more deserving of the mothers' attention later on. Which suited me fine; I love kids.

The film crew had wrapped and they were making their way en masse towards the pub, opposite the basketball court. It turned out they'd been hearing about us for a while too. Many of them stopped to say g'day and before long there was quite the convivial atmosphere going. Dusty crew members, little Aboriginal kids whizzing about the place, the barbie on full tilt, cracked cans and feet. This dusty little outpost was proving well worth the pedal.

Sister June was an absolute marvel. She was at least a septuagenarian but age seemed to have had the reverse effect on her. She beavered away with an upbeat doggedness that was easy to admire. She's devoted her whole life to this little desert township.

There's no family of hers here. The townsfolk are her family. She's the only nurse in town and there's been no doctor here for years, so it pretty much starts and ends with her. She'll look after you to the end and even then, she'll cover the post-mortem stuff too, through her backyard mortuary. She was the second person in 24 hours to completely inspire me. I was starting to think that if shit got any more profound I would have to do a moon dance to stave off all of the meaning floating about the place.

The Indigenous women tolerated my intrusions. There's a mobile screening unit that comes to town once every two years and Sister June always makes sure the ladies get checked. Indigenous women often fight breast cancer silently, so I'm glad that Sister June has taken to policing the issue. I wonder what will happen after Sister June dies. Who will take care of her in her backyard mortuary?

The crew filming *The Rover* took us in as one of their own and shouted us dinner. David gave me a hug and a big rap in front of the crew. He put a fifty in his own hat then passed it on. Between the basketball court and the hat work, we raised a couple of grand.

After dinner, the crew mingled for drinks and stories. Sure enough, Guy Pearce sat down with us and locked in. He drilled me with questions. He wanted to know everything. We chatted for hours. When the bar area closed he disappeared and re-emerged with a cheeky grin and a bottle of Grey Goose. There was more to learn and he was not going to be thwarted!

Guy has a childlike curiosity about him. He enquires constantly, hungry for detail. My own family aren't this interested in Love Your Sister. To many people Love Your Sister is just an oddity, but Guy seemed to actually *get it*. He'd spent weeks out in the desert, he knew exactly how hot it was, and he couldn't quite wrap his head around *how* we were doing it. He talked of his own experiences with his sister who lives with disability. He showed me some home movies on his laptop. We got to know each other. We carried on like old mates. But most of all, he reminded me to be *curious*. Much of our curiosity gets trampled on as we grow up. So many of us lose it and never get it back. Actors never lose it. Not the great ones.

I stumbled back to Sister June's backyard and smiled at the Mortuary shed. What a day. Andrew the legendary Desert Truckie had opened up on the tracks of the famed Old Ghan. Sister June, the bush nurse from a bygone era, had given everybody a lesson in true stoicism. And Guy Pearce had so clearly reminded me what curiosity really looked like.

I thanked Connie in my head, like I did every night, and hurtled towards sleep with stars in my heart. I slept well, knowing I was a small piece in this magnificent puzzle.

CONNIE

Between Adelaide and Darwin there is a lot of outback, a lot of desert, and not many people. Sam was doing a lot of kilometres and had fundraisers every couple of days, because there weren't many towns to stop in. While he was out in the heat of the desert, I was back in Canberra organising a line of merchandise, which I planned to sell online.

It sounds like an easy thing to do, get 'merch' made then sell it online, but Love Your Sister has been a massive learning experience for all of us, and this was another one for me. The Garvan Institute had already organised pens, tattoos, ribbons and wristbands, but we wanted more.

We wanted to provide hats and so we had to find a cap that was adjustable so it fitted everyone, was the right shade of pink, and could be embroidered with our logo. I searched high and low for a suitable cap and I couldn't find it. Then one night I walked into a servo and saw the perfect hat! It was Love Your Sister pink, made of light sporty material and it was adjustable. I bought it on the spot and took it home to do some research. It turned out it was made by a company called Aerial Designs and I tracked down their contact details and gave them a call. I explained who I was and why I would like to buy the hats. I asked if I could get the name of the manufacturer because we couldn't afford to buy them at the retail price. A lovely lady called Joanne Murrell took my number and said she'd call me back.

I thought that would be the end of that, but the phone rang later that day and it was Joanne. She'd searched their inventory and tracked down every last existing hat in that colour. They had 108 left, and as the line was being discontinued, she was happy to donate 50 and sell the rest to us at cost price. Amazing.

Then I started calling and emailing embroidery companies to get quotes for the hats to be embroidered. The costs came back at anywhere between eight and eighteen dollars per hat. We couldn't sell the hats for more than $30, and it would have been better if they were $25, so this wasn't going to work. Then an email came in from Emma at Countrywide Embroidery in Queensland. They were happy to do all of the embroidery, not just for the hats but also on patches for us to sew onto the crew uniforms, for free! Because of Aerial's and Countrywide's generosity, after the first 50, only eight dollars would come off the sale price to cover costs. We could then donate a hundred per cent of the merchandise sales to research. I can't tell you how excited I was that it had all come together. We had balloons, with help from Money Now, t-shirts with help from Copperhead Screen Printing, stickers, notepads, postcards and bookmarks with the help of Print Design Australia, and drink bottles and stubby holders, again with help from Money Now.

Once all that was sorted Em and I had to set up an online shop. Needless to say, it was more complicated than we first thought. Just taking photos of the merch with a clean white background and the right light took us hours. Each item of stock needed to be measured and described accurately, so people understood exactly what they were ordering. All of the stock had to be categorised and easy to find; we didn't want people to leave our online shop because it was too difficult to navigate.

With some help from Tony at Clever Bits, and Louise Munnoch, we finally got the shop online, and it was worth all the work. I launched the shop at ten o'clock at night, and before the clock struck midnight we had had 101 orders. I was so proud of myself because I'd been in charge of the merch lines and online selling, and with lots of help from many generous contributors, I'd done it!

I knew how hard Sam was slogging it out on his unicycle and it made me twice as determined to push myself back at home base. There are no slackers in the Johnson family – it just isn't allowed!

SAM

After 2000 clicks we rolled into Uluru, suspecting it might be special, but with no real idea of just how special. Remarkable people, breathtaking surrounds and spiritual experiences abounded.

I was kinda lost for words, but will try to find some that go part of the way towards explaining what we went through.

One of the first things I did was visit the Wakagetti Cultural Dancers. Before each dance a story was told to help explain the origins of the dance and its cultural significance. I was struck by the humility with which they thanked the creator of each piece. They flipped from being spiritual to funny, to dramatic, to insightful, to inclusive. They invited the crowd up to dance with them and that was all the encouragement I needed. I was terrible, of course, for I don't have that rich and ancient culture coursing through my veins, but I found it to be a most uplifting experience and I was very grateful for the opportunity. My thanks to Michael for welcoming me so warmly, promoting our cause and inviting me into his circle of friends. What a privilege.

The next morning I did a sunrise tour of Kata Tjuta (which translates as 'many heads'), formerly known as The Olgas. I toured with a terrific group of Americans. I worded them up on the whole Love Your Sister fiasco and they loved the idea of our challenge system . . . so much so that they dared me to stealth-kiss Michael for the princely sum of 200 bucks, for the cause.

While I had reservations about infringing on someone's personal space, I was assured that everything would be okay. So, around the brekky table, I pounced and planted a big pucker on Mike's lips. He was an absolute sport and his travelling party were only too happy to part with the money. Laughs aplenty, for sure. It was interesting, in hindsight, that I kissed a man in Kata Tjuta, which is a men-only space for the Indigenous.

Uluru Camel Tours invited us out to ride camels in front of the great rock. I was assigned Conner, a true character to be sure.

While some consider camels a pest, I love all animals and have a new appreciation for these beautiful beasts, thanks in no small part to the devotion, professionalism and passion of Chris, Kel, Roscoe and the crew, who are an impressive outfit, to say the least. If you're ever at Uluru, please do visit them and say hi from me. They'll look after you an absolute treat. We all became pretty tight-knit while I was there.

Meeting Michael from the Wakagetti Cultural Dancers led me to meet Justin Majid, a beautiful and quietly spoken young man from the Torres Strait Islands. Just before we left, he presented me with a beautiful work of his, titled *Kazi Koedal* (Baby Crocodile). Crocodile-breeding season is between November and March. The mother crocodile lays her eggs in small mounds along the banks of the Torres Strait Islands. She will guard her young until they hatch and venture into this world. In Justin's work, the baby crocodile is coming out of its egg to begin its life. The design within the egg showed the habitat where it would grow up for the next few months, avoiding predators and catching its prey. It's an amazing piece and Justin was happy for us to auction it off for the cause.

After that it was back on the bike on the road to Darwin, for lots more road, desert, roadhouses and incredibly welcoming Indigenous communities. I was hanging out to see Connie and she was flying there to meet up with us.

CONNIE

Sam was approaching Darwin and I was off to meet him there. I was a bit worried about this trip. Before the launch in February I was so much more energetic than I was at this point. Back then I was able to run on adrenaline and sleep after it was all over. When I went to visit Sam in Adelaide it was the same – even though I was still not fully healthy, I was able to go to all the events and managed to get to all the media. After the launch in Melbourne, and the Adelaide visit, I slept for two days solid, waking to eat and take medicine, then going straight back to sleep. But I was still able to go, and to work while I was there.

This felt different. I wasn't sure I had it in me and I was a bit scared about that, but I had to keep going. Well, I arrived in Darwin and had a – let's say – eventful time (read – disastrous!). I started to feel quite unwell and was in a bit of pain. When I arrived I slept for five hours. That refreshed me somewhat, but I was very disappointed when Sam came to wake me up because I had missed the whole evening with my family and some of the Darwin crew.

I wasn't awake long before I started to feel really sick and then I passed out. I ended up in hospital for the rest of the evening and in the morning I felt dreadful and looked even worse. I was told I could leave hospital but it would be against medical advice. I must have still been high from the adrenaline they'd given me when I arrived, and had some sort of super human strength/invincibility thing going on because I decided I didn't want to miss the visit to Wulagi Primary School. We had some media lined up so I did a runner from the hospital, promising to come back a bit later to finish treatment and rush back if I started to go downhill again.

With some help, I ventured off to the radio stations. These interviews are strange things, sometimes they're all fun and jokes, and in others they can pull on the heartstrings and you never know whether you'll be laughing or crying. It all happens so quickly that you hardly have time to process what has happened until much later.

I met up with Sam just before the first radio interview, and the expression on his face told me how terrible I looked. When we were on air he tried to explain how he felt seeing me with all the tubes hanging off my arms and diodes stuck all over me. Since he was a kid, he'd never been good with hospital stuff, and times like this reminded me just how hard it was for him. He really was facing his fears in so many ways on this journey, and his fear of hospitals was one of the biggest ones.

My brother is a brave man, and so strong in the way he was embracing the challenges on the road while also trying to be supportive of me and dealing with the physical demands of turning that wheel.

Darwin and the Territorians really got right behind Love Your Sister, and Sam and I were overwhelmed by the generosity of the communities we met and the support we received.

Thanks to Darwin City Council, we were able to use Raintree Park in the centre of town for fundraising and meeting people and spreading the booby-trap awareness message. I struggled to get up that day but I eventually summoned up the energy to go along and I was so glad I did.

When I arrived Sam was talking into the microphone, addressing the crowd. I went up and stood next to him while he was talking about me. He was so happy to see me, but then suddenly, he handed the microphone to me. I wasn't expecting it but I had a chat with the crowd and the day progressed nicely from then on.

One mob there was a group of dancers from different tribes around the Northern Territory. They danced and played music and were wonderful. The dance and music was so expressive and it was great to have some custodians of the land welcome us to Darwin. I felt honoured to be welcomed in this way.

After that a champion whip cracker called Mick challenged Sam to give it a go and he mastered it after about ten tries. Then they made it more difficult and challenged him to crack the whip while riding a unicycle – and he did it! When he completed the challenge everyone screamed and clapped madly; there was a real sense of achievement amongst everyone there, it was a triumphant moment. I had a go and it was, let's say, pitiful – no whip cracking for me.

Sam's phone never stopped ringing, and that day I was reminded that he would answer it whenever possible, even when he was busy. Someone presented him with a snake at Raintree Park, and at first he recoiled (as anyone should when someone puts a snake around their neck!), but he became accustomed to it after a little while. He was even answering the phone and conducting business as usual – with a snake wrapped around his neck. I love that he will try anything in the name of Love Your Sister.

In between fundraisers, Sam and I went and had a dip in the pool at the hotel where the boys were staying. We had the pool to ourselves. It was serene and peaceful and I was sitting on the edge dangling my feet in when two guys, Scott and Liam, came along for a swim. They were young, probably in their twenties, maybe early thirties. I don't know why, but I was surprised when one of them recognised Sam and said, 'Aren't you that guy on the unicycle?'

This started a lovely conversation. They were so interested in Love Your Sister, so lovely to Sam and me, just all-round nice guys, and it was so good to see that young men were interested in Love Your Sister as well. Before we left they gave us a huge donation. I think they gave us everything in their wallets, it was so touching.

Later, when I was talking about it with Sam he told me that I'd be surprised by how often this sort of thing happened on the road, where people gave donations, small and large. He called them doughies, and said there were various types of doughies – mostly roadside doughies, but Scott and Liam's was a poolside doughie. I felt privileged to witness this.

—

The school visit to Wulagi Primary was the first one I'd done with Sam. Sam gets to meet heaps of kids in schools but what a privilege it was to talk to children about Love Your Sister. I don't know the statistics but I guarantee that a good number of the kids would have known someone who had been diagnosed with cancer. All the kids had dressed up in pink and they'd made welcome posters that were simply adorable. While I was talking, a little girl ran up from her class group and gave me a huge hug. It made me teary.

After a special Love Your Sister assembly, we were lucky enough to meet a small group of students who were experiencing grief. We had a very touching chat and I felt honoured that they talked to us about their loss. It gave me a glimpse into what my children will experience, and it affected me profoundly. I cried with these kids and later when I was alone I cried for them and for my own boys, who, sometime soon, will lose their own mummy. I wish there was something I could do to ease their pain, some way that I could prepare them for what they're going to have to experience but all I can do is spend as much time with them as I can and make sure I write letters and books for them to read after I'm gone. It's why writing this book is so special to me.

When I walked out of the school gates at the end of our visit I knew I'd left a small part of my heart with all those kids!

—

The next day I woke up at 8.30 am and realised that I had missed my alarms (I'd set three the night before) and missed two calls from Sam. I was so disappointed. Again, I'd slept through stuff I really wanted to do. Sam and I had been booked to do a live cross to *The Today Show* and he'd had to do it on his own. *The Today Show* and Karl Stefanovic had been so incredibly supportive of Love Your Sister. They'd helped us raise awareness and money for vital research. I was just getting up when my phone rang again and it was a private number. I nearly fell over with excitement when the voice on the other end was Karl Stefanovic! Karl had called to see how I was feeling. I was gobsmacked and I don't think I could string a sensible sentence together I was so starstruck. It was such a lovely kind gesture and it really got me inspired to try to attend some of the functions planned for the rest of the day.

Those days in Darwin were huge but before I knew it, it was time to say goodbye to Sam (and Jonno and Leighton) again. I didn't want to because this time I really didn't know if I'd see them again. I'd really battled to stay involved in everything and it hit me hard when I was so sick I couldn't do all that I wanted to. Determination, willpower and adrenaline weren't enough. Maybe I'd been in denial a little but the brutal reality was that I was living with terminal cancer and my body had reminded me of that fact.

Watching Sam disappear from view was too much and I was a sobbing mess. After our emotional goodbye, I spent the rest of the day recovering. I'd been staying with Michelle Teather and Steve Ellis while in Darwin and that night we talked, we laughed, we cried and then we laughed some more. When I started crying I went and got a roll of toilet paper to use as tissues, and Michelle exclaimed, 'We do have tissues here, you know!' She'd been finding rolls of toilet paper all around the house the whole time we'd been there, 'cos Sam and I grabbed a roll whenever anyone teared up. We joked that I was crying so much that I needed a string around my neck to hang the roll on. Steve disappeared for a minute and came back with a camping toilet roll holder on a string. It was so funny I cried tears of laughter, and needed the toilet roll again!

SAM

It's funny, you can be talking to someone, their spittle will fly straight into your face and you'll pretend nothing ever happened. You'll wait until they look away before you go the wipe. You carry on as normal, as if you don't have a care in the world, when all you can think about is their bit of spittle near your eye. It's the same when you hug someone and they're all sweaty. You pretend you haven't just hugged a lump of soggy flesh. You don't want to offend them, even though their sweat is all over your well-intentioned limbs. You would rather feel their sweat dry on your skin than pipe up and wipe.

So, somehow, according to some social mores that were created however many centuries ago from wherever the fuck, you're allowed to spit in strangers' faces and sweat all over them, and they won't do a thing about it, they'll smile at you right through it as if nothing could be finer. It's like feeling that you shouldn't tell someone that their nostril is full of snot, or that their tooth has a polka dot on it. Isn't not telling them more offensive? If someone goes in for the hug and I'm all sweaty, I don't want to be rude and say 'don't touch'. What kind of an inconsiderate wanker would I seem then? There's no way out. You can't block an advance of kindness, nor can you shield them from the impending sensorial reality. That sweating, toxic, heaving reality, holding his breath because he doesn't want you to smell the rollie he just smoked in the caravan. Smile!

I'm doing this whole unicycling thing for a great cause and everyone wants a hug. I mean, I'm basically the go-to guy for hugs. But I'm a profuse sweater. I know what it's like to hug me, because I'm also an avid hugger, and I really don't want you to have that feeling like you've just copped an armful of yuck. I've watched enough people try to slide out with grace, attempting to subvert the whole process, but the problem is, photos and selfies are *de rigueur* and I've no chance against a cultural phenomenon this size. Couple my profuse sweating with my uncontrollable bursts of paranoia and social discomfiture and I don't stand a chance on most days.

I'm two days out of Fitzroy Crossing and we are well and truly between community engagements. None of us has showered; it's all festy and twisted. My inner Big Mother is running the place with particular zest today; her mood is Zing Pow Bam in your face, with a splash of sarcasm to finish. Every time I break, Leighton finds a few roadside bottles and sets them up in a row and we piff rocks at them till they're all smashed. Hoots and disappointed groans accompany each direct hit, as you would expect from three blokes in the desert. We are masters of distraction. We know that just sitting in the heat during breaks doesn't help. We rock toss bottles when it's too hot for a kick of the footy or a push-up competition, and we've been rock-tossing for days on end now. I've taken my usual bye and am somewhere between my magnesium drink, a snack and a smashed bottle when two attractive young women pull over to shower us with praise. Tough gig if you can get it, right?

Thing is, and I don't realise it at the time, Henry the bear is on the couch. He's been rude and come in without asking again. As the two women approach I worry about how sweaty I am, which of course makes me more sweaty. Henry calls me Mr Puddles. I'm convinced I'll fail to meet expectations, because so often that's what happens. I'm never as cheery as on the telly, or as funny; I've had the chance to craft my answers when I'm on *The Project* or *The Today Show*, but in real life I'm no whip. When it comes to the Love Your Sister narrative I'm somewhat of a tone-freak, a spin-prince on a good day, but when I'm off-message I flap about rather pathetically, especially when Big Mother is making herself known. I haven't had a chance to remind myself to be me.

I tell myself to smile with my teeth if they want a photo. I have a complex about my teeth and I've been smiling with a closed mouth and both of the boys have had a word with me about it and told me to cut it out so I have to 'proper smile' this time. I think she said her name was Ally but I can't remember because I'm not thinking properly. I blame the heat but really it's Henry's fault. I think she donated $50, maybe because Henry told her to – they seem so nice.

I can't spare them the torture of cuddling a wet sponge, for sweaty selfies are on the menu no matter which restaurant I'm in;

they smile through it and say they don't mind when I apologise for dampening our huggle.

CONNIE

Whenever I spoke to Sam on the phone we had so much to tell each other. Love Your Sister united us in so many ways, because we were working on the same project, but ironically it also separated us. There were times when I missed him so much.

It wasn't just missing him that was hard, though. It was also that I felt like he was able to experience all the things we'd planned together, while I was back at home, having to stay close to a hospital. I'd missed out on Uluru and the Ord River, and that was particularly hard because those were both places I'd really wanted to visit and we'd talked so much about going there while we were planning this massive adventure.

Sam told me that he thought of me every day and sometimes he felt like he'd told me things that he hadn't because he's told people he met along the way instead. So when he rang, he'd tell me all the things he'd told people on the road. He said that he'd thought of me every time it got hard to pedal. That he hated that there is no cure for my cancer and that it made him mad as hell. That he felt helpless, and realised from time to time that no matter how far he rode, how much money we raised or how much awareness we spread, my cancer would still not go away. That it would still kill me, and that it made him feel very empty inside. But on the upside, we were doing something, at least we were trying to make a difference, and we were doing it while I was still well enough to enjoy it, and follow what was happening.

And I still didn't think Sam understood what saying yes to this crazy idea had given me. Because of him I experienced things I'd never dreamed were possible. For instance, things like making a speech in front of thousands of people and appearing on TV.

A guy called Ged Williams was on holiday in the outback with his lovely partner, Sue, when they came across a guy in pink on a unicycle, beating the drum about breast cancer awareness. Ged was inspired by Sam and Love Your Sister, and he wanted to take a piece of it back to the Gold Coast with him. As a director of nursing for the Gold Coast Health Service, he was in charge of the Nurses and Midwives Day celebrations, and when he got back to work he contacted us and asked me to come along and talk to his staff about my experiences as a patient.

I was honoured to be asked, not as Sam's sister, not because Sam couldn't attend, but to give my perspective of my experiences as a patient. It was going to be my first speech without Sam by my side and I was nervous but excited at the same time.

There were about 200 people there, mostly women, mostly nurses and midwives. I'd stayed up until 3 am the night before writing my speech. I'd broken it down into five parts: My first cancer, second cancer, my babies being born, my third cancer and Love Your Sister. This was an incredibly important moment for me because it was my chance to prove that I was worthy of being *the* sister in Love Your Sister.

As I spoke I looked at the audience regularly, and it seemed their eyes were glued on me. I had their attention. They nodded when I mentioned the nurses who looked after me when I was a child, and they smiled in acknowledgement and understanding.

I talked about my second cancer and how I was misdiagnosed. I mentioned that I was told by one doctor that I wasn't taking my health seriously, and being told by another doctor that he didn't understand what I was so upset about – after all, it was never a real baby. I talked about the district nurses who saved my life by allowing me to have my treatment at home because, after all the bad experiences I had had at that hospital, I really didn't want to go back there.

Then I talked about the midwives and nurses involved in my care, and the care of my premature baby boy, when he was born at 32 weeks, and then again with my second born, who threatened to come into the world at 23 weeks. The audience came on the journey with me. They sighed when I told them of my heartache, gasped at some of the horrors I experienced and nodded and smiled with understanding when I talked about the help given to me by the excellent staff at the Canberra Hospital.

By the time I started talking about my breast cancer and my terminal diagnosis, many women in the audience were in tears. When I talked about Love Your Sister they smiled and clapped. At the end I couldn't believe it when they gave me a standing ovation. The clapping seemed to go on and on and I felt such pride and gratitude that I had connected with these people. They'd heard the Love Your Sister story and been touched. I knew they'd check their breasts, and that they'd tell their friends to be breast aware and that was why I was doing this.

After that experience I felt worthy of the title of 'The Sister' and I knew I didn't need Sam to always be with me to make an impact. We were a team, and a strong and competent team at that, but individually we were strong too.

Ged came up to me after my speech and hugged me, thanking me for getting involved. I felt good that a friendship that had started on the side of the road in the outback had developed into something that made such an impact for all of us. Doing that speech gave me the confidence to take on more. But I wasn't quite prepared when Em called, practically shouting down the phone, 'This is all about you, baby. They want you!'

'Who wants me? What are you talking about?'

'*Insight*, on SBS, they want YOU, not Sam. They're doing a show on living with a terminal illness. You wanna do it?'

That was scary! Jenny Brockie is so smart and can make an issue as controversial as she wants to make it. She has mad skills and I didn't know if I could handle it. They had proposed I would be one of four panellists with the audience made up of people living with terminal illness, doctors who diagnose and treat terminal patients, and family members of terminal patients. This would be interesting. I said yes.

I flew to Sydney with Em for the filming and I was so nervous. I remembered what Sam had said on launch day. It's good to be nervous, it means you care. I tried to rationalise why I was there. I deserved to be there, I had a story to tell and I wanted people to know about it. This was my first TV appearance without Sam and I was worried I would blow it. I called Sam to get advice and he said with a laugh, 'No pressure or anything Con, but you better be good, people are going to be watching.' Thanks, brother! Great help.

There were huge cameras, lots of crew and the audience was instructed on how to speak and act during the filming.

I sat there and felt too hot. I coughed to clear my throat. I started to think when it was my turn to speak only a little croak would come out. All I could think of was if I stumbled or said anything stupid it was going to be on film forever. It wasn't the most helpful thing to have running through my brain. I wanted to run.

As soon as Jenny started the questions though, I suddenly felt at ease. It became an interesting conversation about something I knew very well. One of the panellists, Penny, was unable to join us on the stage so she was linked in via a camera at her bedside in hospital. She had breast cancer and was terminal too, but she was closer to the end of her journey than I am. It was like a knife in my chest. I knew that I would be in her situation one day, probably in the not-too-distant future, and I could only hope I'd have the grace and strength that Penny showed.

Another panellist didn't consider himself terminal. He said they just hadn't found the secret to his cure yet. We all cope with our terminal diagnoses in very different ways and I found myself thinking that I was glad I'd found some sort of peace; that I'd found some sort of acceptance of my future. I am not fighting it anymore. I just want to make the most of the time I have left. It is a confronting issue and Jenny explored it adeptly. After it was over I was even more in awe of her; her intelligence is jaw-dropping.

I had to wait a week for the show to air and I was asked to be involved with Twitter and other social media during the screening and after the show. I was honoured and felt very privileged to have that opportunity.

I called Sam the day after it had aired. 'Did you see it? What did you think?'

'Oh Con, I want to lie and tell you that I watched it, but I couldn't, I can't deal with it. You know I don't want to think about you being terminal; it's too hard for me to watch.'

I understood, but I was a little bit disappointed nonetheless.

'But the boys watched it and they said you were awesome, and people stopped me on the street and said you were amazing, so congratulations.'

I wondered if he'd ever be able to watch it. Would it ever get any easier for him to deal with the truth?

A few days after the show was on television I was recognised down the street. I couldn't help laughing at the irony of it all, fancy being famous for having cancer? Of all the things!

I had well and truly had my fifteen minutes of fame and I have to tell you, I liked the taste of it. I was lucky, because I was not hassled, but we did get a lot of press to promote Love Your Sister and it helped us raise money and awareness. People often acknowledge me in the shops or down the street, but they stop themselves before they say anything, wanting to respect my privacy. I am so grateful that we got press to promote Love Your Sister, and that we were respected and given space. Any people who did stop to talk to us were kind, loving and generous; they often shoved money into our hands, donating whatever they could afford.

Sam told me that he was so much prouder to be recognised as a unicycling breast cancer advocate than a TV star. It felt real and worthwhile. We had the best of both worlds and we revelled in every precious moment of it.

—

After Darwin, I wasn't sure that I would make it to Perth, but the whole time I had been hoping I would. I couldn't commit, because I never knew how I'd be feeling in advance, but then *The Project* offered to fly me over for a surprise visit to Sam. I was so excited.

The only catch was I had to keep it a secret from Sam, which was tough. Every time he asked if I was coming to Perth I had to say that I wasn't feeling strong enough. I hated lying to him, but I really wanted to surprise him. The plan was that Carrie Bickmore would ride into Perth with Sam (on a two-wheeler) and then she would present me as a surprise once they got there. When Sam heard that Carrie would be joining him on the road, he rang me up and said, 'Con, you have to come to Perth now, Carrie Bickmore is coming and riding with me. You have to come, you can't miss this!'

I felt like such a phoney when I said that I would love to, but I just couldn't do it.

The flight over to Perth was awesome! I got to fly business class and they had these pods to sit in. The chairs extended and I could lie flat, and the chairs had an inbuilt massager. I had a big sleep and when I woke up there was a cupcake beside me. I can see why people fly business class now; I had always thought, why would you spend all that extra money when the flight will be over soon enough, and then you get off and forget about it? Now I understand! You get to be comfortable, spread out, sleep and eat at your leisure.

After this flight I was ready to surprise Sam. I wondered how he would react when he saw me.

—

Well, I guess having to bleep out Sam's reaction on *The Project* tells it all. He was so surprised and so happy he swore then bent over as if he was going to fall before steadying himself and giving me the biggest hug. It was magic!

I was in Perth for six days and I was pretty sick because I was in the middle of chemo but it was the milder sort, which meant I kept my hair. I tried to keep up with Sam but as we drove around to all the media we kept having to stop so I could throw up. Sam would pat my back and help me walk. There were lots of events and lots of media. A huge highlight for Sam was meeting Danny Green. I don't think I'd ever seen him so nervous and so starstruck but Danny was a true champion and gave us a lot of his time. He gave Sam boxing tips and they had a pretty serious spar. I got in the ring as well at one point but I couldn't stop laughing and sadly my sporting prowess is about as good as it was when I was a kid. I had a go but then left Sam to it. After that we visited Ikea and they donated $25,000 to Love Your Sister. Danny was with us and we had a chair-building challenge. Danny didn't try hard and taped his chair together so that when he sat on it, it collapsed, but Sam and I were as competitive as ever. I was determined to beat him and he was just as determined to make sure he beat me. I am proud to say that I whooped him and my pink chair was strong and sturdy!

We had a high tea scheduled at the governor's mansion but that morning I was really sick and Sam had to go without me. The Governor of Western Australia, Malcolm McCusker, his wife Tonya and their little girl, Mary, were so supportive of Love Your Sister. I wish I'd been there to see Sam ride into that grand building on his unicycle. I don't think that's something that happens too often there. With a generous personal donation in his pocket and a spring in his step, Sam had experienced another first; meeting the Governor.

Saying goodbye to Sam after we'd spent so much time together was tough. Sam was really emotional because he hadn't expected to see me again until Melbourne and seeing me so fragile gave him a bit of a shake-up. I cried like a baby as I watched him ride away.

SAM

Since the very beginning of Love Your Sister, when Connie and I decided that we'd combine our challenge system with her own personal bucket list, Connie was adamant that I experience the tree-top walk in the Walpole Wilderness on her behalf. It's a series of boardwalks strung 40 metres above the ground, snaking through the tops of a beautiful tingle tree forest. These are no ordinary trees – they tower higher than any other trees I've seen before, reminiscent of *The Magic Faraway Tree*, one of our favourite books. The trees are so tall and majestic; it felt unreal. So it was with mixed feelings that I embarked upon Connie's challenge – to ride through the tree tops atop my one-wheeler. It felt wrong that she wasn't there, but at the same time it was impossible not to appreciate the majesty of the place. I recorded this little vid to try to help capture the experience. A great reward really, for enduring the most challenging undulations of the trip thus far. Sorry to rub it in, Sis!

To watch Sam's video to Connie go to:
http://vt.tumblr.com/tumblr_mpripoQ0TbIsI1jtw.mp4#_=_

CONNIE

When the crew were making their way down the Western Australian coastline, Em discovered a little fact that would have a huge impact on Love Your Sister. It turns out that 85 per cent of the population of WA live south of Perth – and we weren't going there! We had to think quickly if we were going to remind women from the area not to fall into the booby trap. We actually had to meet them, so a route change was needed, and fast. We realised that we had allotted weeks to the Nullarbor, where hardly anyone lived, and we were about to miss out on the majority of the WA population instead. It didn't seem right, so we changed plans, and re-routed so we could visit south-west WA, including Esperance, Bunbury and Albany.

By now Love Your Sister was used to short deadlines and organising events with very little notice, so it was more of the usual for us. Em sent emails out to every school, hospital, council and community group she could find on 'The Google'. In this way, as we did all over the country, our community events and fundraisers were organised locally by people who Em had found. They donated their time and resources and whipped up events quickly and happily.

Sam rang me nearly every night from the South-West. It seemed like each day couldn't get any better; that he was floating on a high, then he would get to the next town, and more love, more compassion and more generosity flew his way. He was gobsmacked, constantly ringing and reporting in on the latest news.

I was just about to go to bed one cold night in Canberra, but somehow it didn't feel as though my day was complete.

Was there an email I'd forgotten to send? A phone call I'd forgotten to make? Then the phone rang. It was Sam.

He shouted down the phone at me, 'Hi Con, did I wake you?'

There was a lot of noise in the background. It sounded like he was in a pub or a nightclub. He was at a cocktail party in Bunbury, and he held the phone up to the crowd while they all shouted, 'Hi Connie' down the phone at me. The vibe was infectious. I found myself sitting alone on the phone with a grin from ear to ear, awaiting the next update.

'We wanted to ring you to tell you that we made so much money tonight. I'll let them tell you.'

'Twenty-four thousand dollars!' the crowd screamed down the phone line.

He put the phone up to the microphone and I thanked them. I couldn't believe how much they had made. Wow. But more than anything, Sam just sounded so happy.

In the South-West, Sam also found himself a mum. After years of searching, it happened at the family fun day in Esperance, where Sam stumbled across a woman named June Gribble who hugged him in only the way Aunty Marg knew how, and Sam was immediately a son again. The day was a family fun day at the Foreshore. There were sandcastle competitions, sausage sizzle and bake sales; the kids had a blast on the mini-bikes and trick bikes. Fun was had by all, young and old, and one of the many highlights of the day was when they built a big pair of boobs in the sand.

SAM

Sometimes the kilometres all disappeared into themselves and I was nowhere near my unicycle. I'd snap out of my reveries and wonder what happened to time, like you often do on long drives. All the right bits were strapped on and I was pursuing the road with the trademark willingness that only the night can bring, but the night's kilometres amalgamated in an indistinct gaggle, muted by the voices in my head, in the middle of one of their more raucous caucuses. It was made all the worse by Henry, playing chieftain and postulating like a right twit. Even the moon was hiding; the odd star appeared, hoping to form a chorus somewhere. The Boobmobile's headlights were on overtime, struggling to rob the dark of its mystery on an indistinct night where nothing was matching up. At least it wasn't the boring numbers game in my head.

My periphery sounded high alert. Jeopardy at three o'clock. There was a little creature scurrying straight across the road and towards where I'd be. It was a field mouse with an impressive tail. She had somewhere very urgent to be. Or she was very aware of the perils of the open road. Either way, she wasn't mucking around.

At first I thought, 'hold fast'. I didn't know what was behind me as I was focused on the she-mouse, I didn't have time to check. My gut was telling me that we'd connect. But I'm committed. The field mouse was committed. Time slowed down, like it does before most every accident. If I changed tack suddenly I might inflict a horrific, event-ending injury. If I held my course I might run over her and inflict a horrific, event-ending injury. My brain screamed Lose–Lose.

I'd much prefer to say that I surrendered to destiny, but in truth I just ran out of time to decide. The field mouse scuttled underneath my wheel as I rode past. I swear I didn't miss her by the merest of squidgeons. I swear I didn't roll over her tail, for her speed remained unchanged. She dead-set snuck her tail through the grooves of my turning tyre, scout's honour. I was never a scout actually. I'll swear on whoever you like until my dying day that I witnessed, first hand, the grooviest tail in the world.

I pedalled away and imagined if things had been different, if things hadn't turned out quite so smoothly, she may have ended up in field-mouse heaven, making new friends around a table, playing cards, smoking ciggies and them all discussing how they got there. Most of the field mice say 'wedge-tail got me', or 'fox got me' or 'feral cat got me'. I imagine my field mouse piping up with, 'Got run over by a long distance unicyclist.'

The other field mice would all think she was having a lend. It would create for a livelier card game, that's for sure. What a way to go. What a stupid way to die. Being run over by a unicyclist . . .

Thank golly she didn't cause me injury. Imagine trying to explain that you couldn't finish your trans-national unicycle ride because you ran over a mouse and broke a vertebra.

CONNIE

By the time late October rolled around we were a pretty tight little operation. We had raised well over $900,000, the online shop was going great guns, the merch was popular on the road, and we'd already had some reports that women were actively looking after their breasts because of our message. The world record was within Sam's reach. Things were going stunningly well.

Of course, there was a catch. There were four months left on the Ride Year calendar, and that would mark the end of a three-year period during which Sam had not been able to work due to his Love Your Sister commitments. He was broke, and likely to stay that way until he came home. When the call came from Big4 Holiday Parks for Sam to give the keynote speech at their annual conference, he couldn't really afford to turn down the opportunity to earn a little cash. They'd generously offered to cover travel costs to get him back to Melbourne, so he hopped a little flying tin can out of Tamworth and dashed back to Crown.

He sat at the back of the room in the last session on the last day of the biggest event in the Big4 year. The conference participants were tired, and some of them didn't know what Love Your Sister was, or even why they were about to listen to a mad unicyclist for an hour, but they dutifully clapped as the MC announced his session.

Sam made friends with the entire room in the first ten minutes. He spoke to them from the heart. He told them as much of our story as he could fit into one measly hour, and invited them to share all of it with him. Every tear, every giggle, every blister and all the silliness in between. By the time he was done the conference attendees were just as crazy about their new little brother as he was about them.

The crowd jumped up from their chairs, applauded and whistled. The MC, Scott Williams, was back at the microphone, and announced that he would donate $5000 to Love Your Sister. What? It wasn't meant to be a fundraiser! It was meant to be grocery money. Samuel turned back to thank him, and another man stepped in front of him.

'I'm a director here at Big4, and I've just sold one of my caravan parks. I've got plenty to spare, and I'll donate $10,000 as well.'

Utterly gobsmacked, Sam shook hands and thanked him too. Such a spontaneous moment of generosity. The CEO, Ray Schleibs asked Sam and Em to join them in the Palladium Room later that evening for dinner at their awards night.

The Spring Carnival theme saw Palladium decked out in thousands of bright spring blooms. It looked absolutely stunning. Seated at the edge of the dance floor, Sam, Em and Sarah had a lovely dinner. When all the awards had been announced, Sam called it a night. He had a dawn o'clock flight the next day and his unicycle was waiting for him.

As Sam said goodbye, Ray said, 'After you leave I'm going to talk to the room a little bit. I think we could raise $40,000 tonight, considering we already have pledges for $15,000. I'm going to try. If I call you, can you come back?'

As they strolled back to the hotel, numbers were rushing around Sam's head. What was the current total? What fundraising did we know about that hadn't hit Garvan's accounts yet? Was $40,000 enough? If it was enough, was it about to happen right now? If it wasn't enough, it was DAMN close, maybe a couple of thousand off the $1,000,000. So close . . .

The call came in much less than an hour later. It was one of the Big4 team, positively yelling down the phone to *get back here now*. Sam, Em and Sarah ran back from one side of the Crown complex to the other.

Everyone had big grins on their faces. What had happened after they'd left? Conspiracy was in the air. They stopped the music and Sam, Sarah and Em all stepped onto the stage.

The CEO was at the microphone. 'Well, Samuel, we have a surprise for you. We've done rather well for you tonight. The Big4 family has come up with a hundred k for you.'

The crowd went absolutely berserk, screaming and cheering. Sam's jaw dropped, Em had her hands on her face and a woman shoved a crumpled piece of paper at her, a scratchy list of all the pledges they'd be donating to Love Your Sister. Those lovely, generous, big-hearted Big4 peeps had no idea what they'd even done.

$1,000,000.

Tick.

Sam regained his composure and grabbed the microphone. He yelled his thanks over the crowd. The crowd screamed and cheered even more. This must be what it was like to be in a successful rock band. When Sam, Sarah and Em finally left the stage, the dance floor crowd mobbed them with hugs and kisses and congratulations. The band started up again, and they played 'Rain' by Dragon. Of all the songs in the world to play. In the dark flashing lights, with the band so loud the bass went right through you, Love Your Sister had raised $1,000,000.

They may have run across the entire Crown complex to get back to the Palladium less than a couple of hours before, but on the return trip they didn't run. They floated.

—

The Gold Coast and Brisbane visits were particularly exciting for me, because this time my kids were coming. They had been missing their Uncle Long Legs, and although they'd been tracking his progress around the country, I was not sure they really understood just what it was that Sam was doing, and just how far he had travelled. They were looking forward to going on a plane, they were looking forward to seeing the crew, and they were most definitely looking forward to seeing their uncle.

We couldn't have planned a more exciting arrival to the Sunshine State than what Daryl Agnew from NAK haircare organised for us. He was there at the airport to meet us, and showed us out to our limousine! Me and the kids climbed in and were chauffeur-driven to the hotel, which NAK had also organised. In the foyer of the hotel there were some pastry chefs building a huge gingerbread house, and they were French. I was delighted to have a small chat with them in French, and very proud when Willoughby joined in, showing me up! There wasn't much time to relax though, because we were going out to have our hair cut. Purple Daze in Brisbane opened up on their day off just to cut our hair, and I got a dark pinky-purply colour put in mine. We were given the star treatment and were totally spoilt!

Daryl had organised for NAK to make Love Your Sister one of their beneficiary charities, and they organised a big breakfast for us the next day. While Sam rode in on his usual mode of transport, the kids and I were treated to another trip in a limo. For kilometres approaching NAK headquarters there were pink balloons lining the streets – it must have taken ages to set it all up – then when we arrived all the staff were there for a great, fun brekky. Daryl announced that NAK would contribute a massive $10,000 to Love Your Sister, and that was on top of the fundraising they had already done, but Sam was going to have to earn it. He would have to put his pink heart to the test. He had had pink nail polish done before, and ridden through the desert in pink lycra, but would he go the whole hog and dye his hair pink?

Kristy Smibert from NAK took on the challenge and kindly did the deed for Sam. She wielded that pink hair dye with no fear, and Sam was her (almost) willing victim. Sam always said that he was willing to do anything for a donation, and he had more than proven himself over the year, especially when it came to that poor unsuspecting huntsman spider, but this was a new level of commitment. I loved it, but unfortunately Sam did not, though he did persist with it for a number of weeks. I think he finally had enough of the teasing and funny looks, and gave himself an army buzz cut about two weeks later, removing all evidence.

After what seemed like a really fleeting visit to Brisbane we were off to the Gold Coast for further adventure and fundraising. Ged Williams, who had previously invited me to speak at the Nurses and Midwives Day celebrations, had been working hard with a committee of dedicated volunteers to organise a cracker show for the Gold Coast. Ged was not going to let Sam forget their neck of the woods. They organised a lot of events and fundraisers, back to back, completely filling the schedule for our time on the Coast.

A charity bed race, where local celebrity 'bed jockeys' were pushed around the lake on hospital beds by the local fire fighters, ambos and nurses, was a cracker, not to mention the *Phantom of the Opera* evening, the golf day and the PJ party. There was also a fundraiser and speeches at the hospital.

The PJ party was a classic! Hundreds of people showed up dressed in their finest pyjamas. Bridge, from the Bridge and Spida show on 92.5 Gold FM on the Gold Coast was the MC for the night, and she devised a devilish dare for the evening. Sam had to get into her onesie pyjamas with her (she, of course, had clothes on underneath). We passed a bucket around and clearly, everyone wanted to see two people in a onesie, because hundreds of dollars were raised just to see this little trick of contortionist cheekiness. They actually pulled it off, though they might have been a bit bruised and battered the next day. It was a bag of laughs and the onesie was stretched to its very limits.

The Gold Coast also offered us a very rare treat. A day off together. Sam had been pedalling every single day for the previous 200+ days and attended community events nearly every day. Some days he squeezed in a couple, or even three. He was on the trip of a lifetime, but gee, he must have been tired. A normal day in the office for him was riding about 80 kilometres on the uni and doing a fundraiser at the end of that, and he'd been doing it seven days a week since February! I was absolutely chuffed that when he finally did get a day off, it was to spend it with me and Willoughby and Hamilton.

We were special guests at Wet'n'Wild water park, and Sea World. We felt rude, getting straight to the front of the queues, but a lot of people recognised Sam, and stopped him to thank him for what he was doing, and people were very kind about us cutting in. Willoughby and Hamilton got a first-class experience at the theme parks with their Uncle Long Legs. We got to go on so many rides, though I found all the stairs to be a challenge. I have some metastases in my right knee, from when I'd had the bone cut out of my left leg, so my legs aren't the strongest, and it did get to a point in the day when I was happy to just go and float in the rubber tubes on Calypso Beach. The kids were so happy to be there, not just with Sam, but with the crew – so many big boys all together, having fun at a theme park. It was innocent. It was fun. And it was a well-deserved break for Sam.

When we visited Sea World, Sam went home for a nap, and unfortunately missed the opportunity to meet Henry, the polar bear cub. Sam couldn't believe that his name was actually Henry, the one and the same name that Sam has given his bi-polar bear mate. We got to feed the bears, hiding food around the enclosure while they were out the back, then we got to watch them hunt out all the food and toys we had left for them to find. Polar bears are my favourite animal, without question, and I felt like a teenager at a Justin Bieber concert. I couldn't wipe the smile off my face. I remember thinking that night, after I had read a book to the kids and kissed them goodnight, that this would be one of those days they remembered forever, long after I was gone, and it was certainly one of the moments with them that I would treasure until my last breath.

As with all things Love Your Sister, the NSW coast was a whirlwind of activity and excitement. Coffs Harbour lit up the Big Banana in pink for our visit. There was a huge fundraiser at CEX with The Matty Devitt Band providing the entertainment and the Bendigo Bank crew and the Love Your Sister crew dancing up a storm. There were raffles and auctions and $5000 was raised. But that wasn't all Coffs had in store for us, Marine Magic had Sam and the crew over for the day to play with baby dolphins and seals. Sam even got taken for a ride by a dolphin. I don't know who was happier, the dolphins or the Love Your Sister crew. It was a once-in-a-lifetime opportunity.

On the way out of town the boys stopped by the Coffs Harbour Racing Club. They had held a Pink Silks Race Day, raising money for breast cancer, and kindly donated $10,000. I found myself constantly amazed, surprised and humbled by people's generosity.

Newcastle was next, and this was a different sort of fundraiser – a tattoo day. Diabolik donated their time and helped organise the event. Matt and Mel who own Diabolik had been personally affected by breast cancer, as Mel's mum is a survivor, so they were more than happy to help. The idea was that each artist designed exclusive breast cancer tattoos that would only ever be used once, and anyone who came along on the day could buy that tattoo and know that it will never be reproduced, it would be a genuine one-of-a-kind.

Eddy-Lou was amazing! She worked all day without pay and designed several of the one-off designs – she also gave Sam a tattoo with my initials, CJ, in a beautiful geometric pattern on his back. There were so many people waiting to get breast cancer tattoos that not everyone was able to be seen! There were many people who had fought the disease and won, and wanted to celebrate the victory with a tattoo, and there were also people who had loved ones fighting the disease, who wanted to show their support that way.

Then came my challenge to Sam, to get a nipple ring. It was the closest he'd ever get to the pain of losing your breasts, so it seemed fitting that he shared my pain! I wasn't there, but there were reports that his screaming could be heard for miles around. I didn't actually expect him to go through with it, but he did, and more power to him. I think he is quietly proud of that challenge, because he never got rid of the nipple ring. He wears it to this day.

Diabolik raised over $6000 for breast cancer research, which was a fantastic result!

Kincumber is a gorgeous little place on the Central Coast, and the Kincumber Hotel put on a family fun day that sure was a cracker. They had fire engines with sirens blaring escorting Sam to the event. It was the perfect place for a family fun day, because the hotel sits atop huge grounds with a playground and lawns for the kids to play on while their parents have lunch. It was packed with 350 people for the day. The police and firies were there, as well as the Bendigo Bank staff and a reptile-petting zoo. The local surf lifesavers put on a sausage sizzle using pink bread and there was a jumping castle and face painting. Live music was provided by Hats Bennett and Dear Monday, Alan Phillips MC'd the event and the stars of the show were the Athol Children's dance group, who did the welcome to country. They made a pink ochre and used it to paint the breast cancer symbols on their back and did some traditional dancing for the crowd.

Athol made a Love Your Sister boomerang and presented it to Sam with his blessing for safe travels. Sam rang me that night and said, 'It just keeps happening, Sis. I think that I've seen it all, and experienced everything, then this happens. To be given a blessing for safe passage down the east coast by a true local means so much!'

When we first started planning Love Your Sister, Sam wanted to visit a jail. Cancer doesn't discriminate – people from all walks of life are affected. If cancer doesn't discriminate, neither should we, and we wanted to include a jail visit as one of our community engagement activities. Sam and the crew visited the Frank Baxter Juvenile Justice Centre where Sam got to talk to a few guys who have had hard lives.

Family is something that is very close to a lot of people in the justice system. Missing their families is often what drives them to change their lives and make better choices in the future. These guys were no different. At first they weren't interested, Sam was just another person coming to talk to them, but when they saw the Love Your Sister video and realised what Sam was doing and why, they sat up, shut up and took notice.

Over the course of the afternoon they participated in lots of fun activities and by the time Sam left, they were all calling each other brother and sharing stories. One of the activities was to see how many people they could fit in a huge, inflated truck tyre tube. The previous record was nine, and Sam was hell bent on beating it. Sam and Leighton were the first ones in, then the kids joined them, one by one. It was a confronting exercise, because everyone was jammed into a confined space, but even boys who were at first hesitant joined in, and they smashed the record, fitting a massive 13 people into the tube at once. Victory!

St Philips Christian College in Narara is a K–12 school. One family was in the same boat as us. Lu Munnoch is terminally ill with breast cancer and she has two young daughters, Charlotte and Alex, who attend the school. Their school community have been most supportive throughout Lu's illness and when they heard that Love Your Sister was coming to town, they were determined to be the biggest school fundraiser in the country. With just 470 students in the whole school, they set about the challenge with a very serious, can-do attitude. They set up the Pink Run, where each child paid an entry fee and then collected sponsorship money from their families, friends and neighbours. One child, a foster kid, went round his neighbourhood and knocked on every door with his foster carer, and this little eight-year-old raised $1100. Incredible! They also had a bake sale, and between that and the Pink Run the school managed to raise a record breaking $17,500! Schools are very often the very centre of our communities, as families gather together and deal with issues that face them in their lives. I was so impressed by what the St Philip's school achieved. It made me want to live in Gosford so our kids could go there. Schools all over the country have raised money for Love Your Sister, and had visits from Sam. I would like to extend a huge thank you to every school who accepted us, embraced us, fundraised for us and let us bring some Love Your Sister cheer and breast cancer awareness to your families.

—

Wherever you go in the world, there is rivalry between towns, cities and countries. Melbourne and Sydney are famous for their rivalry, and this rivalry definitely came into play with Love Your Sister. Locals in Adelaide wanted Adelaide to be the town where the most funds were raised; many smaller towns tried to top the leaderboard for the amount of money raised. Their primary aim, of course, was to raise money for research, and to raise awareness, but there was certainly a bit of healthy competition going on as well. (Just like me and Sam at Ikea!)

I can honestly say that every single one of the fundraisers coordinated in each town, capital city, regional centre or state was special. Every one was unique, and every single fundraiser had dedicated, community-minded people driving it. No state outperformed another state, and no city stood out, except Sydney.

Sam and I were both absolutely despairing at our failure to penetrate this huge city. We allocated a week for Sydney, and it truly felt like we'd failed miserably. We did some press, like *The Today Show* and some radio, but we failed to get a successful event happening in the biggest city in the country, and it caused us to reflect. The smaller the community, the easier it was to get people's attention, and the more that was donated as a result. In a town like Harden, NSW, with a population of about 2000, we raised over $6000, which is an average of $3 per person; Esperance in south-west WA raised a whopping $24,000, with a population of 13,000. That's nearly $2 per person. Then we hit a big city and the work got a lot harder. There was so much competition for attention, and it was insanely difficult to get anybody to hear us, and this is where it came down to true community spirit.

Just when we felt it was all too hard we received an invitation to meet the Governor of New South Wales, the Honourable Marie Bashir. I felt about two feet tall as I walked into the grand old building on its immaculately manicured grounds near sparkling Sydney Harbour. At first I thought we didn't deserve the attention but then I realised I shouldn't underestimate what we were doing for women's health and research. We'd worked hard, and the opportunity to meet with the governor validated our hard work. Once I let go of my insecurity I felt honoured and proud but it didn't stop the nerves. We had champagne and canapés and the Honourable Marie Bashir made a lovely speech. From that point on Sydney was all good!

The fabulous women of Cronulla in the Sutherland Shire, or 'The Shire' as it's affectionately known, organised a cocktail party fundraiser for us. It was our last night in Sydney and we turned up to find about 200 people there. The Body Shop staff were giving out little hand massages, the local gym had their Zumba group there performing, and at the end of the night I had had enough wine to try to join in. The dare for Sam was to see how many marshmallows he could fit in his mouth and still say 'Chubby Bunny'. Nikki Cousins was truly the hostess with the mostest; she was hilarious, pledging $50 to the cause herself if Sam would give her an autograph on her body. I won't tell you which body part, but it all stayed relatively decent and tame, but very funny. A jar went around the room and $500 was raised to see Sam sign Nikki's . . . well, you know.

The women of 'The Shire' shone, and because of them we left Sydney with plenty to smile about. But that wasn't the only thing that made us grin from ear to ear. The Garvan Research Foundation, the recipient of all the money raised by Love Your Sister, is based in Sydney, and while we were in town we visited the labs to see how it was all going there. We were welcomed with a cake the size of a small car that took eight people to carry into the foyer. Every researcher, administrator, manager and clerk was packed into the foyer and up the staircases and on the balconies of each level, all crammed in to hear about what Garvan were doing with the Love Your Sister money, to catch a glimpse of Sam on his unicycle and to hear us speak.

The CEO, Andrew Giles, made an amazing speech about how Garvan was moving forward on breast cancer research with the money from Love Your Sister, then Professor John Mattick stood up and explained the science behind it all. Sam and I made a speech and then the biggest surprise of all, 'The Connie Johnson Fellowship in Breast Cancer Research', was unveiled.

I was overwhelmed. There is going to be a scientist employed, just to work on breast cancer research, in my name. They're putting the call out worldwide, to attract the best breast cancer researchers in the world, and that person will be able to be creative and think outside the box with the money we have raised. They won't have to spend half of their time applying for funding, or justifying it; this scientist will be able to concentrate fulltime on the genes and molecules of breast cancer and work towards a cure. It was incredibly exciting, and I was very honoured. I cried. This is what it was all about and why Sam had accepted his sister's challenge. I think Sam was even prouder than I was. We both had to pinch ourselves. This was really happening!

After such a huge high it was back on the road for Uncle Long Legs and back home for me. With 298 days of riding under his belt, he was on the home run. Well, almost!

—

Besides Daylesford, our hometown, and Melbourne, the city where we grew up, there is probably nowhere else in the world that Sam feels more comfortable than Canberra. He has lots of good memories here, and home really is where family is, so he enjoys his visits to Canberra to catch up with family very much.

People say all sorts of bad things about Canberra, mostly how boring it is, but in our family, only boring people get bored, and we have never been bored here, we love it. It isn't far between Canberra and Sydney, where I'd seen Sam last, but the boys hadn't seen him since the Gold Coast and were eager to catch up with him again. It was approaching Grinch season, so we were planning an early family and crew Christmas in our local park while he was here. There was a lot to look forward to both personally and for Love Your Sister.

The team at Eden Monaro Cancer Support Group and Kim Burnett, volunteer extraordinaire, had been planning a gala night out in Canberra. As with the many fundraisers that had been held in every corner of this wide brown land of ours, local businesses had been really supportive and donated lots of auction items, door prizes and raffle prizes.

Unicyclists from all over the country and the world gathered in Canberra for the Asia Pacific Unicycling Championships, which meant that for once, Sam wasn't the best unicyclist in the room. Jamey Mossengren, a professional unicycling performer and stunt unicyclist and Chris Huriwai had both volunteered to perform, and both put on cracker shows. There was a band, raffles and auctions, and a three-course meal. Sam was dared to wear some gear from Fyshwick, a district famous for its fireworks (before they got banned here too) and it was, let's call it, adult entertainment. Dressed in a tutu and a corset, with some lovely high heels, Sam went onto the stage to meet the winner of the mystery prize – which was the opportunity to smash Sam in the face with a cream pie. Like it wasn't enough that he had egg on his face, metaphorically speaking, he had to wear a cream pie as well! Canberra, why were we so mean?

A great time was had by all, and a massive $30,000 was raised. But that wasn't the end of our Love Your Sister engagements. We had the usual array of media opportunities and we were to meet the Governor-General, Quentin Bryce. Dressed in our polo shirt uniforms, and driving onto the grounds in our beaten-up Commodore wagon, we felt a bit too shabby to be entering such a regal place as Government House in Canberra, but the staff, Al Charry and Joe Kabalan, immediately made us feel welcome. In fact, they made us feel like it was only right for us to be there. Our appointment with the Prime Minister had been cancelled due to the very sad death of Nelson Mandela, but our visit to Government House was not. Her Excellency, Quentin Bryce, Australia's first female Governor General, was at once powerful and gentle. I found myself thinking, 'How is it that we got here? To be sitting with Quentin Bryce, sharing tea and biscuits and tales of community and causes. Wow!'

As part of the Asia Pacific Unicycling Championships Sam competed in a long distance event, a 10 kilometre ride around Lake Ginninderra. I assumed his travels over the previous ten months would have prepared him well for the event. But I was surprised to find him nervous. He didn't want to come last at something he was supposed to be good at. The competitiveness that I saw so much of as a child came out again. He willed himself to win. He convinced himself he could win.

There are many different types of unicycles. Weird, I know – how many variations can there be? They only have one wheel, for crying out loud! But there are geared and fixed-wheel unicycles, and then there are different sized wheels. The bigger the wheel, the further the rider gets in one rotation of the pedals. Then there is another factor, the length of the cranks. So, to cut a long story short, there are lots of different unicycles out there, but only one race. Sam didn't come first, but he was the first competitor on a 36-inch fixed-wheel uni to finish, which was a great result!

The last event in Canberra was our private little Christmas party, held ten days before Christmas 2013. Over the Christmas–New Year period people would be celebrating with their families – obviously not a good time for fundraising – so what better time for Sam and the crew to have a break? They had a week without unicycles, without community events and without living on top of each other in the Jayco.

Sam needed some time out and I could see no better way to celebrate than with the whole crew. We shared a roast, a barbecue and lots of fruits and salads, but of course the company was the highlight. The kids had their beloved Uncle Long Legs there, as well as the crew, who had all become like cool, fun uncles and aunties between the Gold Coast and Canberra trips. We sat in the park eating, laughing, playing soccer and reminiscing on the incredible year we had all shared.

It was a very special day, but the show had to go on, and the boys headed off to Jindabyne next, for the highest of all the challenges, climbing Mount Kosciuszko on a unicycle.

—

It would be easy to think that ten months on the road would be sufficient training for conquering Kosciuszko, but riding at altitude presented its own set of challenges. The altitude robs the body of oxygen, and all the riding up hills that Sam had done to date wasn't enough to prepare him for this. The lactic acid kept building up in his muscles, causing burning pain, and he simply couldn't catch his breath. The higher he got the more he had to stop, until near the top when he was stopping every 5–10 metres to regain his strength. But my brother rather liked his title of the World's Most Determined Unicyclist, and he definitely earned it. Despite never having trained at altitude and the fact that he had been on the road for ten months straight, he did it. He actually rode his unicycle to the highest point in Australia. He could now say that he had ridden to the eastern-most and western-most edges of the country, and to the lowest and highest points (Lake Eyre being the lowest). We had it in our heads, from the first night in the kitchen when I dared him to ride his unicycle around Australia, that he had to achieve these goals, or he couldn't really say he'd done the whole country. He was getting ever closer to reaching his goal of riding 15,000 kilometres around the entire country.

Any endurance athlete will tell you that a massage really helps your muscles recover, and all around the country massage therapists had visited Sam and given him a therapeutic rub-down after many kilometres on the uni. The Australian College of Massage (ACM) coordinated this along the whole route, even in the most remote areas, and ACM massage therapists all donated their time, happy to help a road-weary Aussie. Massages occurred on the roadside, poolside and even on a pier, but I think that the massage Lisa Green gave him in Jindabyne after climbing Mount Kosciuszko must have been the best. It was certainly the most deserved.

Before that east coast leg of the trip Sam came back to Melbourne and put on the biggest fundraiser yet. We had a committee of dedicated volunteers who helped us organise a gala ball 'Paint the Town Pink'. We had auction items, silent auctions, raffles, live music, speeches from some amazing Love Your Sister contributors and, best of all, we had an excuse to get our glad rags on (yes, Sam had to wear shoes!).

A Melbourne-based band, Hey Frankie, played in the foyer while the guests arrived, all 300 of them, dressed to the nines and ready for a big night out. There was a three-course dinner, plenty of wine, and music to dance to, but at the business end of things we had a heap of live and silent auction items that had been donated to the cause, and there was lots of interest. It was very exciting to see people checking out the items, putting their names down and watching the prices going up and up. We had set a target of $30,000 to raise for the night, but to pull that off would take a lot of things going right for us.

Among the auction items donated were a signed Alice Cooper jacket, a Michael Leunig painting, a trip to the *Offspring* set and lunch with the cast, tickets to *The Project*, a guitar signed by Powderfinger and multiple other high-profile Australian acts and a painting by Gus Leunig. I immediately fell in love with Gus's artwork and put in a bid. I knew I probably wouldn't win it, but I thought it was worth a try. I could just picture it on the wall at the top of the stairs at home; it would match the colour scheme of our apartment perfectly. Measuring nearly 1.5 metres by 3 metres, I had no idea how I was going to get it home to Canberra if I did win it, but I wasn't thinking logically. All I knew was that I wanted it badly.

All throughout the evening I got to meet lovely people who had come along to help raise money for Love Your Sister, usually because they felt a personal connection to our story. Guests shared their own stories of love and loss, and emotions ran high because everyone was so honest. Then a lovely couple came up and asked if I was seriously interested in the Gus Leunig painting. I found it to be an odd question but, in the spirit of the evening, I answered honestly, that I loved it but that realistically I couldn't afford to keep bidding on it. My poor husband had already had to put up with me spontaneously buying a church. (Can you see a pattern forming here?)

There were some speeches made by people who had touched our hearts with their fundraising efforts, including a very moving piece by Lily, who was just 13 at the time. She explained how Love Your Sister had inspired her to go to her school community to raise money. She'd baked a heap of cupcakes and sold them at a stand at her school and raised $241, which she presented to Sam on stage. It was these stories that really captured the spirit of giving that we had seen so much of throughout Sam's trip.

Then came the live auction. With whiz auctioneer Peter Kennet donating his time and expertise, we had high hopes of making a stack of cash out of this. Auctions are so thrilling, it usually comes down to two bidders who really want the item and they go higher and higher, pushing each other to the limit, and sometimes beyond. You never know where it is all going to end up. People were bidding big money on very special items and experiences, and they were spending more because it was for charity. People just wanted to give, and I was very moved as I saw all of this unfolding in the room.

Sam and I were displaying the items, walking them around the room so people could see them while the auctioneer worked his magic. There was one very personal item. It was a scrapbook of photos of the Love Your Sister journey that I had handmade. It was really thick, absolutely chock-full of photos, with a huge Love Your Sister heart on the front. Sam and I had signed it, and I was nervous as it went under the hammer. I wanted it to sell for a good price, because I was emotionally invested, but I was totally gobsmacked when it sold for $2500! The whole room clapped, people were crying, then the most incredible thing happened. Therese Hennessy, who had bought the scrapbook came up to the stage and donated it to Lily, the 13-year-old who had raised money for Sam, and had spoken earlier in the night. Therese's big heart and gesture caused a lot of people to start crying even more, myself included, and everyone in the room stood up and clapped and cheered.

Just when I thought the night couldn't get any better, I was properly introduced to Darren Rumble. I had spoken to him earlier about the Gus Leunig painting. He had won the auction for the painting for $2400, and he had done it for me! After he had spoken to me and saw how much I wanted it, Darren was determined to buy it for me, raising money for a great cause to boot.

It was such an emotional night, with so much compassion in the room. Sam and I were reminded once again just how generous and giving people are, and how much people want to see an end to breast cancer killing their mums, sisters, wives and friends. Through the kindness and generosity of Therese, Darren and many other people at 'Paint the Town Pink', we exceeded our target and raised $64,000. I went home that night exhausted but absolutely amazed at the kindness of strangers.

—

Sometimes I felt like the challenge I set Sam had been a great thing. He was given the chance, over an entire year, to see Australia. Granted, he had to work pretty hard to get around the country given that I insisted he do it on a unicycle, but still, it was a pretty great way to spend a year.

Then, other times, I felt like the challenge was just plain cruel. Really, Con – 15,000 kilometres on a unicycle? What were you thinking? The Nullarbor was one of those times. I couldn't help thinking about the heat and the endless straight road that stretched out for hundreds of kilometres with unchanging desert all around him. I hate blowflies, and yet I'd sent him out into blowie territory, where he had no choice but to find his peace with them and stop bothering to swat them away.

Because of the routing error we'd made in WA, we'd had to find time to go back and do the Nullarbor. And what better time to do it than in the height of summer, right?

Wrong, but we didn't have a choice. And, Sam, I know I didn't do this enough, but I apologise. I'm so sorry I sent you out there on your unicycle, and I'm lucky that you have such a big heart, that you can find forgiveness in there somewhere for your bossy older sister.

I guess it wasn't all bad. It rained a lot while he was riding across it, and so the heat didn't bother him initially, though

I'm not sure what was worse – to be soaked by rain, trying to protect yourself with wet weather gear, or being soaked in sweat.

Note to Sam: The fact that after ten months on the road, you were able to go back and take more punishment on the Nullarbor was yet another reason that I was so proud of you, bro. You were incredible, strong, determined, and had just the right amount of crazy in you to make it all possible. Thanks, Sam, and sorry.

—

Just because Tassie was the last state we visited did not mean that Sam could relax and put his feet up. We had already made the million and broken the record for longest distance travelled on a unicycle but that didn't mean that we could forget our primary aim: to remind every young mum in the land to be breast aware. So Sam headed over to Tassie for a lap of honour around the island before returning to the mainland for the finale.

The *Spirit of Tasmania* was a trip of a lifetime for Sam. He loves boats, and this was the biggest, most impressive boat he had ever seen. What better way to finish a year on the road than a boat trip to the Apple Isle?

Tassie is somewhere Dad and Hilde had both visited and loved. Their raving reports of it have left me with an appetite for the place, but as with many things Love Your Sister, this was one that I had to do vicariously through Sam. I'd been away from my kids so many times throughout the year, and I really wanted to be with them as much as I could be. It was school holidays, and time with family is important.

As soon as they landed in Devonport Sam texted me a photo of a poster out the front of a newsagent. It was huge and yellow with black lettering: LOVE YOUR SISTER ARRIVES ON THE COAST. He called shortly afterwards. 'You know you've done your job when you see that, don't ya, Sis?'

We were both so proud, and so happy. Fancy that, making headlines! Little old us.

Tasmania was chock-full of events, mostly coordinated by the talented (and well connected) Bron Hogan. There was a welcoming party at Salamanca Square in Hobart; a radiothon conducted by Sea FM in Hobart; a sparkly pink circus party; a Bendigo Bank morning-tea fundraiser; Sam played netball in a skirt on his unicycle in Launceston; there was a laser skirmish, and Sam had his fear of heights challenged when he abseiled the Gordon Dam, the highest commercial abseil in the world. It was a flurry of activity, with many people attending fundraisers in multiple cities. Sam joined the Janelle McMillan fan club when he arrived in Hobart and met her at Salamanca Square. Janelle is a local artist and very community driven, and she loves a cause, especially Love Your Sister. She became another huge fundraiser for Love Your Sister.

Tassie communities got behind the cause and raised a heap of cash for research. It looked like we might even reach $1.5 million before we finished – wow! Sam had been welcomed warmly all over Tassie, as on the mainland, and by the time he was ready to take the boat back to Melbourne I thought his heart must be full to bursting with love and beauty.

On his trip around Australia Sam met amazing people each and every day. People opened their hearts, their communities and their wallets to him, and his life was so much richer for it. I felt like I had also achieved one of my goals – to help

Sam see the good in people again, to help him find peace and happiness.

Love Your Sister had given me back my brother.

SAM

To be honest, coming home into Melbourne was hard. I think I was grieving in advance. I loved being on the road. I had a constant stream of meaning and purpose. I was exercising enough to keep Henry at bay and I was away from all of my personal responsibilities, which I've always (mistakenly) found a little onerous. I had a golden ticket straight into the heart of every community I travelled through. I met colourful and kind people all the time, I was given the best of people because of what I was doing. I was inspired on the daily. I felt like I had something very important to do. What would I do when I got off the bike?

The real world was waiting after a year of heightened living. I'd have to find some cash to survive. I'd have to re-enter the mainstream and face Connie's illness. I didn't think I wanted to go home. For the last year, every day I'd woken up and felt like I had something important to do. What would I do now? Where would I live? Oddly, although it was an epic grind at times on the road, it had never been close to the kind of grind that everyday life offers, because what I'd been doing was, frankly, much more gratifying. I was now going to have to look after myself, instead of having duties to focus on every waking hour, and I was worried about the vacuum. As a performer, you can get into a bit of a lull after a gig. You've established bonds and been on a creative journey with people, then it's all over and you scatter. It can leave holes. And Love Your Sister felt much more real than any 'gig' I'd had before. What kind of hole would it leave? There was no way there wasn't going to be a full come-down. What goes up, right? The few people who knew me well were really, really worried about how I'd go after I got back. I'd had to trot out the usual lines, detailing my however-many-pronged strategy to cope with life off the road, but I knew it was all bullshit and that a rut was unavoidable, no matter what measures I'd put in place.

I was excited to have finished the ride safely. Someone getting hurt had always been my biggest fear. I'd looked forward to bringing this puppy home since it began, but while I was proud of everybody, and the anticipation was real, I couldn't help feeling that I was closing the most thrilling chapter in my life. How was anything going to compare with this? I was not sure I could neatly slot back in to a life I had been so keen to escape from in the first place.

I had hatched plans for when the ride was over. We'd decided to keep the Love Your Sister juggernaut going long beyond my return, so the hoped-for respite no longer countered my dread about returning to normal life, because this thing wasn't going to finish like I thought it would.

I'd been reflecting on the year that had been for several weeks. I'd entered pip-spitting competitions, I'd chomped on arachnids, mounted steers, sheared sheep, had Vegemite fights, delivered $50 coffees on my unicycle, run into random guys on penny farthings, swum in croc-infested waters. I'd climbed the Gloucester tree, all 50 metres up, I'd unicycled a kilometre underground in a nickel mine, I'd kissed carp, I'd cross-dressed, I'd shared onesies, I'd stripped at a ladies night, I'd sparred with Danny Green, I'd danced with the Wakagetti Cultural Dancers, I'd sculpted massive boobs in the sand with a whole town of kids, I'd had tea with governors and the Governor-General. I'd been flour-bombed by an entire school, I'd faced altitude sickness and scaled the great Mt Kosciuszko. I'd met with women and their families all around the country and we'd shared our stories and sent love to each other through hugs and words and gifts and smiles. I'd ridden around Uluru, horse tracks, golf courses, speedways . . . Hell, I even got a standing ovation from 35,000 people when I rode around Subiaco Oval during a Freo game. I'd visited dozens of schools, attended hundreds of events and spoken with half the country about not falling into the booby trap. I'd done 1600 media calls and thousands of selfies with the most encouraging and inspiring humans you could ever hope to encounter.

I'd ticked off Connie's bucket list and about a hundred other things. My life was finally just overflowing with colour and beauty after years of wondering what was missing. Connie had gifted me with a life I didn't want to throw away. I'd finally found the pot at the end of the rainbow. But the destination doesn't provide the riches, the gold is in the journey itself. There was no fucking golden pot. I'd be nothing again.

The problem with realising your dreams is that they become real. I imagined a footy player finally winning that elusive premiership, the thing they'd worked their whole life for, only to realise that it was just a medallion. I'd fantasised about crossing the finish line every day since this thing began. It was probably my most powerful motivator. Whenever shit got tough I'd imagine Connie there at Fed Square, alive and well, hugging me upon completion and being more proud of me than anyone has ever been. It had taken almost three years to get to this point and the whole time I'd been terrified of bungling it all, as I'd done with so many other aspects of my life. Barring some freak accident at the final hour, I knew I was going to make it. All of my dreams and aspirations were coming true, but it didn't feel like a fairytale. Quite the opposite, really.

I finally got there, to that place I'd strived for almost three years to get to, and it was packed. People were everywhere. I knew Connie and my family and all of our key supporters were waiting up on stage for me. I was truly excited to see Con, but the rest felt fake. I pedalled up on to the stage and rather than enjoying the moment, I was obsessed with getting this final bit right. A media pack converged and it quickly became about *the narrative*. It felt like the set piece that it was, constructed to fit in with what we thought the public and the media wanted to see.

Don't get me wrong, it's not like there was no joy in the occasion, but I didn't even cry, and I'd cried nearly every day on this thing. There was no tide of relief, or great sense of achievement. I just pretended. It felt like an act . . . partly because Henry came and coat-hangered everything. As soon as I got back and before I'd even left the stage, he was in my ear. He gatecrashed my homecoming something chronic, the silly little prick. I'm not going to dignify it too much, but he made sure that I crumpled before I even had a chance to revel in the success of it all. Henry owned the day, much to my devastation. He paid me back proper for shutting him out.

And so it ended, with Henry triumphant and me in a manic wilt.

I wish there was a happy ending I could give you, but it was funereal for me. The day I got back and hugged my sisters was the day everything got real again. I was relieved and happy, sure, but mostly I was sad, to be perfectly honest. And I was scared about Henry becoming loud again. After all that effort and all that time, it felt like the fight was only beginning . . .

CONNIE

By some freakish occurrence, I had only been in hospital once the whole time Sam had been on the road, and that was in Darwin, when we were together anyway. All of my trips to hospital since then had been day trips for chemo, scans, hormone treatments, oncology appointments, prescriptions, cancer psychiatrist appointments or just to have my port flushed (an implanted catheter used to give intravenous drugs). Everything had gone remarkably well, and been complication free.

I couldn't believe it when I got a fever and started to feel very weak and dizzy in late January. Sam was almost home and a fever always means a trip to hospital – sometimes it puts me in ICU – so I knew it was bad news and that I needed to be careful.

There is always a part of me that thinks, 'If I ignore it, it might just go away.' I wondered at the timing of it all. I'd got through the whole year and, now, two weeks before Sam's return I was going into hospital. Sam had told me he'd been picturing the moment when he rode back in to Federation Square in Melbourne, and fell into my hug. This was what he'd been using as a positive visualisation to get him through those endless kilometres, the flies, the heat, the wind and the driving rain. I had to be there. I had to be.

I felt weak. My blood pressure was low, and I felt like I was going to faint every time I stood up or turned my head too quickly. I was nauseous. The fever was abating but I still felt sick. I had a sore throat and my glands were sensitive. Normally I wouldn't worry about little things like this, but when you have advanced cancer the most innocuous things can bite you hard. I was so scared that I wouldn't make it out of hospital and be well enough to travel to Melbourne for the return event.

'Con, just get out of there, go home, get better and I'll see you at Fed Square,' Sam had said matter-of-factly over the phone, like I was in control of what happened. But then I decided if he could ride 15,000 kilometres around the country for me, the least I could do was be there when he got back.

Em was working almost around the clock getting things ready for Sam's return. She had a team of volunteers who were working so hard to make this day as special as possible.

Sam and I were the stars of the show, and it just wouldn't work if I wasn't there. Em was calm on the outside, but I knew inside she was anxious about me, and hoped that I would be okay, not just because Sam's return date was approaching but because it caused her pain whenever I was sick and hospitalised. As best friends we knew each other well enough to know what the other was thinking, without uttering a word.

The plan was for Sam to come in on the *Spirit of Tasmania* in the morning and be met by Nova Radio with a masseuse to treat his road-weary body and a recliner chair for him to relax in while he had a mini-manicure. Sam was going to do all of the media on his own because we didn't want to see each other until he rode onto the stage and finished for real.

The morning of his return was eerily quiet for me. Despite my concern, I'd been able to fly down and was staying at a friend's place. I was determined to finish the little unicycles I was making for the crew, to say thanks. I'd fashioned them out of wire and they sat on wooden frames. The wheel was connected to the pedals and when you turned the pedals, the wheel rotated. They were about ten centimetres high and looked homemade, but there was no better gift I could think of that would say thanks to everyone. The entire crew had dedicated a year of their time to my cause – breast awareness and breast cancer research. They had put their careers on hold, stored their personal possessions and gone on the road, following a unicycle at 10 kilometres an hour around the country. I know that the experience is one that they'd never have again, and that they'd be bound together for life by this trip, but I still needed to try to say thanks somehow. So I sat in my friend's living room making wire unicycles, listening to Sam on the radio and thinking about the year that had been Love Your Sister.

It was strange that it was all finishing because it felt as though it was too big to finish. We had done everything we set out to do. Sam broke the record for longest distance travelled on a unicycle. We raised well over $1 million and we reminded young mums to be breast aware, not to fall into the booby trap.

At the start of this ride I thought it would be impossible to measure whether we had achieved our most important goal, but I now knew that we had. We had countless emails and Facebook messages telling us that women had been and had a breast exam at the doctor, or had a mammogram if they were eligible for the service. Some gratefully told us that they were given the all-clear, others, sadly were told they had breast cancer.

All of the women we've heard from who were diagnosed with breast cancer after being checked out as a consequence of Love Your Sister, have been diagnosed early and, as a result, have a good prognosis and a good chance of recovery.

Let me tell you about Natalie. Her daughter, Olivia, came home from school one day and asked her, 'Mum, have you checked your boobies?'

Natalie asked her daughter why she was asking such a random question.

Olivia answered, 'A pink man came to our school and asked us to ask our mums to check their boobies.'

So Natalie checked her boobies, dutifully following her daughter's advice. She found a lump, and it turned out to be early breast cancer. Thanks to early detection Natalie has a good chance of seeing Olivia grow up. And that 'Pink Man' has told thousands of women to be breast aware, and continues to do so.

Early detection is the best protection we have against this disease. We don't want to scare people into thinking that they are going to get breast cancer, we just want people to know that if they check regularly and are proactive about their health, then they don't have to end up like me, with a terminal diagnosis, trying to figure out how to tell my children that I'm going to die and they'll have to grow up without their mum.

Sam and I had dedicated the last three years to this project, and now it was coming to an end. I felt exhilarated and incredibly fulfilled, but I also felt a bit empty. I didn't want it to end but the good thing was I would get time with my brother. We would finally get to hang out, not working, not planning, not strategising, just hanging out. It had been a long time coming and I was looking forward to that. I was also a little worried about how Sam would cope with the re-entry into real life. He had claimed back his happiness and I didn't want him to lose that. I was worried Henry would bully him again.

I had my make-up done so I looked fit to face the world and the media. We hoped to trend on Twitter, and to make at least one of the news programs. Sam was riding through Melbourne, pedalling the last kilometres towards Fed Square, and it was time for us to leave. Everything felt oddly calm.

When we arrived in Fed Square there were thousands of people waiting to welcome Sam back. There was a Money Now tent selling Love Your Sister merchandise, and Dominos were giving away pizzas. There were cameras everywhere. I recognised many faces from news and current affairs programs, and was taken aback that they were there for us! The sight of it all was overwhelming and I felt like I was going to cry. I had to stop myself because if I started I doubted if I could stop. And I didn't want to ruin my make-up!

Jo Stanley from Fox FM hosted the return, and there were plenty of celebrities there to celebrate with us: Claudia Karvan, Michala Banas and Guy Pearce among them. The stage was filled with Love Your Sister supporters, people who had gone above and beyond to do fundraisers, donate contra, or help in some huge way, donating time, skills and resources. And there was family; my sister and her children were there; some of the crew were there and the rest would come in with Sam when he arrived; my wonderful husband, Mike, was there with our beautiful little boys, Willoughby and Hamilton. The stage was buzzing with excitement and anticipation. Willoughby kept jumping up searching for his Uncle Long Legs.

The crowd was chanting 'Sammy, Sammy, Sammy!' and Jo Stanley announced that he was just 300 metres away. We hooked up with him on the loudspeaker and I spoke to him as he rode closer and closer. I was shaking, I felt sick, I felt nervous, I couldn't wait for him to arrive. I craned my neck over the front of the stage watching for him, then the crowd let out an almighty scream and I knew he must be in sight.

I saw him snaking his way through the crowd, high-fiving everyone. Then he came up the ramp, and all of a sudden he was on the stage, he dropped his unicycle and collapsed into a hug with me, which Willoughby jumped up and joined. The three of us hugged, celebrating a year on the road, celebrating making the million, celebrating helping other families not to have to say goodbye to their loved ones, but most of all just celebrating being together. A year on and we'd both survived, we were both still here. The rest of our lives started right then.

PART IV
THE NOT-QUITE-LAST CHAPTER

CHAPTER 27

THE REST OF MY LIFE STARTS NOW

Sam will tell you this crazy quest didn't end when he hopped off his unicycle and it won't end when I die. This ends when a cure for breast cancer is found. I know that will be too late for me but I like to think that because of what Sam and I have done, we will have helped get closer to a cure.

Throughout my illness I've been absent from my children for long stretches while I've been in hospital. It's tough. On a few of those occasions I questioned whether I would ever be home again, if my boys would ever get to see their mum again. So when Sam and I started planning Love Your Sister I was hesitant to be too free with my time. I am living with an expiry date, and I am acutely aware of it. So I worried about missing out on time with Hamilton and Willoughby because I was spending all of my time and energy on preventing other families from having to go through what we were going through.

I really wrestled with this. Was I being selfish in wanting to make my own death more meaningful?

In the desperate search to show people the difference between early and advanced cancers, to remind people of the impact of early detection – it could literally save your life – and to raise money for breast cancer research so advanced breast cancer may one day be treatable, I made a conscious decision. That decision involved balancing the benefits that Sam and I could bring to other families against the benefits of spending all of my remaining time with my children and husband. I did sacrifice time with my family to spend time and energy working on Love Your Sister but I still see my kids every day (except when I'm away for volunteer work) and we have a great life together.

And in some ways I think that I have more energy, and have perhaps even extended my life expectancy, by embracing Love Your Sister, so maybe I have gained time with my family due to what Sam and I have done. We will never know for sure but I am so thankful to my husband for his never-ending support and patience. I adore my kids, value them and cherish them. I try not to get bogged down in the everyday, and make the most of every moment we have together.

This whole Love Your Sister 'thing' has amazed and surprised us, delighted and excited us, made us laugh and made us cry. It has been just as amazing as we ever thought it would be, and more. It has started people talking about boobs, which we were determined to do from the outset, but it has also appealed to people in ways we never dreamed of.

Love Your Sister was always a story about breast cancer, but we didn't realise that we would be tapping into an under-publicised love – the love between siblings. There is something special about the love between brothers and sisters. It's there before we meet our spouses and it's there long after our parents are gone. Siblings can pull each other up and say things to each other that friends wouldn't dare think, let alone say out loud. It is competitive between siblings, but protective in the wider world. There is no obligation to protect or nurture, but nothing hurts more than a falling-out between siblings.

We didn't realise that people would connect with us because of our sense of family, that we would tap into that feeling between other siblings out there and draw them closer, or cause them to try to rebuild burned bridges. And that feels nice – because of us, brothers and sisters have reached out to each other and tried to rebuild their relationships.

But it goes further than that. Because people have seen what Sam has done for me, they have decided to make real change in their lives. One woman vowed to lose weight and to raise money for Love Your Sister with every kilo she lost. A pack-a-day smoker we met threw them away forever, another started volunteering at the local refugee service. Nikki Cousins even tried stand-up comedy after hosting the Cronulla fundraiser. Sam has inspired people to change their lives for the better, and together we inspired people to appreciate what they do have; to stop and smell the roses.

As this book goes to print we have about 240,000 likes on The Facebook (as my dad would call it), and a recent post generated 24,000 comments; another yielded 100,000 likes. For a couple of luddites who were basically allergic to social media and a little bit scared of it too, we have built a community, one where people wait for our posts because they like the pick-me-up. Who would have thought that a page about breast cancer could be so uplifting? That's because of my brother. It comes down to the tone that he insisted on from the very beginning. We have done what he aimed for, made the story light, irreverent and occasionally funny. This was never going to be another hard-luck story, this story was about love.

Thank you to everyone who has followed us on 'The Facebook', liked and shared our posts. It's one way for us to know that we are succeeding in our goal, to remind every young mum in the land to be breast aware. People are talking about boobs, and it's great!

Over the year we had over 1600 media hits, we did about 20 appearances on *The Today Show* and a similar number on *The Project*. Sam did regular interviews with radio stations all over the country, we had print media articles including many local papers as Sam travelled through different communities, but also big pieces in *New Idea* and *Who Weekly* as well as the major papers syndicated across the country.

Sam is so magnetic and engaging that every interview he did was funny or entertaining and he never got down and out, never pitied himself and graciously answered the never-ending stream of questions about the wellbeing of his butt/balls. He laid himself completely open, and the press went on his epic journey with him. Because of that we could achieve our number-one goal, to remind women to be breast aware, and the press helped us reach the people we didn't meet in person along the way. Even when he got home and was emotionally and physically exhausted he kept going all day.

Sam visited over 150 towns but he couldn't visit every community in this huge country of ours, so the press helped us reach those people, and I will be forever grateful to the many personalities who followed our story from beginning to end, and into the future. And without the hundreds of Love Your Sister road warriors who just took on the biggest of tasks, no questions asked, we would be nowhere.

We were so fortunate to get the coverage and support we did. People do amazing things for charity every day, and there is only a certain amount of press this kind of story gets. Some people who have done long rides and walks have had no press at all and still managed to raise tens of thousands of dollars for one cause or another.

Jimmy Harrington is a young man, just 18, who walked around Australia at the same time that Sam was riding around. He did it because he met the family of a beautiful little girl who sadly passed away from a brain tumour. Jimmy, with the support of his family, walked and walked, and it wasn't until the end of his trip that the mainstream media picked up his story. He is just one example of the many people who conquer incredible endurance feats for charity. Often we don't hear about them at all. So for us to get the coverage we did was very gratifying, but it also contributed in a huge way to the total of $1.8 million raised, and counting.

I have been blown away by the people I've met and because of my brother I have done things I never thought I could. Writing this book has been a huge thing for me and I only wish Dad was here to share this achievement with us. He'd be so proud.

I have met the most inspiring people during the past few years of Love Your Sister, everyday Australians like Sophie Weston. While Sam was out pedalling around Australia, a Year 12 student from Victoria decided that she would ride from Canberra to Melbourne on her two-wheeler to raise money for Love Your Sister. Sophie Weston went to St Margaret's College in Berwick, and clearly she is going to be the next female prime minister. While completing Year 12 and volunteering for charity, she had decided she could do more, and used her school holidays to raise money for Love Your Sister. At just 17 years of age, she has accomplished more than I have in 37 years on the planet. And she's done it with such grace and commitment.

I went along to her school for the cheque presentation ceremony. I remember feeling so intimidated, these youngsters were so together, driven and community-minded, it put me to shame. But I thought to myself, if these are the future leaders of this country, we are going to be okay – the future looks bright. We hear so much in the press about youngsters being socially disconnected and too obsessed with their mobile phones to engage on a real level, but throughout Love Your Sister I have found the reverse to be true. So many young people Sam and I have met have a social conscience, are engaged with their communities, and are willing and determined to help others.

Sophie rode the interstate bicycle odyssey with her sister and parents as her supports. She coordinated and organised the whole event herself. She could relate to Sam riding around the country for his sister, as she and her sisters are very close, and she loved what we were doing, totally talking down her own achievements.

Sophie raised $7020.80 and she became our single biggest individual fundraiser! But she was one of so many who stepped up to help me and Sam achieve our goals and I will never be able to thank them all.

I've met governors, politicians, celebrities (okay, and Karl Stefanovic!) and I couldn't believe it when Sam and I were invited to a Royal function at Government House in Canberra to meet Prince William and Princess Kate in April 2014. That blew my mind. I chatted to Kate and she was lovely and listened carefully when I told her about Love Your Sister. Later on when she met Sam she said, 'This must be the amazing brother.' She is right about that!

Sam is amazing. We lost our mum when we were young, and things were different back then. There were no mobile phones to take photos and videos on, so we don't have a lot of photos of Mum, and we don't have any footage of her. Neither of us has any memories of her at all. When I was diagnosed, my children were the same age, and I feared that I would die and that my kids wouldn't have memories of me. Because of Sam we made a documentary about Love Your Sister and so I know that even if the memories of me fade, my kids will always be able to watch the documentary and read this book and remember their mum and how much she loved them.

Because, after all is said and done, the most important people in my life are Willoughby and Hamilton, my darling boys. It breaks my heart to think I won't be here to watch them grow up. I can only hope that their sibling bond is as strong as my bond with Sam. I know how special that is.

Though our charity and this book are called Love Your Sister, it has all only been possible because of one man. My brother, Sam. I love you, Sam!

Death is a profound part of everyone's life, which we all have to face one day. I have been incredibly lucky lately. My cancer has been stable. It is responding to treatment after being very aggressive and non-responsive in the early stages of the disease. It went from running rampant to being under control, something none of us expected. I was so close to death a few times that my family were called in. My kidneys and my brain shut down. I was in ICU on machines and drugs that were keeping me alive in the hope that I would get better with support, and eventually be able to support myself again. I remember many doctors and nurses telling me that they were doing everything they could to keep me alive, and to keep fighting.

Being that close to death and living with a terminal prognosis every day means I've learnt to live my life in the present and make the most of my relationships. I have come to realise that that is all that matters in this life. I read something that Michael J. Fox said: 'Family is not an important thing. It's everything.' He's a smart man and they are wise words.

I am so happy that I have survived this long. I've seen Hamilton and Willoughby grow from toddlers into big primary school boys. And I got to see Sam ride back into Federation Square triumphant. I am so happy that Love Your Sister has achieved what it has. And I want to thank everyone who has reached out and shared their stories and their own battles with me. I have been inspired by so many of you. I hope sharing this story does the same and reminds everyone to love your families – sisters, mothers, fathers, brothers, husbands, wives, children and friends.

Hold them close.

Every day is a gift.

ACKNOWLEDGEMENTS

In thanking everyone who has made Love Your Sister possible, and who has made *Love Your Sister*, the book, happen, I simply cannot thank you enough, I would need a whole other book just to do that. Please accept our sincere thanks, and know that we are very grateful, and extremely humbled by the support we have received for these projects.

Thanks to Sam, there are not enough words in the English lexicon to describe my feelings about what you have done for me, so I will stick to the one word that tries to say it all – Thanks. I think I must share you now, as you are not just our brother anymore, you are the brother of all Australians.

Thanks to Mike, Willoughby and Hamilton, and Dave for understanding that I couldn't always be at home and for sharing me and Sam with Australia. You have been very patient and understanding, and you are the best family ever.

Love Your Sister couldn't have happened without our amazing road crew, thanks to Jonno, Al, Leighton, Stuey,

Mando, Dion, Nato, Gemma and Sarah for donating your time to help make our dream a reality, I can only hope that you had enough fun along the way to compensate for all you've sacrificed. I know that time on the road meant time without income, away from your jobs, your family and friends and I am incredibly grateful for all you've done for Love Your Sister and breast cancer in general. Please know that each and every one of you can make the claim that you raised a million dollars for breast cancer research, and saved many lives through early detection and awareness.

Em, you are the reason we made it at all. Without you we wouldn't have known what to do, where we were going, where to stop, who to contact or how to even start. You are a force. Not only did you work fulltime hours at nights and on the weekends, while employed in a 'normal' job, but when you finally became a fulltime staff member for Love Your Sister, you continued to work fulltime hours, then nights and weekends, always working so much harder and longer than we could ever pay you for. Thanks so much, we love you very dearly. And Em, just so you know, you are not only my best friend, but you are THE best friend anyone could ever have. Thanks.

Thanks so much to John and Jamie Johnson. You have been mentors from whom we have learnt so much. You helped us get this thing off the ground by guiding us through the process as well as providing backing when all else failed. Sam owes his whole Love Your Sister experience to you two, and I owe you the extra years I have lived as a result of Love Your Sister. You have seen me go from my deathbed, to leading a full and happy life with my family. Thanks also to Sue, Alison, Peter, Abby, Abby-Lee, Jarryd, Corey, Zoe and Sarah, Michael, Bill, Kim,

Julie and the rest of the Johnson clan, as we all know we have got to have one of the biggest families in the country, I cannot name you all, but you are in our hearts and have our thanks.

Thanks to Uncle George and our dear departed Aunty Marg for always being there for us, and rescuing us when we needed it, for being like a mum and dad to us not just through Love Your Sister, but all through our lives. Uncle George we love you, and Aunty Marg, we miss you.

Hilde, my dear sister, I love you. I am sorry that I took Sam away from you not just for the ride year, but also in the years leading up to it. I know you must miss your chats on the porch, but you remain close to both of our hearts. We are so proud of you for finding your way in a difficult time, and love you for being you. I can't believe you found time to run the Love Your Sister online shop with everything else going on. You are a champ, and we thank you for everything you have done for Love Your Sister, and for being such a guiding light for both of us, your younger siblings.

Sully and Aussy, thanks for your support with Love Your Sister and we are so very proud of you both. Growing up is the hardest thing you ever have to do, and you are both growing into such amazing young men. Be proud. We love you.

When I met Mike, I was immediately welcomed into his family, and have felt a true part of the family ever since. To Chris, you know what it is I'm going through, thanks for being there for me, especially when I have been at my lowest. To Chris and Ray, thanks for raising such an amazing person as Mike, I know you are proud of him, and I see why every day. To Andrew and Penny, Xavier and Ava, Dale and Sacha, Campbell and Miller, thank you for including me in your family. To all of the extended John/Harvey clan, thanks, you are an amazing group of people and I love you all.

During Love Your Sister my friends and family have been remarkably understanding that I have not had time for things like going out, so thanks for your patience with me as a friend, I have neglected you all during the Love Your Sister ride year, and while writing this book. I can't believe you still want me as a friend, but I guess that means we are true friends and will be for the rest of my life. Thanks to Nancy, Robert and Silas Waites, Lloyd and Steph and family, Sue and Jeff Lyons, Garance Deterring, Moira Byrne Garton and family, Sue and Alice McIntosh, Scott Stone, Ilinka Budisic, Andrew Rich, Majah Brooks, Kim Burnett, Kim Lamech, Emy Aylisse, Ruth Monty, Joan and Peter Clayton, John and Julie Sheather, Denis and Joan Halpin, and all the Halpin clan, Juzzie Rozniak, Kirrilee, Amy Luke and family, Yasmine Grey, Ron and Susan Gale, Zoz and Heather, Ben Abrahams, Tony Vacarro, Winnie Salamon and our new friends Allan and Deb Sparkes, Matt and Gen, Alex and Millie Bolger, and Craig Coombes.

My medical team and palliative care team. Without you all doing such a great job of keeping me alive, I wouldn't have been able to share Love Your Sister with my brother. Thank you for the life-saving and life-prolonging work you do everyday for cancer patients like me in and around Canberra. Every day you give so much, and you treat me like a person not a disease, which makes every difference in me being able to turn up for treatment. Thanks to Kerryn Ernst, Dr Anna Burger, Dr Nicole Gorddard, Amanda, Kate Maher and Dr Zekrya and all the staff at oncology, 14A and 14B, radiation, pathology and radiology at the Canberra Hospital.

ACKNOWLEDGEMENTS

To Eden Monaro Cancer Support Group. Thanks for the support that you have given me and my family. A lot of people don't think of the impacts of a cancer diagnosis on a family, and you give practical, real help to families in need. I am appreciative to have been a recipient of help from Eden Monaro. You do great work. Thanks.

Community Options and ACT Nursing Service. Thanks for providing ongoing support for our family, it makes a huge difference, and because I am not spending the little energy I do have in the day on daily tasks, I am free to pursue fundraising activities which is incredibly fulfilling. Your support is invaluable.

Thank you to Sandra, Glenda and the whole Captial Chemist team for managing my medications so well and also for your generosity with Love Your Sister fundraisers.

To the Garvan Research Foundation and Institute, thank you for your groundbreaking work in cancer research. It is a long hard slog, and is often faceless and thankless. To every single staff member at the Garvan we thank you. In particular huge thanks go out to Andrew Giles, Mara-Jean Tilley, Dr Alex Swarbrick, Kylie Sherwood-Kelly, Bec Hassler and Leonie Walton.

Spoonful, to Andre and Kit, Lordo, Paul Winstanley and Rob Broberg, your music has gotten me through some tough times in my life and always manages to put a smile on my face. You have treated me like a little sister, protected me and been my mentors. Thank you for being there for me, you guys rock!

To Mia Kate Russell, Gina Militia and Ferne Millen for doing our make-up and photos before anyone had heard of Love Your Sister, thanks for donating your precious time.

To Kate Radford, you are a shining light my friend, always willing to help, thanks for doing my make-up throughout Love Your Sister, and to Paul, Kit and Darcy for always being there for our family. Lots of love from our family to yours.

Thanks to Alistair Marks for the stills photography.

Thanks to Nick Marks and the whole Soundtrack team. Lu Munnoch, thanks for doing our blogs, as a cancer patient yourself I know it is hard to concentrate on volunteer work while you are sick. Thanks so much also to your little helpers, Alex and Charlotte, for their help with fundraising. You are a cracker family, thank you.

Thanks to Dr Robert Waites for being the Official Love Your Sister dentist.

Thanks to the crew at Hachette Australia for making this book what it is. Vanessa Radnidge, thank you for 'getting' us. Thanks to Kate Stevens, Isabel Staas, Alice Wood and Chris Kunz for your work on the book, you are amazing and ever helpful. Thanks to Christa Moffitt for your design work, not just on this book, but also for *From The Road*.

Thanks to Merran Giddens, Jan Ham, Andre Warhurst and of course Hilde and Dad for your encouragement of my writing.

Roger Harvey, thanks for running around town, usually at the last minute, to help with everything Love Your Sister.

Natalie Clemmet and Natalie Fielding, your strength and determination have been a source of inspiration to me for many years, since we were all sick together in the Royal Children's Hospital. Thanks to Nat and Nat, Helen, Fiona, Kylie, Christian, Travis, Kimberley, Carly, Brooke, Sally, Shaun, Luke, Toby, and all the crew from RCH, Canteen and Challenge. Remembering our fallen friends, Matt, Sherryn, Renee, Fiona and all children who have passed away from childhood cancers and blood disorders.

Ceri Hinton, thanks for shaving your head and making me feel less alone.

Thanks to our Branch Manager, the late Ralph Hawkins for getting us an audience with the Bendigo Bank senior team, and for helping us get Love Your Sister off the ground. Our sympathies to Sharon and your family.

To the individuals at Telopea Park School who have gone above and beyond for our children, Mrs Millar, Mrs Solomko, Sue Forrest, Ellie and Corinna.

Thanks to Richard Selesnick for accepting us, getting in touch, and for coming all this way to see us. I hope that we can see each other again soon.

Sponsors – we have tried not to plug directly to you about our wonderful sponsors, but truly, without them Love Your Sister wouldn't have happened. So next time you need a loan, please consider the Bendigo Bank or Money Now, both huge supporters of Love Your Sister and if you feel like supporting the companies who support breast cancer research, please consider these guys when next you have occasion to use them.

Love Your Sister is all about community, and what made it so special everywhere we travelled was the people we met. To all the Bendigo Bank Community Branches, schools, local councils, hospitals, business owners, police and emergency services personnel, community groups and every single person who organised, attended or donated at a Love Your Sister fundraiser along the way, we send our sincere thanks. We have tried our darndest to compile a list of everyone who contributed, but the nature of these things means that we will have missed some people, but please know that every single person who contributed, even if we don't know you personally has our thanks.

Thanks to Nancy Stroop, who designed and made love your sister heart cushions, selling them online and donating a percentage of proceeds to Love Your Sister and to Lucas Loves Cars, internet business run by Helle and Mark Warming, who not only sent great toys for Willoughby and Hamilton, but ran an online campaign, donating a percentage of sales to Love Your Sister.

To everyone who applied for a Love Your Sister tin and raised money through your business and personal networks, thanks for making the effort. It all adds up, and your help is invaluable.

Every media outlet who helped us announce our arrivals in towns and helped us thank communities after our visits, newpapers and radio stations mainly, as well as local TV in some of the bigger regional centres, thanks for covering our story, and helping us with our breast awareness goal.

Bendigo Bank Community branches, you held innumerable fundraisers all over the country. The participation of each branch came down to local enthusiasm for the cause, and we thank you for helping us on a community level in hundreds of local areas around Australia.

Thanks so much for all of the kind and thoughtful gifts that Sam and I have received. From flowers to chocolates, framed photos to jewellery, quilts and homemade gifts. We are very thankful for the gifts, and haven't always been able to send a personal thank you letter, so thanks to everyone who sent a gift. The gesture is simply beautiful.

ACKNOWLEDGEMENTS

And last, but most definitely not least: Thanks to every single Australian who donated or bought merchandise to help us raise money for breast cancer research. Together, we have made a difference! Thank you.

THANK YOU

Money Now

Solitaire Paul, Callum Wright and all at the Bendigo Bank Community Enterprise Foundation

Justine Bloome and The Village Agency

Nicole Honig at End to End Creative

Dion Beasley and the crew at Print Design Australia

Jayco

Coles Express

Tony Hayes of Cleverbits

Uberglobal

Ark Construction Group Pty Ltd

Domino's Pizza

Vodafone

Brian Heaven and all at Pivotel

Big4 Holiday Parks

NAK Hair & Daryl Agnew

Creative Legal

iSentia

Deventer Public Relations & Mel & Jodie

Mark Brewster

ProduceIT

Andy at Kaos Custom Bikes

John Grauduszus & Antique Motorcycle Unicycle.Com

Gatorade

Asics

Swisse

Fitness First

Kelloggs

Sheppard Cycle & Park Tool

Swalbe

Garmin

Oakley

Andrea Lindsay and all at Australian College of Massage

LateNite Films

Chemical Media

Gina Milicia Photography

Ferne Millen Photography

Paul Simmons Photography

Jim Kellam Photography

Kelly Gardiner Photography

Wicked of Oz

Kate Radford MUA

Copperhead Printing

Prop-A-Ganda

Fighters Factory

Pacific Optics

Robyn Grove Graphic Design

Andrew Mara

Madeleine Burke

Jo Scard at Fifty Acres

Twig Marketing

Julian & Lucas Rutten

Monica at The Sticker Family

Countrywide Embroidery

Alicia at Print On My

Karen Ristevski & Bella Bleu

Dez Stallard at The Graphics Department

Nicole Graham at Emergency ID Australia

Jen Mulholland at Fancy Shoe Land

Briony & Leanne at Thoroughbred Park

National 4x4 & Outdoors Show

Andrea Cross

Lucy Freeman

Amanda Freeman

Georgie Morrison

Kris Dalgleish

Kristie McInerney

Susan Clavin

Liz Garrett

Lauren King

100.9 Sea FM

1830 Restaurant

ACKNOWLEDGEMENTS

5 Senses
Aamies Photography
Aardvark Adventures
Aaron Crump
Aaron Wilson
Abel Tasman Airport Motor Inn
AccounTech Solutions & Tencia & Peter
    Beckerleg
ACT Unicycle Riders Society
Adam Hills
Adam Ziino & Shout Media
Adventureland Park
Agatha Fonesca
AJ Hackett Cairns & Jacqui Flack
AJA Restaurant
Alan Brown
Albany Harbourside Apartments & Mark
    & Louisa
Albert Clark
Alex Howroyd
Alexandra Thomas
Alicia Dewberry
Alicia & Glass Lake
Alison Karafilis
Allie Cooler
Allphones Arena
Alyssa Braithwaite
Amanda Keller
Amber Turner
Anada Jones
Andrea Cross
Andrea Lindsay
Andrew Mara
Andrew Meats
Andy Hood
Andy McGarvie
Angie Cowen
Anita Demopoulos
Annabel Gay
Anne Little
Annette Anning
Apple Blossom Cottage & Robert
    Ebenestelli

April Conforti
Ararat Primary School & Christine Fiscalini
Arbonne
Arianne Thornton
Ariel Shaw
Ash & Natasha Brennan
Ashwin Bhoina
Astrid Cooper
Athol and his Mob
Augusta Hotel
Augusta Lighthouse
Australian Unicycle Society
Auto Barn
Bakers Delight Claremont
Bank Hotel (Newtown)
Bar Nosh
Barb Pinter
Batters Fish N Chips and Glen & Susan
Bazlec Ba Rompa
BCF
Beachside Medi Spa
Beautiful Valley Café
Bec Willis & Shadow Lust Designs
Bee on Boardwalk
Beck Hardman
Belinda Fithie
Belinda J Hendriksen
Bella at Lil Miss Macaron
Bellicious
Ben Brown
Ben Coles & the Super Wrestling Heroes
Ben Joss
Bennetts Steel
Ben Praccus
Bernie Tanner
Better Read Than Dead
Bev Ardagh
Beyond The Sea
Beyond The Sea & Kylie van Wanrooy
BIG4 Cairns Coconut Holiday Resort
BIG4 Noosa Bougainvillia
BIG4 Toowoomba Garden City Holiday
    Park

Bill Johnston
Bill Kalajdziovski
Billabong Zoo
Billiard Blitz
Black Duck Brewery
Blossy Bloom
Bob Robertson
Bohemian Diva
Bondi Beach Cruisers
Bonnie & Clydes
Bordertown Speedway & Michelle Jenkin
Brad Berlin
Braden Walters
Bradley Heathcote
Brady Denehey
Brae Grimes
Brandi Crouch
Brave Hearts on the Murray
Bree Russell
Brendan Tsui
Brendon Pavey
Brenton Matulick
Bret Perkins
BridgeClimb Sydney
Bridie O'Reilly's
Brigitte Duclos
Briony Kidd
Brittany Sheahan
Brock Mathers
Bron Hogan
Bruce Hintz
Bunbury Trotting Club
Bunnings Alexandria
Bunnings Morayfield & Jenny Fourez
Bunyip Preschool
Buyin Time & Kelley Adamo
C.ex Staff & Carrie Skinner
Caboolture Family Network & Bron Emerson
Caboolture Riverlakes Motel
Caerwen Martin
Cafe Jas & Sharron and Mat Keating
Café Martini

Cam Batten
Cameron & Liz Francis
Campana's
Canada White
Candice Marshall
Cape Leeuwin Lighthouse
Capital Chemists
Carlton United Breweries
Carly Findlay
Carmel Kennedy & all at Hibiscus Tavern
Carpethire.com & Julie Singh
Carrie Bickmore
Cassandra Kun Body Therapy
Cassegrain Winery
Cassie Matthees
Cath Roberts
Cathy Allen
Cathy Freeman
Ceduna Community Hotel & Stefan Thiselton
Ceduna Koonabba Aboriginal Health Service
Challenge Fitness
Chapter One Clothing
Charlie Allum
Charlie Pickering
Charity Rose Turner
Chel Cherie
Chelsea & Deanna & Kambalda Garden Services
Cheryl McLeary
Chris Bailiff
Chris Hallet
Chris Huriwai
Chris Walker
Chrissy Swan
Christian Puusep
Christian Read
Christophe Domergue
Cindy Clarkson
City Golf Club
City of Ballarat
Claire d'Este

ACKNOWLEDGEMENTS

Claire Hooper
Clare Woolcott
Clarke Rubber
Claudia Karvan
Coastwide Concrete Pumping
Colin Christensen
Colin Lane
Colin McHardy
Colleen Cox
Collette McCool
Commercial Hotel Murrumburrah
Community AXIS Enterprises & Viv
    Watson
Conrad Mace
Coolaroo Umbrella
Coolum Beach Real Estate
Coolum Beach Shoes and Accessories &
    Joanne Hampson
Coolum Beach Surf Club
Cooma Ex-Services Club & Kade Morrell
Coonabarabran High School & Jenny
    Sullivan
Coral Coast Tourist Park
Corona Beer
Cowra Police & Cath Sutherland
Craft Design Realisation
Craig Coombes
Craig Nicholls & PFD Food Services
Craig's Royal Hotel
Crossfit Logic
Damien Flegg
Daniel McKuride
Danila Dilba Health Service
Danny Green
Darren Bottom
Darren Rumble
Dave Biggin
Dave Hughes
Dave Starr
Dave Thornton
David Buchanan
David Jones
David O'Meara

Deb Deidricks
Deb Hallyburton
Deborah Botica & Travelworld Kalgoorlie
Deborah Mailman
Della Mano
Demi Fox-Jones
Dendy Cinema Newtown
Denise Scott
Deniz Tek
Deny Kirkwood
Devonport Advocate Newspaper
Di Richards
Di Wright
Diane Tipping & Katies Cakes
Dina Karamaloudis
Divers Tavern & Robin Strauss
Dog Pack
Dog Show Prizes
DollFace Hair & Body
Dolphin Discover Centre & Jan Tierney
Donna Hughes
Dr Garden
Dragons Abreast
Drawable
DXN Solutions
Dylan Lewis
Eagle Farm Racecourse
East Coast Photography & Craig Mason
El Questro Station
Elaine Duffy
Electrical Project Solutions
Ellis Remedial Sports Therapy
Eloise Gregorias
Em Anders & Murals & Art Décor
Emerald Lakes Golf Course
Emily Agostino & THE MAC
Emily Elkhoury
Emily Heathcote
Emjays
Emma Crethary
Emma Tunstead
Emma Wilson
Emmanuel & Cox

Emmetts
Endota Spa
Erin Davey
Erskineville Deli
Esperance Driftwood Apartments
Essa Trend
Eucla Motel & Amanda
Eve Nightclub
Evo Hair Care
Exquisit & Shana Miatke
FDC Group
Fern Anderson & the Sydney Swans
Final Sound
Finishing Touch
Finucane Island Club & Uncle Tom &
    Aunty
Flax Flowers & Amanda
Flying Penguin Toy Store
Focus Magazine
Forage & Ken Villa
Frances Watts
Frank Baxter Juvenile Justice Facility
Frank Woodley
Frankie Bush
Freddo's Meats
Fullthrottle Flyboarding & Jackie &
    Shannon Rostron
Gaza Sports & Community Club
Gecko Red Restaurant & Kodi Brady
Ged Williams
Genevieve House
Georgia Bolton
Georgie Strong
Giant Steps
Gilgandra Jockey Club
Gillwinga Public School
Ginny Bolger
Ginny Tooth
Gino Piombo
Glasshouse Hair & Beauty
Glen Osborne House B&B
Glen Steveson
Glenferrie Hotel

Glenn Cairncross & Elouera SLSC
Glenn Koek
Glenn Ridge
Glenno Smith
Gloria Moyle & Goldfields Women's
    Health Care Centre
Gold Coast TAFE
Gold Coast University Hospital
Gold Mark Jewellers
Golden Guitar Motor Inn
Goldfields Physiotherapy Services
Gone Bonkers
Graham Thompson
Great Southern Grammar
Greens Quality Meats
Greyhound Australia & Nick McDonald
Grant Higgins
Griffith University
Growers Market & Rebecca & Mike
    Cusato
Guerilla Zingari
Gus Leunig
Guy LeCouteur
Guy Pearce
Halls Creek Home Electrical
Halls Creek IGA
Hand Of Law
Hands of Imagination & Leanne Carroll
Hannah Gadsby
Hannah Jeffers
Hansen Print
Harvest Food Store
Harvey World Travel & Nat Henry
Haylee Doring
Heather Yarker
Heidi Watter
Her Excellency Marie Bashir
Hey Frankie
Hiatus Kaiyote
Hired Gun Productions
Horsham Amcal Pharmacy & Carlie &
    Bianca
Horsham Aquatic Centre

ACKNOWLEDGEMENTS

Horsham Lanes and Games
Horsham Sports & Liesure
Howards Storage World
Hugh Pavitt
Hungerford Hill Wines
Ian Clough
Ian Roberts
Ibis Styles Hotel & Jason Green
Ibis Styles Kalgoorlie
IKEA
Intimo Café & Winebar
Ithaca Cottage, Mudgee
Itsy Bitsy Baskets
Jacqui Nicholson
Jake Toivonen
Jaklene Vukasinovic
Jamie Mossengren
Jana Tallon
Jane Perkin
Jane Ramsay
Jane Taylor
Janet Devenney
Janet Parkhouse
Janine Grover
Jasmin Boyd
Jason English
Jason James
Jay Osbourn
Jayna Gibson
Jayne Coombes
JCB Carpentry
Jeff Jones Plants & Produce
Jennifer Hansen
Jenny Brockie
Jenny Kollman
Jeremy Rogers Photography
Jess at Buggy Boo
Jess Dix
Jess Palmer
Jessica Marais
Jessica Marunui
Jetty Café & Tearooms
Jill Gregory

Jill O'Brien & Shire of Coolgardie
Jim & Lenka Henry
Jindabyne Central School & Kirsten Farmer
Jo Stanley
Joanna McGrow
Joanne Saunders
Joao Dujon Pereira
Jodi Topping
Jodie Green
Jody Beven
Joel Moore
John Wood
Johnny Gee
Johnny Thunder & the Lightnings
Jon Barrie
Joico Hair Products
Jonathan Schuster
Josh Roelink
Josh Thomas
Jules Pascoe
Julia Zass
Julian O'Brien
Julian Wilson
Juliana Chambers
Julie Ross
Julie-anne Hassall
Justin Majid
Kain Borlass
Kapunda High School & Andrew Mickan
Karden Disability Support Foundation &
    Steph Wallace
Karen Beale
Karen Fysh
Karen Marshall
Karen Nettelfield
Karen Orchard
Karin Karafilis
Karin Little & Oil & Spice Café
Karl Dentong
Karl Stefanovic
Karyn Hogan
Kass Hall
Kate Candlish

Kate Kelsey-Sugg
Kate Langbroek
Kate Pickett
Kate Wood-Foye
Kath Hunt
Kath Taylor
Katherine Dodd
Katherine Eden
Katherine Moore
Katie's Cakes
Katrina Woolcott
Kawaii Kids
Kaye Few
Kaz Humphrey
Keith and Shane Urban
Kellie Rosenthal
Kelly-Ann Bunney
Ken Healy
Ken Hose
Kerri Nichols Naturopath
Kerry Ratcliffe & The Koru Studio
Kevin Martin
Kevin Nugent
Kim Bitossi
Kim Burnett
Kim Gilliott & family
Kim Lennon
Kim Steinbeck
Kimberley Air Tours
Kimberleyland Holiday Park
Kincumber High School
Kincumber Hotel Staff
Kir Corney
Kleenheat
Kmart Horsham
Kmart Charmaine
Koru Framing Specialists
Kostas Trakas
Kris Johnstone
Krissie McDonald
Kristian Murphy
Kristina Echols & Channel 7
Kununurra Skate Park

Kununurra Speedway
Kylie Obst
Kylie Sessa
Lacey Paperone & Leash Dog Grooming
Laconda Italian Steakhouse
Lake Crackenback Resort & Spa & Scott
   O'Neile
Lake Imaging
Lake View Hotel
Lakelands Caravan Park
Lancelin Primary School
Landy's Bistro & Grant Howard
Laura Hess
Laura Purcell
Lauren Davine
Lauren Glezer
Lauren Reading
Leadership Ballarat and Western Region
Leanne Jones
Lehmo
Leigh Courtney
Leisa Young
Lena Seeto & Dog Pack
Lidia Cosla
Lighthouse Beach Resort
Lighthouse Tattoo
Lily Mays Hair
Linda Carroll at Ambleside on The Lake
Lindy and Shelly Horton
Lion
Lions Club & Vince Nocente
Lisa Bleakley Professionals Kalgoorlie
Lisa Gervasoni & Family
Lisa Green
Lisa Wilkinson
Litisha van der Weert
Little Black Booth
Little Caesars Pizzeria & Theo Kalogeracos
Little Fish Café
LiveLife Pharmacy
Liz Matulick
Liz's Open Cut Café
Lizzy Welsh

ACKNOWLEDGEMENTS

Lloyd Remedio
Loma Simmons
Lorna Roberts
Lou Moxey
LouLou Merchant
Lovelight Kingdom & Rain Magrin
Lucy Dwyer
Lucy Paplinska
Luella Moore
Luke Campbell
Luke Mullan
Luke Spalding
LUX Bread
Lyndel Sutton
Lyndon Bartholomew
Lynne & Ron Lemon
Macchia Jewellery
Macksville Ex-Services Club
Macleay Hotel Potts Point
Malcolm East
Mandy Whitwell
Mansfield Cottage Barrington
Margaret River Hotel
Marie & George Lancaster – Gascoyne
    Hotel
Marilyn Ward & Gold Fields St Ives
Mark Hayes
Marked Hair & Mark Harrigan
Marni Jenkin
Mars
Masterchef
Matt Bolger
Matt Hayes
Matt Mannix
Matt, Mel and the Diabolik Team
Matthew Coulsen
Matthew Deller
Matthew Gnech
Matthew Lincoln
Mawunyo Gbogbo
Max Gillies
McFarlanes Plumbing
McDonald's Karratha

McGrath Real Estate Agents
Mean Fiddler Restaurant & Pete &
    Michelle
Megadeck Staging Systems
Megan Callus
Megan Marwood
Megan Reeve
Mel White
Melbourne Pub Group
Melinda O'Brien
Melissa Cue
Melissa Gardiner
Melissa King
Melissa Stewart
Melrose Primary School & Gail Murphy
Mercure Hotel & Klaus Kinateder
Mercure Hotel Perth & Mandy Rodgers
Metro Hotel Ipswich International
Michael Chamberlin
Michael Fountain
Michael Leunig
Michael List
Michala Banas
Michelle Day
Michelle Kelly
Michelle McIntosh
Michelle Roderick
Michelle Shannon, Oscar Grigg, Lewis
    Grigg & George Grigg
Michelle Teather
Mike Watt
Mitre 10
Moe's Mexican Bar & Grill
Moira Lye & Family
Molly Meldrum
Momentum Financial Group & Mark
    Ainsworth
Monique Galloway
Monkey Mia Dolphin Resort
MooMedia – Chris & Shannon Bryan
More Than Paws
Mornington Secondary College
Moroccan Oil Hair Care

Morven Gemmill
Mount Zero Olives & Neil and Jane
Mudgeeraba Special School
Mundaring Primary School
Nadia Ali
Nadine Barry
Nadine Shiells
Nambour High School
Nambucca Valley Breast Cancer Support
   Group
Natalia James
Natalie Paatsch & Family
Natalie Thomas
Nature's Formula
Neridah Zlatnik
Netball Tasmania
Nial Townsend
Nic Vevers
Nick Cooper
Nicholas Marks
Nick Martyn
Nicole Naylor
Nicole Parry-Leahy
Niki Tunstall
Nikki Atkinson
Nikki Grieve & The Alan Walker Cancer
   Centre
Noah Rosenbloom
Noelene McWhirter & Cobham Aviation
   Services
Noni Hazelhurst
Noosa Bakery & Patisserie
Normandie Meyer & Normandie Meyer
   Photography
North Ballarat Sports Club
North Coast Holiday Park
Northern Beaches Unicycle Club
Northern Blues FC
Norton Estate Wines & Chris Spence
Nu Fitness
Ocean Addicts
Office of Environment & Heritage & Trish
   Swain

Omar Chicho
Optical Alkemi Studios
Orange Primary School
Ord River Dragon Boats
Origin Muscle Clinic & Cath Eather
P.B.A.C.
Pacific Brands
Palmwoods Caravan Park & Simon
Pam & Terry Foye
Pam Watkinson
Party Rocket Icecream
Paterson Stadium
Paul McCarthy Advertising
Paul Shanahan
Peta Thomas & Motorcycling Victoria
Peter Buchstaller
Peter Carrodus
Peter Marks
Phil Collins
Phoebe Lindner
Pia Miranda
Pinctada Cable Beach Resort
Pink Roadhouse & Lauren
Pink Silks Team & Simon Chladil
Pisces Big 4 Apollo Bay
Platform 28
PM Electric
PMQ Golf Driving Range
Pompeos Family Italian Restaurant
Port City Commercial
Port Jet
Port Macquarie Surf School
Portland Hotel
Prairie Hotel
Preston Market
Publican Group
Quality Hotel Wangaratta Gateway
Queensland Bulls Masters
Quorn Area School & Sarah Bury
Quota International of Coolum Beach
Rach Doney & her amazing family
Rachael Allan
Rachael Bean

ACKNOWLEDGEMENTS

Rachael Comte
Rachael Miller
Rachel Edwards
Rachel Pascoe
Ralph Downer
Randall Medd
Ray Ahn, John Needham & The Hard Ons
Ray Dally
Ray White Karratha
Rebecca O'Connell
Rebecca Thomson
Red Symonds
Rhys Passmore
Richard J Watkins
Richard Stolz
Rick Grossman & the Hoodoo Gurus
Rick Nicholson
Rick Scarfone
Rik McCaig & Bendigo Madison
Riva Restaurant
River Angels
Rob (Paw Paw) Moore
Rob Armstrong
Rob Hurst from Midnight Oil
Rob Kinninmont & Yahava KoffeeWorks
Robb Tickner
Robbie Gard
Robert Musgrove
Robertsons Furniture & Lisa & Roger
    Sordello
Robyn Cole
Robyn Shanks
Rocks Brewing Co – Mark Feathers & Tim
    Fishwick
Rod Lambert
Romina Di Federico
Ron & Susan Gale & Talk About Hair &
    Beauty
Ros Lovell
Rose Ottavi-Kokkoris
Roses Vineyard
Rotary Caravan Parl
Royal Flying Doctor Service

Royce Hotels
Rubi Hair
Ryan Lim
Ryans Hot Bread
Rydges Hobart
Rydges Port Macquarie
S & D McNamara & MCM Security
Sails Resort PMQ by Rydges
Sam Hirschfelder
Samantha Wantling, Ella Archibald-Binge
    & the staff at the Stanthorpe Border
    Post
Sammi Whang
Sammy McPherson
Sandra Robinson
Sarah Edwards & Kambalda Hair
Sarah Keith
Sarah Little & Breastscreen NSW
Sarah Marinos
Sarah Parkes
Sarah Tancred
Sarah White
Sarah Wilson
Savage Seas Adventures
Savannah Nickel Mine & Sahn & McGaw
Savons d'ailleurs & Marie-Helene
    Blackmore
Scampis Restaurant
Scott Elkington
Scrapbooking Memories Australia &
    Vanessa Cavassini
Sea FM Hobart
Sea World
Sean Dugan
Selkirks
Sharee Dew
Sharon Ayres
Sharon Broad
Sharon Chapple & Uno Amore Coffee
Sharon Gambrill Laughter Yoga
Sharon Lewis
Sharon Vanderkaay Golotta
Sharyn McKitterick

Shelley Beach Caravan Park & Brownie
Sheridan Wright
Sherry Fitzgerald
Sherryl Robinson
Shire of Roebourne
Sigrid Thornton
Silver Star Café & Restaurant
Silverdome & Rebecca Hardman
Simon Carter
Simone Reid
Simone Richards
Sindy Sinn
Sister June
Skydive The Beach Sydney &
    Brooke Grudy
SLC
Snap West Melbourne
Solotel
Sophie Switajewski
Sophie Weston & Family
South Grafton Bowling Club
Sovereign Hill
Spirit Radio
Sporties Club Tuncurry
Spotlight Theather Ashmore & all the cast
    of Phantom
Sprent Primary School & Rachael Watt
Spring Hill Farm
St Philip's Christian College
Stawell West Primary & Sarah Howard
Steph Farmelo
Stephen Babbage
Steve Ellis
Steve Hari
Steve Lambrinos
Steve Marshall
Steve Moneghetti
Stone & Wood Brewery
Strata Professionals
Suanne Sykes
Subway & Shari Knox
Sue Gray
Sue Morris

Sun Dial Dental
Suncorp Stadium
Sundowner Caravan Park
Susan Hughes
Susan Kilgour & Wulagi Primary School
Susan O'Loughlin & Crocosaurus Cove
Sutherland Shire Women
Suzanne Oakley
Sweet Decadence
Switch Café & Bar
Sydney Buddhist Centre
Sydney Harbour Tall Ships
Sydney Pub Tours & Gary West
Sydney Swans
Sydney Tall Ships
Symbio Wildlife Park & Michelle
T2 tea Wholesale
Tallangatta Rotary Club
Tamara Dyson
Tamara Knapp
Tanya Kerrison
Tanya Singleton Events
Tas Laser Skirmish & Jonathon Simonetis
Taylor Nealon
TEAMS & Stefanie Morgan
Tender Touch Landscaping
Terrigal High School
The Advocate Newspaper & Julian
    O'Brien
The Alpine Inn & Steve
The Bank Hotel
The Chantoozies
The Chocolate Room
The Cocoa Tree Café & Trish & Pauline
The Courthouse Hotel
The Cruise Terminal
The Elephant & Wheelbarrow
The Erko Hotel Sausage Sizzle
The Erskineville Hotel
The Fremantle Dockers
The Gables & Susie Perrott
The George Hotel

ACKNOWLEDGEMENTS

The Goose Café
The Hon. Quentin Bryce
The Hon. Malcolm & Tonya McCusker
    (and Mary!)
The Insight Team
The Kahuna Daddies
The Liddell family
The Little Brewing Co
The Long Yard Pub
The Marks family
The Milk Bar
The Next Grind Café
The Observatory & Chris Denny
The Offspring Cast & Crew
The Old Bastards
The One Mile Jetty Committee
The Palmwoods Hotel
The Project Family
The Purl Bar
The Reardon Family
The Shop Coolum
The Spirit of Tasmania & Sonia Fernandez
The Thomas family
The Tiger Box
The Today Show Family
The Weirder The Better & Graham &
    Pinning
Threadmill Market
Three Mile Hill Mine
Tim Champion
Tim Coller – Coller Rathgeber Real Estate
Tim Minchin
Tim Watkins
Tina Baker
Tina Hasiuk
Tina Seirlis
Tish van der Weert
Tom Gleeson
Tom Lambert
Toni Hayes
Tonic Beauty Therapy
Tooheys New

Touched by an Angel
Towong Shire Council & Lauren Elvin
Toy's Restaurant
Tracey Cook
Tracey Cosgrove
Tracey Rathbone
Tradelink Kunda Park
Trading Faces Beauty Salon
Tree Top Walk & Julie Ross
Tri & Rob Dunne
Trudi O'Donnell
Tuncurry Beach North Coast
    Holiday Park
United Artworks
Upwey High School &
    Christopher Hadfield
Valerie Koch
Vanessa Waters
Vanity Room
Vibi Harris
Victoria Ballard
Victoria Brooking
Victoria Kaczkowski
Vincent Taylor
Vivian Bryant
Walkers Arms Hotel
Walpole School
Warrick Sinclair
Wauchope Travel
We Work Out
Wester Hotel
Wet 'n' Wild Waterworld
White on One Coffee
Whitegum Park
Wild Mango Café
Wild Saffron & Heather Pretlove
Wilmington Primary School
Wilmington Progress Society
Wolf Ink Dog Grooming
Woodstock Audios
Wrapped In Paper & Gail
Zebu Restaurant

ALL THE COMMUNITIES LOVE YOUR SISTER VISITED

Adelaide	Daly Waters	Jindabyne	Parachilna
Aileron	Dampier	Kalgoorlie	Pardoo
Albany	Darwin	Kambalda	Pemberton
Albury Wodonga	Daylesford	Kaniva	Perth
Alice Springs	Denham	Kapunda	Port Augusta
Anmatjere	Denmark	Karratha	Port Hedland
Ararat	Derby	Karuah	Port Macquarie
Armidale	Devonport	Katherine	Quorn
Augusta	Dimboola	Kempsey	Rockingham
Bacchus Marsh	Dongara/Port	Kempton	Seymour
Ballarat	Denison	Khancoban	Stawell
Beaufort	Dubbo	Kununurra	Sydney
Benalla	Elizabeth	Lancelin	Tailem Bend
Bordertown	Elliott	Larrimah	Tallangatta
Brisbane	Esperance	Launceston	Tamworth
Broome	Eucla	Leeman	Tennant Creek
Brunswick Heads	Fitzroy Crossing	Leigh Creek	Tenterfield
Bunbury	Forster	Lismore	Thredbo
Burnie	Geraldton	Margaret River	Three Ways
Busselton	Ghan	Marree	Timber Creek
Byron Bay	Gilgandra	Mataranka	Tintinara
Caboolture	Gladstone	Melbourne	Toowoomba
Callington	Glen Innes	Melrose	Turkey Creek
Caloundra	Gold Coast	Monkey Mia	Two Rocks
Campbell Town	Gosford	Mooloolaba	Uluru
Canarvon	Goulburn	Moss Vale	Victoria River
Canberra	Grafton	Mt Kosciuszko	Wagga Wagga
Ceduna	Gunnedah	Mundaring	Walpole
Cervantes	Halls Creek	Nambour	Wangaratta
Clare	Harden	Newcastle	Warragul
Coffs Harbour	Hawker	Nhill	Warwick
Cooma	Henty	Noosa	Willeroo
Coonabarabran	Hobart	Northcliffe	Wilmington
Cootamundra	Horsham	Oodnadatta	Wollongong
Cowra	Ipswich	Orange	

. . . and all the communities in between.

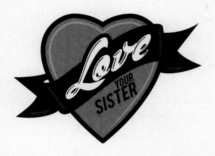

For more information on LOVE YOUR SISTER,
to donate and to keep in touch with Connie and
Sam, you can go to their Facebook page, Instagram
or go to the website:

www.facebook.com/loveyoursister
www.instagram.com/loveyoursister

www.loveyoursister.org

If your wardrobe is lacking a bit of pink the
Love Your Sister online store can help you out with
some fab merchandise:

www.loveyoursister.org/shop.php

⊏⊐ hachette
AUSTRALIA

If you would like to find out more about Hachette Australia,
our authors, upcoming events and new releases you can visit
our website, Facebook or follow us on Twitter:

www.hachette.com.au
www.twitter.com/HachetteAus
www.facebook.com/HachetteAustralia